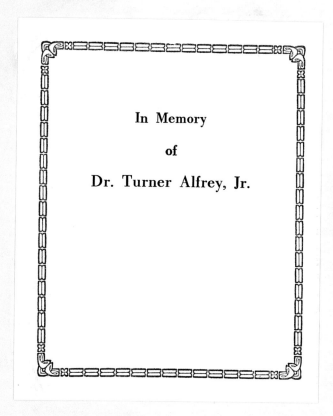

In Memory

of

Dr. Turner Alfrey, Jr.

The Chemistry
and Reactivity
of Collagen

The Chemistry
and Reactivity
of Collagen

By K. H. GUSTAVSON

Garverinäringens Forskningsinstitut, Stockholm, Sweden

ACADEMIC PRESS INC.
Publishers, New York 10, N. Y.
1956

Library of Congress Catalog Card Number: 56–7047

PRINTED IN THE UNITED STATES OF AMERICA

Preface

This monograph gives an outline of the chemistry of collagen, its structural organization and behavior, particularly in reversible aqueous systems, in the light of the modern concepts of proteins and protein reactions. The nature of the stabilizing forces in collagen and their alteration on various pretreatments of collagen, including the hydrothermal shrinkage, are comprehensively discussed, as are problems of importance in biochemistry, medicine, and technology. Special attention is given to reactions forming the basis for the processing of skin prior to tanning, and for the making of gelatin. Although the monograph has been developed around the problems which the author considers to be the outstanding and actual ones at present, the various aspects of collagen are probably more widely and extensively covered in this text than in any other book on this important class of proteins. The available books on collagen are limited in scope, principally treating the physics of collagen, its structure and the solubilized collagens, whereas the chemistry and reactivity are given scant attention only. These last are the principal issues of this book. The presentation has been arranged to suit the nonspecialist as well as the specialist.

The problem of cross-linking of collagen is covered comprehensively, since it forms the foundation for the tanning processes. As to tanning, only an outline of the modern physicochemical approach to the chemistry of the tanning processes is given. The fundamentals of the important field of tanning processes are comprehensively discussed in the accompanying volume on "The Chemistry of Tanning Processes." Although the present volume is a complete and independent treatise, the monograph on tanning, to which frequent references are given in this book, should be a useful adjunct for supplying information on the behavior of collagen in irreversible systems.

The background for this monograph is the author's work with collagen, in the form of hides and skins, for nearly four decades. This book, which is the result of the ardent efforts of a "one-man team," would not have been possible without the kind help of the publishers. The patient and critical editing of the manuscript is sincerely appreciated.

Stockholm, Sweden
October, 1955

K. H. GUSTAVSON

Contents

CHAPTER 1

An Outline of the Nature of the Proteins

1. The Chemistry of Proteins

Proteins are products of the living organism, and they are of fundamental importance for the processes of life and its sustenance. Further, they provide raw material for everyday necessities. The water-soluble proteins of the blood and the organs show great versatility in their various functions in the cells of the organisms and are intimately connected with the vital processes. Thus, they function as the essential constituents of multiplying cells, as enzymes and hormones of the body, such as the respiratory pigments and insulin, and as antibodies and toxins (1). The molecules of the water-soluble proteins, which are rather labile chemically, are folded, forming spherical particles, as is indicated by their name, *globular* proteins.

The other main type of proteins, which serve to support the organs and to protect the organism, form rather stable structures and are insoluble. These proteins form fibers and are therefore called *fibrous* proteins. From the point of view of tanning processes, this class of proteins is particularly interesting, since the chief substrate in tanning, the main constituent of the corium of skin, collagen, belongs to this group. Their ultimate units, the polypeptide chains, were conceived to be more or less stretched, forming chains; in the light of the present conception, these chains take the form of spirals, i.e., the helical structure which appears to be the common form for the architecture of the proteins generally. A great deal of our present knowledge of the molecular architecture of the fibrous proteins is due to the pioneering researches of Astbury and his school (2). The classification of proteins on the basis of the shape of the molecules was also suggested by Astbury.

The great variety of the properties of proteins and the diversity of the functions they fulfil may be studied from various points of view (3, 4). As already mentioned, consideration of the form of the protein molecules constitutes one type of approach. This molecular morphology of the proteins is instructive and didactically valuable in outlining the principal issues of protein behavior from the point of view of tanning. In such an outline, information relative to the forces exerted by the individual groups of the protein molecule on each other and on other molecules is of primary interest, as are the effects of these forces on the properties and reactivity of the proteins, particularly collagen.

a. Structural units and linkages

The peptide theory of protein structure, suggested by Hofmeister (5) and further enunciated and established on a sound experimental basis by Emil Fischer (6) more than fifty years ago, still remains unchallenged in principle. The principal covalent linking of the various amino acids constituting the protein molecule is one aspect which has emerged with clarity in recent years and is universally accepted. According to this concept, the proteins are built up of α-amino acids which are linked by the condensation of the amino group of one acid with the carboxyl group of another, with the formation of the keto-imide bond (the peptide linkage, —CO—NH—). The resulting structures are long chains of high molecular weight, represented by the general formula

$$-CO \cdot NH \cdot CHR_1 \cdot CO \cdot NH \cdot CHR_2 \cdot CO \cdot NH \cdot CHR_3-$$

On hydrolysis the polypeptide is broken down into its constituent amino acids, forming strong evidence for the polypeptide concept. The general formula for the amino acid residue is —CO·CHR·NH—, in which R denotes the group specific for the amino acid. The nature of the lateral R groups, particularly their chemical nature, including their electrochemical state and their size, has important bearing on the properties of the proteins. The amino acid formula also shows that the carbon atom is asymmetric in all α-amino acids, except the one with R = H, i.e., glycine, as four different groups are attached to the carbon atom. The hydrogen atom, the R group, the amino and carboxyl groups are arranged in exactly the same way in each related compound, and all the natural amino acids belong to the L series (1). For some exceptions, see reference 7.

There are about twenty different amino acids which form the building stones of the proteins. These amino acids are of widely different chemical character, classified by the R group, which is the individual, distinctive portion of the protein molecule. These R groups may consist of a simple hydrogen atom as in glycine, or of large, strongly polar groups as in arginine. Four types of R groups are recognized:

1. *Nonpolar*, as in glycine, alanine, and proline.
2. *Cationic*, as exemplified by lysine and arginine.
3. *Anionic*, present in the free carboxyls of aspartic and glutamic acids.
4. *Polar nonionic*, represented by residues of serine and hydroxyproline.

The problem of the structural characteristics of proteins is in itself not so easy. The difficulties of isolating the various amino acids from a protein hydrolyzate are small compared to the difficulties of determining the structure of the intact protein, but nevertheless they are considerable, because the amino acids in such hydrolyzates form a complex mixture of components of similar physical properties. Further, the behavior of any particular amino acid is profoundly affected by the presence of other amino acids or salts in the solution. Hence, the separation of a mixture of twenty different amino acids by means of the classical approach, which was mainly limited to certain classes of amino acids, presented a most formidable task.

New possibilities of more exact fractionation and determination of the individual amino acids have been provided by the developments of recent years, mainly by the Chibnall group at Cambridge (8), the Martin-Synge group (9), and the group of the Rockefeller Institute for Medical Research (10). The classical methods of Fischer (6) and Dakin (11) were very tedious and required large amounts of the protein, about 10 g. for a complete analysis. By means of the Moore and Stein methods (10), employing chromatographic separation on columns of starch and ion-exchanging resins, a complete analysis can be performed in a few hours. Only a few milligrams of the protein are required. The accuracy has also been greatly increased, the values being within 2 % of the true value.

In Table 1 the structure of the natural amino acids is given by their R groups, arranged according to their chemical nature, similar to the aforementioned electrochemical classification.

The degree of polarity of the side chains is an important factor for the affinity of the proteins to other compounds and for their internal structure. Apart from the electrochemical nature of the R groups, their size is a important feature, since the packing of the protein chains depends on the bulk of these groups; small side chains, such as the hydrogen and methyl groups, allow close packing of chains, whereas large groups, such as the lysine and arginine residues, prevent the approach of elementary chains. This will be evident from the discussion to be presented later on the intermolecular linking of silk fibroin and collagen.

Since the development of the polypeptide hypothesis of protein structure by Emil Fischer in the early years of this century and the introduction of methods for the synthesis of polypeptides, including the preparation of large polypeptides having molecular weights of the order of thousands (12), the peptide chain concept has been further strengthened by a huge volume of research in the protein field. It should be remembered, however, as aptly remarked by Sanger (13), that it is still a hypothesis and has not been definitely proved. Probably the best evidence in support of its validity is that no facts have been found to contradict it during the fifty years of its existence. Certainly other types of covalent links, besides the cystine link, have been demonstrated in certain uncommon proteins, and a smaller number of such links may be present in some proteins, for instance, an ester link in collagen.

The main classical evidences in support of the peptide link concept of protein structure are: (1) Fischer and his school found that amino acids

TABLE 1

STRUCTURE OF THE R GROUPS OF THE MOST COMMON AMINO ACIDS FOUND IN PROTEINS

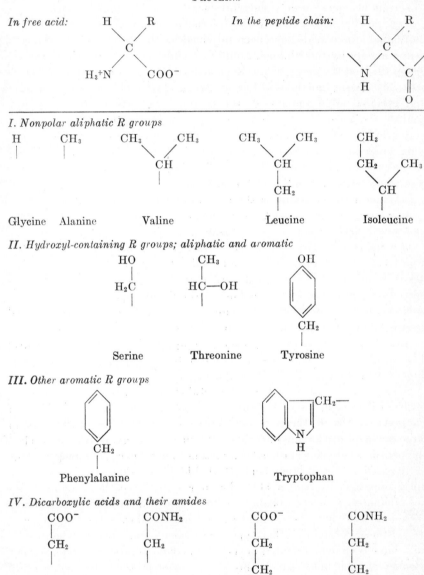

In free acid:

In the peptide chain:

I. Nonpolar aliphatic R groups

Glycine   Alanine   Valine   Leucine   Isoleucine

II. Hydroxyl-containing R groups; aliphatic and aromatic

Serine   Threonine   Tyrosine

III. Other aromatic R groups

Phenylalanine   Tryptophan

IV. Dicarboxylic acids and their amides

Aspartic acid   Asparagine   Glutamic acid   Glutamine

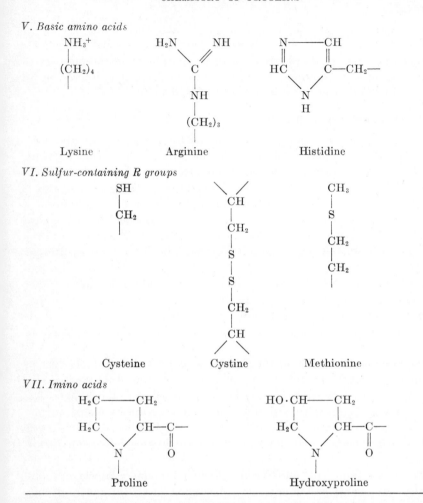

V. Basic amino acids

Lysine   Arginine   Histidine

VI. Sulfur-containing R groups

Cysteine   Cystine   Methionine

VII. Imino acids

Proline   Hydroxyproline

are formed by hydrolysis of proteins by means of acids, bases, and certain enzymes. (*2*) Dipeptides are present in the protein hydrolyzate, glycyl-L-alanine being the first natural dipeptide obtained by partial acid hydrolysis of silk fibroin by Fischer and Abderhalden in 1906 (6, 14). (*3*) Proteins contain very few amino and carboxyl groups, indicating that these groups of the amino acids are involved in the building up of protein chains by condensation (—CO—NH— group). (*4*) By the action of protein-splitting enzymes on most proteins, equal numbers of acid and basic groups are set free; an outstanding exception is collagen and other proteins containing large amounts of imino acids (proline and hydroxyproline), which yield the weakly basic imino groups instead of the strongly basic amino groups on hydrolysis (15). (5) Synthetic polypeptides are split by special proteinases, so called peptidases (16–18). In view of the possibility of the presence of ester links in some proteins, for instance in collagen, it is interesting to know that proteinases are able to split such links (19).

b. Hydrolytic cleavage of proteins

Certain peptide links show greater stability toward acids than others, depending on the residues involved in the link and the environment. Thus, α-amino groups stabilize the peptide bond, and hence a bond adjacent to a terminal NH_2 group is rather stable. An additional consequence of this is the preferred formation of dipeptides on hydrolytic cleavage by means of acids (20). Thus in the hydrolysis of silk fibroin by concentrated hydrochloric acid, almost all the nitrogen present as peptide linkages was in the form of dipeptides (21). The keto-imide links, which are most easily split by strong acids, are those involving the amino groups of serine and threonine residues (adjacent hydroxy group). A more random cleavage at other types of peptide bonds follows subsequently. It is interesting to note that dilute solutions of strong acids and concentrated solutions of weak acids preferentially split the keto-imide group adjacent to the end residue of aspartic acid (22).

The nature of the anion of the acid influences also the rate and type of the hydrolysis of the peptide bonds, and a marked catalysis of the hydrolysis is effected by long-chain anions. These are attached to the cationic protein groups and apparently also to the keto-imide groups by dipolar attraction, which results in the activation of peptide bonds. Thus, dodecylsulfuric acid is about one hundred times as effective as hydrochloric acid. At low concentrations of the former acid, the increased rate of removal of the amide groups from wool and certain globular proteins is especially noteworthy (Steinhardt and Fugitt, 23). According to Cassel and McKenna (24), however, the deamidation of collagen is only slightly affected by the degree of affinity of the anion of the acid, used in deamidation, for the cationic groups of collagen. References can be given only to the most important methods of following the progress of the protein cleavage (25–28).

These methods do not distinguish between *free* amino acids and peptides. For that purpose reagents reacting with the carboxyl and amino groups of the same amino acid molecules are used. The most prominent one is triketohydrindene hydrate, better known as *ninhydrin*, which in recent years has obtained great importance as an amino acid reagent in the paper chromatographic method of amino acid determination. A weakly acid, aqueous solution of an α-amino acid heated in the presence of ninhydrin gives a blue color which can be colorimetrically measured. The reaction involves oxidation of the amino acid to the corresponding aldehyde, carbon dioxide, and ammonia (29). The aldehyde condenses with the reduction product of ninhydrin to the blue dye. Neither proteins nor peptides give this reaction. Imino acids give a brown color with this reagent.

c. Fractionation and isolation of amino acids

The recently developed adsorption techniques for the separation of protein hydrolyzates have become of the greatest importance for the astonishingly rapid progress in protein analysis. By the choice of suitable adsorbents, the various classes of amino acids can be separated quantitatively (30–32).

An almost complete separation is obtained by the method of Moore and Stein (32), employing a column of starch or ion-exchange resins or a combination of both, eluting the amino acids with mixtures of butanol, propanol, and hydrochloric acid. The amino acids are freed at different rates, as shown by the graph in Fig. 1. They can then be determined by the ninhydrin reaction or by micro-Kjeldahl. The paper partition method of Consden, Gordon, and Martin (33) brought about a revolution in the technique of the analysis of protein split-products; in a few years this has become the most widely used method for separation and qualitative analysis of complicated mixtures of natural products. In 1944, Consden et al. (33) applied partition chromatography to separation of amino acids, using cellulose in the form of filter paper as the support of the stationary phase. This method (34, 35) is the most useful application of partition chromatography. The amino acids are fractionated on strips of filter paper, the aqueous phase being held by the cellulose, while an organic solvent which is immiscible with but partly soluble in water is allowed to flow down or up the paper. The development may be carried out first in one direction and then at right angles with the use of two different solvents. This con-

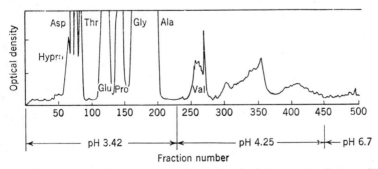

FIG. 1. Ion-exchange chromatogram of complete hydrolyzate of gelatin on Dowex 50 by the Moore-Stein method. The gelatin refluxed in 6 N HCl for 24 hours.

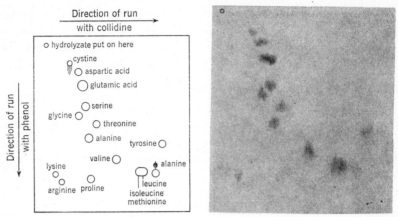

FIG. 2. Two-dimensional chromatogram on a wool hydrolyzate. First run with collidine; second run with phenol; 300 micrograms of proteins used. From F. Haurowitz, "Chemistry and Biology of Proteins," Academc Press, New York, 1950.

siderably increases the resolving power of the method. The position of the different amino acids on the paper is revealed by spraying it with a solution of ninhydrin (36). Each of the spots consists of a single amino acid (Fig. 2). The ratio of the flow of any amino acid to the flow rate of the pure solvent, the R_f value, is a characteristic constant for each amino acid. The most useful solvents are phenol and a mixture of butanol and acetic acid. This excellent method has practically completely replaced older methods of identifying amino acids and is now a standard procedure in chemical research on proteins (36). The intensity of the ninhydrin spots can be measured spectrophotometrically by determining the transmission of the filter paper, making it a quantitative method. A new development in that direction is due to McFarren (37), who uses buffered solvents, each of which separates some of the amino acids in the hydrolyzate on a one-dimensional chromatogram with buffered filter paper. A modification of this method has been successfully applied to quantitative analysis of the amino acids in collagen by Brown, Kelly, and Watson (38).

Important methods for the separation of amino acids in protein hydrolyzates are based on electrodialysis in cells (39) and on paper (40–42). By the isotopic dilution method, developed by Rittenberg (43), an accuracy of 1 % is obtained. The decarboxylase technique of Gale (44) makes use of bacterial decarboxylases, and the microbiological assay depends on the fact that certain amino acids are essential for the growth of microorganisms (45). These methods have been critically appraised by Chibnall (8).

d. Estimation of terminal groups

In this connection some recently developed methods for the estimation of specific groups of amino acid residues of proteins will be briefly discussed (46). It concerns groups which are of importance in identifying terminal groups, and hence methods which are expected to contribute to our knowledge of the order of the various residues of amino acid built into the proteins. For identifying the terminal α-amino groups in the peptide chains, Sanger's method (47) employing 2,4-dinitrofluorobenzene (DNFB) has proved to be of great value for the elucidation of protein structure, notably insulin. DNFB interacts smoothly in moderately alkaline solution (1 % sodium bicarbonate solution) with the free amino groups at room temperature. Hence both the ϵ-amino groups of lysine, more or less completely according to the steric environment of the groups, and the terminal amino groups are inactivated. By subsequent hydrolysis of the treated protein with acid, the brightly colored DNP-amino acids are obtained; these are readily estimated by partition chromatography or by the countercurrent distribution technique.

It is evident that by determining the number of terminal α-amino and α-carboxyl groups information can be obtained as to whether a peptide chain is straight or branched. An unbranched chain will contain only a single α-amino and a single carboxyl group, whereas branched chains, unless the chains form rings, will possess a number of these groups. The classical researches of Sanger (47) on the amino acid sequence in insulin show the fundamental importance of this method. The end-group method applied to gradually split peptide chains has already proved useful for ascertaining the sequence of the residues of amino acids built into the protein chains. Reference can only be given to the recent developments in the estimation of N-terminal groups (48, 49) and C-terminal groups (50–52).

At this point, it can be stated that native collagen does not contain any free terminal groups (50, 53). This may be taken as an indication that its molecular weight is of the order of hundreds of thousands and, further, that the molecule of collagen consists of a straight unbranched peptide chain, since the alternative explanation—the absence of terminal α-amino groups, i.e., the cyclic structure of the chains—is practically ruled out in view of other known facts about this protein. Aspartic acid has been found as C-terminal groups of certain pretreated collagens (54). It is interesting to note that of the common proteins ovalbumin contains no terminal amino group (55). Other methods of inactivating special protein groups will be considered in connection with the chemistry of collagen, particularly the means of modifying its structure.

e. Total protein nitrogen

The most common method of protein analysis is the determination of the total nitrogen of the protein, usually carried out by the Kjeldahl method, which really is a problem of elementary analysis. It gives a very important value, however, since its accurate estimation is the foundation on which depends the calculation of analytical data, irrespective of the way in which the results are expressed. The accurate determination of total nitrogen has long been a subject of investigation and controversy. Its importance for the accurate analysis of leather is obvious, since the amount of some of the tanning materials combined with collagen in various leathers, vegetable tannins for instance, is determined from the hide substance figure of the dry leather by subtraction, and further since the directly determined content of fixed tanning agents is referred to on the basis of hide protein. Chibnall and his school (56) have made fundamental contributions to the problems of estimating the total nitrogen and of expressing the amino acid composition of proteins.

It clearly would be desirable, in order to assist the comparison of the analytical results, to determine the total nitrogen by a standard procedure, such as that suggested by Tristram (56). It is also quite clear that the accuracy of the Kjeldahl method is related to the amino acid composition of the proteins. It appears to be common knowledge that proteins rich in lysine are the most difficult to digest (56).

It is usually assumed that the nitrogen content of proteins is 16%. Actually this value varies within rather wide limits, from 15 to 19% (56). Thus, collagen of bovine skin contains 17.0 to 18.6% nitrogen, and edestine shows even higher values of 18.7%. The average for keratin (wool) is 16.3%. Proteins with an exceptionally low content of nitrogen are ovalbumin, casein, and insulin, which contain only about 15.5% (56). It is necessary, therefore, to have an accurate determination of the total nitrogen content of the protein to be analyzed. In some proteins, such as collagen, the total protein nitrogen is changed in the processing, nitrogen being lost in preliminary processes, by deamidation in alkaline solution for instance. Hence, the nitrogen content of hide collagen at the various stages of the pretanning operations and in the tanning must be ascertained accurately on the particular substrate, in order to yield the true conversion factor of nitrogen into collagen. This detail will be further discussed in connection with the chemistry of collagen.

2. THE INTERNAL STRUCTURE OF PROTEINS

a. The form of molecular chains

If the peptide chains are postulated as the basis of protein structure, there still remain three possible variations of structure: first, the pattern

determined by the order of the different amino acid residues; second, the
geometrical configuration of the chains, involving their folds and twists;
and third, the forces operating between adjacent peptide chains, resulting
in stabilization of the structure.

The conceivable variations of an individual protein molecule are vast,
although limitations exist, since the peptide chains are held in definite configurations by strong intra- and intermolecular forces. In this respect the
proteins differ profoundly from the chains of simple polymers. The latter
are free to assume a great variety of different configurations; all or the
majority of these configurations are shown in a solution of simple polymer
molecules at any moment, and the individual molecule is constantly undergoing transition from one possible configuration to another. A random
distribution among the different forms is evident and is determined by
probability considerations, as is clearly shown in the researches of Werner
Kuhn (57).

Thus, a linear uncharged molecule consisting of n units and a total chain
length of l, being suspended in a solvent, will coil. The average length of
the coiled structure, l_1, will be $l_1 = \dfrac{2\sqrt{2} \times b \times \sqrt{n}}{\sqrt{\pi}}$, where b is a constant
containing the angle of valency and n denotes the number of units of the
molecular chain. The loose coiling means a great increase of the volume of
the molecule. Thus, the volume of a chain of 10,000 units in the state of
the statistically most probable coiling will be about one hundred times as
large as that of the molecule in the form of a solid sphere. Figure 3 gives
an idea of the free molecular folding. Generally, the volume of the most
probable configuration of uncharged molecules of the loose-coiling type increases proportionally with n^3.

If the chain carries free electric charges, quite a different picture is given.
This has been strikingly illustrated by Werner Kuhn and Katchalsky (58)
in their work on polymethacrylic acid. The influence of the ionized groups
on the form of this chain molecule should be expected to have its counterpart in solutions of proteins at pH values at which free charged groups

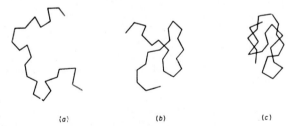

(a)   (b)   (c)

Fig. 3. Different constellations of a threadlike macromolecule. From F. Haurowitz, "Chemistry and Biology of Proteins," p. 50, Fig. 8, Academic Press, New York,
1950.

form on the protein chains (59). It is reasonable to assume that in the ionization of a coiled molecule of a polymer, in which all the charged groups are of the same sign, repulsive forces between the ionized groups become operative. Thus, by the formation of the alkali salt of the polymethacrylic acid, part of the carboxylic groups will ionize and, hence, the carboxyl ions will repel each other electrostatically, as the following structural formula shows:

$$-CH_2-\underset{\underset{COO^-}{|}}{\overset{\overset{CH_3}{|}}{C}}-CH_2-\underset{\underset{COO^-}{|}}{\overset{\overset{CH_3}{|}}{C}}-$$

The originally coiled uncharged molecule opens up and extends under the influence of the repulsion between the negatively charged groups formed. With increase of the number of charged carboxylic groups, i.e., with increasing pH value of the medium, this repulsive force gradually becomes greater until it overcomes the coiling tendency induced by the Brownian movement. Finally, the chain is stretched to its full length. It is thus possible to change the form of a molecule of this type from a spherical, highly coiled structure to a fully extended chain by adjusting the pH of the medium in which it is suspended. Thus, Kuhn et al. (60) have succeeded in preparing foils of oriented filaments of a three-dimensional network of polyacrylic acids. These filaments swell anisotropically in water, very much as collagen does. They contract and expand reversibly on the addition of H and OH ions to the solution. It is also possible to change the chemical energy of the molecules into mechanical energy by balancing the filament with a small weight. The free energy which is gained by the liberation of the polyacid on addition of H ions to the sodium salt is due to the difference in free energy content of the balanced and unbalanced filaments. These models are similar to the simplified structures earlier visualized for muscle prototypes by Meyer (61), consisting of chains with charged groups. These chains are caused to coil by being brought to the isoelectric point and extended by charge or discharge of their polar groups. These models are interesting from the point of view of fibrous proteins, since the swelling of fibers with varying pH values may be of a similar type. However, the behavior of uncharged chain molecules does not apply directly to proteins, since the various types of valency forces operating between adjacent protein chains and larger units are potent factors for the form and shape of the protein molecules.

The changed form of the protein molecules, for instance that of gelatin (59) or collagen induced by alteration of the pH of the environment, may be conceived as involving reactions of the type described by the Kuhn-

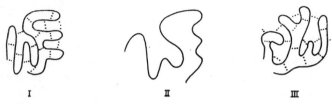

I   II   III

Fig. 4. Form and shape of proteins in the native and denatured states. From F. Haurowitz, "Chemistry and Biology of Proteins," p. 127, Fig. 29, Academic Press, New York, 1950.

Katchalsky model. From Haurowitz' idea of the changed configuration of globular proteins in the process of denaturation (62), the following suggestion seems plausible. In the isoelectric state, the protein molecules tend to take on the coiled form, the molecular chains being bridged by intrachain hydrogen bonds and saltlike links, as shown by Fig. 4, I, with due consideration of the fact that the two-dimensional structure actually represents a three-dimensional system. By partial discharge of the carboxyl ions of the protein by the protons of the added acid, the chain acquires positive charge. The liberated cationic protein groups tend to repel each other, resulting in an extension of the coiled molecule (Fig. 4, II) corresponding to the first reaction in denaturation. Some of the reactive sites of the chain can no longer compensate their valency forces in the same molecule. Spatially and by the Brownian movement, attraction between adjacent molecules is favored, resulting in the formation of interchain bridges (crosslinks) and aggregation of the protein. This is schematically pictured in Fig. 4, III, which represents Haurowitz's final step of denaturation. Stainsby's investigation (59) of the viscosity of gelatin solutions and the research of Pouradier and his co-workers (63) on the reactivity of gelatin in dilute solutions in the isoelectric state and in a slightly acid environment are in harmony with the concept brought out in the diagrams and with the general concept of Kuhn and Katchalsky as to the alteration of the form of polyelectrolytes with the hydrogen ion concentration of the medium. Also the swelling and contraction of collagen in acidic and alkaline solutions may advantageously be described in the light of this concept.

The results of the investigation of the location of the hydrogen bonds relative to the direction of the protein chains by the technique of polarized infrared radiation, reported in the lucid researches of Ambrose *et al.* (64), are of interest in this connection. The results are interpreted to indicate that in the coiled state, the α configuration of proteins, the hydrogen bonds are mainly present as *intrachain* links, with preferred direction parallel with the main axis of the chain, whereas in the fully stretched chain, the β configuration of proteins, these bonds lie perpendicular to the main chain direction and thus are able to form *interchain* hydrogen bonds. The Court-auld group (64a) has been able to demonstrate on some synthetic polypep-tides that the two modifications are reversibly interconvertible, particularly for polypeptides of long chain length with large nonpolar sidechains. The importance of these researches for our conception of protein organi-zation will be discussed below.

The very marked specificity of proteins is difficult to comprehend unless the coiling of the peptide chains is laid down according to a certain definite manner. In contradistinction to the uncharged molecules of high polymers, as the example earlier mentioned, a specific *internal structure* is characteristic for the protein molecule. The individual structural properties are main-tained in the protein molecule even in the dissolved state. The stability of the secondary structures formed by the peptide chains is still greater in the fibrous proteins than in the class of globular proteins discussed. A detailed discussion of the fiber-forming proteins as exemplified by collagen will be given in later chapters. In many respects, this class of proteins provides the best example of the importance of form and internal structure of proteins.

b. The stabilizing forces of the protein molecule

For the simplest arrangement of the peptide chains, the fully extended chain has the structure shown below:

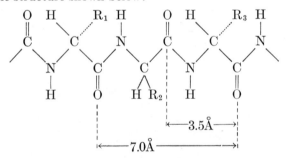

The following principles apply. The atoms of the chain lie in the plane of the paper, and the successive side chains, R_1, R_2, etc., extend alternately above and below this plane, from the carbon atoms to which they are linked. These R groups may consist mainly of H and CH_3 groups which are nonpolar and hence do not contribute to the building up of larger struc-tures by intermolecular forces. However, their small size plays an impor-tant role in allowing close packing of the peptide chains and hence sterically facilitating the close approach of adjacent chains. This in its turn makes for the participation of weaker valency forces between adjacent chains, allowing compensation of the —CO—NH— bonds on adjacent chains and operation of van der Waals forces. Bamford and his co-workers (64a)

emphasize that in synthetic polypeptides the length of the polypeptide chain and the size and nature of the side groups have a definite influence on the relative stability of the α and β forms (contracted and fully extended chains, respectively). As a rule, small side groups favor the β configuration, which is stabilized by interchain hydrogen bonds. Silk is an outstanding example among proteins. Strongly polar R groups, such as the COO^- and NH_3^+ groups, will be able to compensate their charges in the form of the saltlike crosslinks [range up to 100 Å. (64b)]. The distance between interacting protein groups is a primary factor determining the strength and the stability of the bond formed. This is particularly true with the weaker type of bond. The mutual attraction of ionic groups is proportional to the reciprocal of the square of their distance apart; i.e., it decreases with r^{-2}, whereas the attraction of weak dipolar forces decreases with r^{-6} or r^{-7}. Hence, the forces of nonionic nature between peptide chains of proteins can exist over very *short* distances only (<5Å.); further, it is obvious that crosslinking of chains can take place only between closely adjacent electrostatic centra. This type of force includes also the important link called the hydrogen bond or hydrogen bridge (65). In proteins the main part of the hydrogen bridges probably is formed between the imino groups of the keto-imide groups, the —CO—NH— links, on the one hand, and the carbonyl groups of adjacent keto-imide groups, on the other, as shown by the schematic formula:

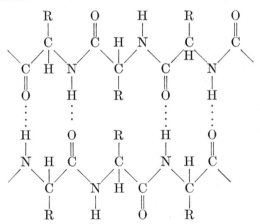

The hydrogen bond will be further discussed later.

To return to the amino acid residue of the extended peptide chain and the geometrical configuration of the peptide chains, it is of interest to ascertain the size of the elementary structure. The most probably values of the interatomic distances in the peptide chain shown in Fig. 5, as given by Corey (66), is in Ångström units as follows: C—C, 1.53; C—N (as in the

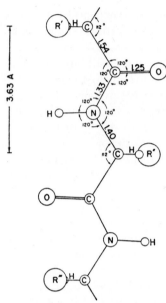

Fig. 5. Diagrammatic representation of a fully extended polypeptide chain based on Corey's data on the crystal structures of diketopiperazine, glycine, and alanine. From R. B. Corey, *Advances in Protein Chem.* **4**, 385 (1948), Fig. 13.

NH—CH—R— link), 1.46 to 1.49; C—N (in the —CO—NH— bond), 1.32. The valency bond angles are probably somewhat greater than the tetrahedral value because of the resonance and the steric hindrance. Then, the distance of the unit along the main chain between successive R groups or carbonyl groups is calculated to be about 3.65 Å. The measured value is 3.57 Å. The fully extended structure is represented in silk fibroin and in the stretched chains (β form) of the keratin-myosin family of fibrous proteins. The characteristic 7-Å. spacing, found in the X-ray diagrams of silk fibroin to be parallel to the fiber axis, is generally conceived to correspond to the interval of the same length for two amino acid residues, given in the figure of the extended peptide chain. The active force between adjacent chains of silk fibroin is generally considered to be weakly polar, i.e., arising from hydrogen bridges, and the last structural formula would thus be an actual picture of silk fibroin, which consists of molecular chains held together by means of the numerous hydrogen bridges between adjacent —CO—NH— groups. The existence of this type of intermolecular bond has been conclusively proved by Corey in his X-ray researches on the crystal structure of the simple diketopiperazine (66), a contraction of the regular bond distance (C—N) between the interacting peptide bonds of adjacent molecules of diketopiperazine being observed. The intermolecular distance between chains forming solid β-glycylglycine (66) has also been interpreted as evidence of the hydrogen bridging of these molecules. Since this type of bond operates only within a very short distance, the N—H$\cdots$O distance being 2.8 Å., it is very likely that the specific internal structure of the globular protein molecule and the coiling of the chains are maintained by the numerous intramolecular hydrogen bridges.

The structure of the hydrogen bond and its connection with the occurrence of resonance between the participating atoms is clearly shown by the electronic formula (67):

$$:\overset{|}{\underset{|}{N}}-H:\overset{..}{\underset{}{O}}=\overset{|}{\underset{|}{C}} \rightleftarrows :\overset{|}{\underset{|}{N}}^-:H^+:\overset{..}{\underset{}{O}}=\overset{|}{\underset{|}{C}}$$

The unshared electron pairs of the electron octets are given by the double dots, and the shared electrons pair is represented by a dash. Obviously, attraction must be set up between the positively charged proton and the unshared electron pair of the oxygen atom. This will result in the formation of a hydrogen bond, as shown by the structure on the right. The bond is unsymmetrical, since the proton forming the bond is nearer the nitrogen atom than the oxygen. The bond energy of the different types of hydrogen bonds varies from 2 to 9 kcal. (67). Since the peptide bonds of the polypeptide chains are the most numerous of all reactive protein groups and the steric conditions for valency interaction between adjacent —CO—NH— groups are favorable, it is probable that the main part of the hydrogen bridging of protein chains involves these groups. Infrared spectral studies of proteins show the presence of NHO— bridges in large quantities in proteins (68). These hydrogen bridges are probably linked together in rings capable both of resonance and of synchronized oscillations of the hydrogens and the mobile electron systems (69). Hence, the C—N bond should possess a marked double-bond character (70). In the afore-mentioned X-ray diffraction studies on diketopiperazine by Corey (66), the distance between C and N was found to be 1.33 Å., which is decidedly less than the expected value for the regular C—N single bond. This shortening of the bond was ascribed to resonance involving a double-bond ionic structure:

$$\underset{\diagup}{\overset{H}{\diagdown}}N^+ = C\underset{\diagdown}{\overset{O^-}{\diagup}}$$

This type of bond was used by Corey for construction of a polypeptide chain model.

The question then occurs as to whether the hydrogen bonds shown to be present in proteins are formed within the *same* peptide chain (*intramo-*

lecular) or between *different* chains (*intermolecular*). Since the formation of hydrogen bonds is not restricted to the peptide bond but can take place with other groups, such as hydroxy, amide, amino, and carboxyl groups, serious consideration must be given to the bonds between these groups, particularly the amide and carboxyl groups. For collagen the linking of hydroxy and keto-imide groups should be considered (71). Hence, a number of various hydrogen bonds are possible. One of these groups furnishes the hydrogen ion, whereas one of the other groups containing nitrogen or oxygen, furnishes the lone electron pair. Its negative charge will attract the positively charged hydrogen. It is to be noted and repeated that there are far more peptide linkages than other groups as prospective sites for hydrogen bonds in the protein. It appears probable from chemical evidence that the majority of the hydrogen bonds in fibrous proteins are intermolecular, linking together adjacent peptide chains. The intramolecular crosslinking is believed to be the principal force in maintaining the specific internal structure of globular proteins (64). In collagen, silk, and quill keratin, the *interchain* type of bond is dominating. However, there are indications that one form of hydrogen bond does not exclude the existence of the other type. The polarized ultrared radiation spectra offer the possibility of differentiation between the α and β configurations present in admixture in any protein (64).

c. Denaturation

Denaturation of proteins is fundamentally a problem of the internal structure of the protein molecule (72). Native proteins are very sensitive to changes in their natural environment and to the action of agents as different as heat, urea, and acids. The properties of the protein—such as solubility, biological activity, and characteristic physicochemical properties—are more or less radically altered in the process of denaturation. Apparently denaturation as a general phenomenon involves rearrangement of the peptide chains in the protein molecule, due to rupture of the weak interchain bonds of the protein by the denaturing agent. It is also evident that the denaturation of globular proteins and that of fibrous proteins both tend to bring the two extremes of protein configuration closer to each other, since the globular proteins are in a state of disorder, whereas, on the contrary, a state of high order of organization is characteristic of the fiber proteins. Since the denaturation of collagen by hydrothermal shrinkage will be given special attention in a later chapter, only a brief outline of denaturation as a general phenomenon will be given here.

Among the denaturing agents belonging to the class of nonionic or weakly polar compounds which exert an effect on proteins by means of their molecular orientation (such as the neutral compounds, urea, acid amides, and certain guanidine derivatives), the behavior of urea is exceedingly interesting and instructive. It has the power when dissolved to increase the dielectric constant of water—evidence of its dipolar nature. The molecule is in resonance between the nonpolar form, $H_2N \cdot CO \cdot NH_2$, and the polar form, $H_2N \cdot CO \overset{-}{=} \overset{+}{NH_2}$. Concentrated solutions of urea (>6 M) are effective denaturing agents. The urea molecule probably competes with the protein groups for the active sites of the hydrogen bridges on the —CO—NH— linkages, cleaving the hydrogen bridges and associating itself with the liberated valency loci on the peptide linkages, as represented schematically by the following formula:

$$
\begin{array}{ccc}
\begin{array}{c}
-\text{N}-\text{C}- \\
| \quad \| \\
\text{H} \quad \text{O} \\
\vdots \quad \vdots \\
\text{O} \quad \text{H} \\
\| \quad | \\
-\text{C}-\text{N}-
\end{array}
& + n\,H_2N \cdot CO \cdot NH_2 \rightarrow &
\begin{array}{c}
-\text{N}-\text{C}\rightarrow \\
| \quad \| \\
\text{H} \quad \text{O} \\
\vdots \quad \vdots \\
\text{O} \quad \text{H} \\
\| \quad | \\
H_2N\text{C}-\text{NH} \\[4pt]
\text{H}-\text{N}-\text{C}-\text{NH}_2 \\
| \quad \| \\
\text{H} \quad \text{O} \\
\vdots \quad \vdots \\
\text{O} \quad \text{H} \\
\| \quad | \\
-\text{C}-\text{N}\rightarrow
\end{array}
\end{array}
$$

Probably the small urea molecule wedges apart the peptide chains and brings about an unfolding of the chains by dislocation of a part of the hydrogen bridges. Phenol in concentrated solution reacts preferably with weakly polar protein groups and does not compete with hydrogen bonds (Alexander, 72a). This difference allows an evaluation of the type of secondary bonds formed.

3. Some Special Properties of Proteins

a. The ionizing protein groups

Since the important problems of the isoelectric point and the physical chemistry of proteins will be comprehensively discussed in separate chapters, only a brief outline of the ionizing protein groups will be given here. The amphoteric properties of proteins are on the whole a composite of the effects of the amino acid residues which they contain. The side chains (R

TABLE 2

CHARACTERISTIC IONIZATION CONSTANTS (pK) AND HEATS OF IONIZATION (ΔH) OF
IONIC GROUPS OF PROTEINS (73)

Group	pK	ΔH_1, cal./mole	Group	pK	ΔH_1, cal./mole
Carboxyl	3.0–3.2	0	Imidazolium (histidine)	5.6–7.0	7,000–7,500
Carboxyl (aspartyl)	3.0–4.7	0	Ammonium (α)	7.6–8.4	10,000–13,000
Carboxyl (glutamyl)	4.4	0	Ammonium (ϵ) (lysine)	9.4–10.6	10,000–12,000
Phenolic hydroxyl (tyrosine)	9.8–10.4	6000	Guanidinium (arginine)	11.6–12.6	12,000–13,000

groups) of the amino acids forming the protein are of three different types, as pointed out earlier (p. 2): (*1*) *nonpolar groups;* (*2*) *polar groups*, not carrying net charge in neutral solution; (*3*) *ionic groups*, positively or negatively charged. The third type, the most important side chains of proteins because of their electrochemical behavior, are those carrying strongly ionic groups. The positively charged groups or cationic groups are represented by the ε-ammonium group of lysine, the guanidyl group, and further by any free terminal α-amino groups. The anionic groups, carrying negative charges, are the carboxyl groups. The characteristic ionization constants of these various groups can be determined from the titration curves of the protein. The corresponding constants of simple amino acids and synthetic peptides are known and have served as primary source material for the determination of the nature of the active groups in the proteins (73).

A number of methods are available for ascertaining the nature of the ionizing groups in the various pH zones of the titration curve of a protein. The simplest and indeed the most obvious method is to compare the titration region of a protein with that expected from the pK value of the ionizable groups of the amino acid residues of the protein, making use of the data of Table 2. In many instances, the pK values of the original amino acid are shifted by the influence of the environment of the chains (73). Ordinarily these changes in pK are small. However, in a number of cases shifts of the order of 2 to 3 pH units are encountered. Thus the acid strength of the carboxyl groups is increased if its α-carbon atom forms part of a peptide link, and still further if an amino groups is introduced, as shown by the structures below. The basic strength of the amino groups is decreased if a carboxyl groups is attached to the α-carbon atoms, and the basic strength is still further impaired if the carbon atom forms part of a peptide link.

For H$\cdot$COO$^-$ → H$^+$ pK 3.7

For H$\cdot$NH$_2$ → H$^+$ pK 9.3

$$\begin{array}{ll} \text{H} & \text{NH}_3{}^+ \\ & \diagdown\,\diagup \\ & \text{C} \\ & \diagup\,\diagdown \\ \text{R} & \text{COO}^- \to \text{H}^+ \quad \text{p}K\ 2.3 \end{array}$$

$$\begin{array}{ll} \text{H} & \text{NH}\cdot\text{CO}— \\ & \diagdown\,\diagup \\ & \text{C} \\ & \diagup\,\diagdown \\ \text{R} & \text{COO}^- \to \text{H}^+ \quad \text{p}K\ 3.0 \end{array}$$

$$\begin{array}{ll} \text{H} & \text{H} \\ & \diagdown\,\diagup \\ & \text{C} \\ & \diagup\,\diagdown \\ \text{R} & \text{COO}^- \to \text{H}^+ \quad \text{p}K\ 4.7 \end{array}$$

$$\begin{array}{ll} \text{H} & \text{NH}_2 \to \text{H}^+ \\ & \diagdown\,\diagup \\ & \text{C} \\ & \diagup\,\diagdown \\ \text{R} & \text{CONH}— \quad \text{p}K\ 8.1 \end{array}$$

$$\begin{array}{ll} \text{H} & \text{NH}_2 \to \text{H}^+ \\ & \diagdown\,\diagup \\ & \text{C} \\ & \diagup\,\diagdown \\ \text{R} & \text{COO}^- \quad \text{p}K\ 9.6 \end{array}$$

$$\begin{array}{ll} \text{H} & \text{NH}_2 \to \text{H}^+ \\ & \diagdown\,\diagup \\ & \text{C} \\ & \diagup\,\diagdown \\ \text{R} & \text{H} \quad \text{p}K\ 10.7 \end{array}$$

It appears that the influence of one group on another can extend over a chain of several carbon atoms. It is also evident from the work of Stiasny and Scotti (74) that the ionization of the carboxyl group is increased by the presence of one or two peptide links, additional links having no further effect. The effect of the peptide link on the strength of the amino group of polypeptides built up entirely from glycine residues is cumulative up to the pentapeptide stage.

The heat of ionization of the various groups presented in Table 2 will give information as to the groups concerned in a restricted pH range. Simply by determination of the heats of reaction at different temperatures in any special case, the classical van't Hoff equation will give the heat of ionization of the protein groups involved.

Some of the tests for proving the dipolar nature of proteins may also be applied for localization of the groups involved. Thus, changes in the titration curve produced by the addition of formaldehyde will give certain indications of the nature of the titratable protein groups, since formaldehyde markedly shifts the titration of the ε-amino and imidazole groups toward a lower pH range, leaving the carboxylic groups unchanged. Use can also be made of elimination of individual protein groups. For instance, the ε-amino group of lysine may be inactivated by diazotization. Another possibility is to carry out the titration in alcohol or acetone for estimation of the carboxylic and amino groups, respectively. Obviously, for proteins such as prolamins, which are soluble in alcohol, the first method is particularly useful.

The insoluble fibrous proteins behave as if they were much stronger acids and bases than the globular proteins or than the free amino acids (23). This is probably due to the electric charge carried by the fibers. The pK values of the acidic and basic groups in amino acids and in soluble and insoluble proteins show this clearly (75). Titration curves of soluble proteins are obtained by electrometric titration of aqueous solutions containing a known amount of the protein, brought to the isoelectric point, by adding strong acids and bases, such as hydrochloric acid and sodium hydroxide. By addition of hydrogen ions to the isoelectric protein, part of the protons will interact with the charged carboxyl groups, converting them into carboxyl groups. Any uncharged amino groups present will acquire protons and hence be converted into NH_3 ions. The reaction is generally complete at final pH values of 1 to 2. The base-binding capacity of the protein is similarly determined by titration with sodium hydroxide. The hydroxyl ions applied in the form of the base are not bound to the protein. Their function is to remove protons from the positively charged guanidinium and lysine-ammonium groups. Hence, there is not a true base binding, only the transfer of protons from cationic protein groups to hydroxyl ions. Since the titration curve of collagen will be discussed in detail in connection with the chemistry of collagen, no example and elucidation of the titration curves will be given here.

b. The hydration of proteins

The hydration of proteins, the interaction of water with proteins, is a vital factor in the behavior of proteins in biological and technical systems, since water is the normal medium for proteins (76).

In an outline of the mechanism of protein hydration, the unique position of water as a chemical compound must first be recognized. Since the water molecule, H_2O, is a dipole, the forces operating between these dipoles are responsible for the mutual association of water molecules and hence also for the irregularities in many of the physical and chemical properties of water. The water molecule can be described as resonating among four electronic structures (77), of which the three dominating ones are

$$
\begin{array}{ccc}
\text{H} & \text{H}^+ & \text{H} \\
\ddot{\text{O}}\!:\!\text{H} & \overset{\cdot\cdot}{\text{O}}\!:\!\overset{-}{\text{H}} & \overset{\cdot\cdot}{\text{O}}\!:\!\overset{-}{\text{H}}^+ \\
\ddot{\text{H}} & \cdot\cdot & \cdot\cdot
\end{array}
$$

representing 44 %, 28 %, and 28 %, respectively, of the total number of water molecules. The presence of these structures and the operation of attraction between the molecules lead to hydrogen bond formation. In the solid state the water molecules form a three-dimensional network of oxygen atoms joined by hydrogen bonds, represented roughly by the structure in which the oxygen valencies are directed toward the corners of a tetrahedron. Even in water the clusterlike ice structure persists. In the liquid form the large-scale regularity of hydrogen-bonded clusters has broken down and the simple $(H_2O)_n$ molecules increase in number. Nevertheless, transient regularities of the ice type remain. The chemical interaction of water with proteins probably involves the dipolar single H_2O molecule mainly. This dipole is attracted to, and combines with, any charged protein groups. In this process of combination, the water molecule loses its free translational mobility. The volume of a hydrated protein molecule is as a rule smaller than the sum of the volumes of its components; that is, hydration of a protein diminishes the total volume of the system. This is in part due to the disappearance of water molecules and shift of the equilibrium between H_2O monomers and polymers in favor of the monomers, which have smaller volume. The change in volume can be measured dilatometrically, if no change in the pH of the system simultaneously takes place (78).

Part of the water associated with proteins is present in a state different from that of water as we know it in bulk, in the form of *bound* water (76). It appears that the cell activities of both plant and animal organisms are in a considerable degree regulated by the equilibrium between *bound* and *free* water, which can under certain conditions of stress be shifted in one direction or the other in order to provide for the preservation of the species. The importance of the water equilibrium in protein systems for the function of the protoplasm of living organisms under conditions of low temperature and drought is an established fact (76).

Calculations of the bond energy of the water molecules bound to dry proteins show values of the order of 3 to 6 kcal. per mole of water bound in the initial water uptake, corresponding to the stage of *bound* water (79, 80). The bond energy of the additional water uptake is very small. The possibility of absorption of multiple layers of water is quite remote, since it has been found that the excess forces of the dipoles present in the first layer are far too weak to hold the additional water molecules in a definite position. The values found for the third and following layers are indeed lower than the energies involved in the thermal oscillation of the water molecules (79). The initial water binding is probably of the nature of an adsorption of an oriented layer of polar water molecules (80). Therefore this process should result in a higher degree of order of the system; i.e., the entropy should be decreased. In the additional association of water molecules with the protein, the water molecules function as a solvent. This should result in a system of a lower degree of order; i.e., the entropy should be increased.

Fricke and Lüke (81) found that dry casein absorbs water with an initial evolution of heat and that the heat evolved, ΔH, is greater than the free energy, ΔF. Accordingly, the entropy decreases. This indicates that the water absorbed initially is bound by forces of attraction at definite points in the protein lattice. When 20 % of water has been absorbed, ΔF becomes equal to ΔH. On further uptake, the free energy change, ΔF, is chiefly supplied by the entropy of mixing. The system gelatin-water behaves similarly as does collagen in its initial water absorption. Figure 27 (Chapter 6) shows some typical curves for water absorption by various proteins.

It is also evident from the marked contraction of the system, as a result of the hydration process, that stronger valency forces than van der Waals forces are involved. Hydrogen bonds probably are formed between the H_2O and the polar groups. As to the nature of the groups of the protein combining with the bound water, opinions differ considerably. It was once believed by some investigators that the ionic protein groups were the main sites for water binding (82). However, some of the present investigators are more inclined to ascribe the additional hydration sites of the protein to the peptide link (83). By the association of one molecule of water on each —CONH— group of the amino acid residue in gelatin, with a mean residue weight of 93, the water content should be of the order found for the degree of hydration of collagen and gelatin—about 20 % water on the basis of the weight of the protein (84). It seems possible that the water molecule forms the link between internally compensated peptide linkages, giving the struc-

ture $\begin{array}{c} \diagdown \qquad\quad \diagup \\ N \cdot H\text{----}O \cdot H\text{----}OC \\ \diagup \quad | \qquad \diagdown \\ \quad\ \ H \end{array}$, thus functioning as an agent for crosslinking

(84a). It is also interesting to note that polyamides such as nylon, in the drawn state, and hence with the chains almost parallelly aligned and extensively crosslinked by means of hydrogen bridges on adjacent peptide bonds, take up very small amounts of water. By rupture of the crosslinks or by introduction of other chains which will break the regularity of the structural pattern and tend to decrease the orderliness of the structure, the modified polyamide will take up considerable quantities of water.

c. Spreading of proteins on surfaces (monolayers) (85)

Soluble proteins readily form surface films on water or on dilute salt solutions (86, 87). Gelatin is best spread on ammonium sulfate solution (88). Solubilized collagen can also be spread into monolayers, by a technique devised by Ellis and Pankhurst (87).

In view of recent applications of the surface-film technique to the study of interactions of proteins with tanning agents (89–92), some aspects of the surface chemistry of proteins will be mentioned. By the spreading of small drops of a protein solution from a capillary pipet on a salt solution with its pH adjusted to the pH value of the isoelectric point of the protein, stable films are obtained. It is a remarkable fact that all proteins form films of the same type. It has been found that 1 mg. of protein covers an area of about 0.7 to 0.8 m.^{2}. Since the volume of 1 mg. of protein is 0.75 mm.^{3}, the height of the protein film, obtained by dividing volume by area (0.75:750,000), is of 10 Å. This very small order of magnitude of the dimension of the oriented film indicates that the peptide chains of globular proteins unfold and that monomolecular layers of the peptide chains are oriented on the solution with their long axes parallel to the surface of the water (86).

It appears probable that the hydrophilic ionic groups of the proteins are attracted toward the aqueous layer, whereas the apolar protein groups are directed toward the air, forming the backbone of the spread molecule. The process of the formation of protein monolayers is generally irreversible and results in partial or total denaturation of the protein. This provides important proof of the two-dimensional structure of proteins. The lateral pressure of protein films is measured by the surface balance, a simple but exceedingly ingenious instrument. The curves obtained show that the protein molecules can move freely in two dimensions, parallel to the surface. No movement in the third dimension is possible.

Schulman and Rideal (89) and Cockbain and Schulman (90) have studied the interaction of polyphenols, including vegetable tannins, with monolayers of amines and proteins. If the polyphenols are injected beneath a protein monolayer, no penetration occurs, since they anchor themselves to the polar protein groups forming the undersurface of the monolayer. Schulman and Rideal (89) found that gallic acid reacts very slowly, whereas tannic acid is exceedingly reactive, even in extremely dilute solutions. Gorter and Blokker (91) have also investigated these systems. Recent papers by Ellis and Pankhurst (92) and by Schulman and Dogan (93) consider the effect of both organic and inorganic tanning agents on protein films. The main findings of the monolayer investigations will be reviewed in Chapter 13.

Although a great deal of work has been carried out on films of globular proteins, little attention has been given to monolayers formed from fibrous proteins until recently. Pankhurst's pioneering work on collagen monolayers is of fundamental importance for the development of views on the mechanism of reaction of tanning processes. Ellis and Pankhurst (94) prepared monolayers of collagen by spreading solubilized collagen on concentrated solutions of ammonium sulfate. Solutions of collagen were obtained by dissolving cowhide split in anhydrous formic acid at 35°C. It should be noted that by this drastic mode of preparation no appreciable hydrolysis of collagen is incurred, although the end-group determinations (95) show that N-terminal groups are formed in the solubilization of the collagen (aspartic acid and glycine), probably by hydrolytic cleavage of keto-imide links.

The solution obtained was spread on 30 % ammonium sulfate solution of pH 4. The surface pressure, II, and the surface potential, ΔV, were studied over a pressure range of 0.01 to 30 dynes per centimeter. Ellis and Pankhurst found that the film formed is heterogeneous, when the area, A, is greater than 5 m.^{2} per milligram of collagen. As the monolayer is compressed to smaller areas, it becomes homogeneous and the value of $\Delta V \times A$ is then constant. Two critical areas were found on further compression: (1) A_1 (1.8 m.^{2} per milligram of collagen) below which the values of $\Delta V \times A$ decrease, indicating a change in orientation, accompanied by a decrease in compressibility; (2) A_2 (1.3 m.^{2} per milligram of collagen). Ellis and Pankhurst suggest that the two areas correspond to closely packed polypeptide chains with their side groups orientated (1) parallel to and (2) perpendicular to the water surface. These areas correspond to about 27.5 and 20 Å.^{2} per mean residue of collagen, respectively.

The clarifying experiments with tanning agents, covered in the researches of Ellis and Pankhurst, will be discussed in Chapter 13. However, it should be mentioned here that this unique method of studying tanning reactions is particularly valuable, since it eliminates most of the undesirable complicating factors of the fibrous structures, namely, the steric factors. Hence, the ultimate chemical reaction between the simple polypeptide chains of collagen and the tanning agent can be studied undisturbed. The surface studies of the Rideal school and of Pankhurst have contributed substantially to a better understanding of the mechanism of tanning.

REFERENCES

1. An excellent introduction is given by Haurowitz, F., "Chemistry and Biology of Proteins." Academic Press, New York, 1950.
2. Astbury, W. T., "Fundamentals of Fibre Structure." Oxford University Press, London, 1933.
3. Edsall, J. T., in "Proteins, Amino Acids, and Peptides" (E. J. Cohn and J. T. Edsall, eds.). Reinhold, New York, 1943.
4. Edsall, J. T., in "High Molecular Weight Organic Compounds" (R. E. Burk and O. Grummitt, eds.), p. 144. Interscience, New York, 1949.
5. Hofmeister, F., "*Naturw. Rundschau* 17, 529, 545 (1902); *Ergeb. Physiol.* 1, 758 (1902).
6. Fischer, E., *Ber.* 35, 1095 (1902); see also "Untersuchungen über Aminosäuren, Polypeptide und Proteine." Springer, Berlin, 1906.
7. Lipmann, F., Hotchkiss, R. D., and Dubos, R. J., *J. Biol. Chem.* 141, 163, 171 (1941); Hotchkiss, R. D., *Advances in Enzymol.* 4, 153 (1944).
8. See Chibnall, A. C., *J. Soc. Leather Trades Chem.* 30, 1 (1946).
9. See Martin, A. J. P., and Synge, R. L. M., *Advances in Protein Chem.* 2, 1 (1945); Synge, R. L. M., *Biochem. Soc. Symposia* No. 3, 90 (1949).
10. See Moore, S., and Stein, W. H., *J. Biol. Chem.* 176, 337 (1948); 178, 53, 79 (1949).
11. Dakin, H. D., *J. Biol. Chem.* 44, 499 (1920).
12. Fischer, E., *Ber.* 40, 1754 (1907); Abderhalden, E., and Fodor, A., *ibid.* 49, 56 (1916).

13. Sanger, F., *Advances in Protein Chem.* **7**, 3 (1952).
14. Fischer, E., and Abderhalden, E., *Ber.* **40**, 3555 (1907).
15. Bergmann, M., *Chem. Revs.* **22**, 423 (1938).
16. Bergmann, M., and Fruton, J. S., *J. Biol. Chem.* **117**, 189 (1937).
17. See Bergmann, M., *Harvey Lectures* **31**, 37 (1935–1936); Bergmann, M., and Niemann, C., *Science* **86**, 187 (1937).
18. Bergmann, M., and Fruton, J. S., *Advances in Enzymol.* **1**, 63 (1941).
19. Neurath, H., Schwerdt, G. W., Kaufman, S., and Snoke, J. E., *J. Biol. Chem.* **172**, 222 (1948).
20. Gordon, A. H., Martin, A. J. P., and Synge, R. L. M., *Biochem. J.* **35**, 1369 (1941)
21. Stein, W. H., Moore, S., and Bergmann, M., *J. Biol. Chem.* **154**, 191 (1944).
22. Partridge, S. M., and Davis, H. F., *Nature* **165**, 62 (1950).
23. Steinhardt, J., and Fugitt, C. H., *J. Research Natl. Bur. Standards* **29**, 315 (1942).
24. Cassel, J. M., and McKenna, E., *J. Am. Leather Chem. Assoc.* **48**, 142 (1953).
25. Sörensen, S. P. L., *Biochem. Z.* **7**, 45 (1907).
26. Willstätter, R., and Waldschmidt-Leitz, E., *Ber.* **54**, 2988 (1921).
27. Van Slyke, D. D., *J. Biol. Chem.* **9**, 185 (1911); **23**, 407 (1915).
28. Linderstrøm-Lang, K., and Holter, H., *Z. physiol. Chem.* **201**, 9 (1931).
29. Retinger, J., *J. Am. Chem. Soc.* **39**, 1059 (1917).
30. Cannan, R. K., *J. Biol. Chem.* **152**, 401 (1944).
31. Block, R. J., *Arch. Biochem.* **11**, 235 (1946).
32. Moore, S., and Stein, W. H., *J. Biol. Chem.* **178**, 53, 79 (1949).
33. Consden, R., Gordon, A. H., and Martin, A. J. P., *Biochem. J.* **38**, 224 (1944).
34. See Martin, A. J. P., and Synge, R. L. M., *Advances in Protein Chem.* **2**, 1 (1945).
35. Gordon, A. H., Martin, A. J. P., and Synge, R. L. M., *Biochem. J.* **37**, 79 (1943).
36. See "Partition Chromatography," *Biochem. Soc. Symposia* **No. 3**, 21 (1950); "Chromatographic Analysis" *Discussions Faraday Soc.* **No. 7**, 128 (1949); Moore, S., and Stein, W. H., *J. Biol. Chem.* **178**, 53, 79 (1949).
37. McFarren, E. F., *Anal. Chem.* **23**, 168 (1951); McFarren, E. F., and Mills, J., *ibid.* **24**, 650 (1952).
38. Brown, G. L., Kelly, F. C., and Watson, M., *in* "Nature and Structure of Collagen" (J. T. Randall, ed.), pp. 117–123. Butterworths, London, 1953.
39. Macpherson, H. T., *Biochem. J.* **40**, 470 (1946).
40. Durrum, E. L., *J. Am. Chem. Soc.* **72**, 2943 (1950); **73**, 4875 (1951).
41. Tiselius, A., and Kunkel, H. G., *J. Gen. Physiol.* **35**, 89 (1951).
42. Tiselius, A., and Cremer, H. D., *Biochem. Z.* **320**, 273 (1950).
43. Rittenberg, D., and Foster, G. L., *J. Biol. Chem.* **133**, 737 (1940).
44. Gale, E. F., *Biochem. J.* **39**, 46 (1945).
45. Snell, E. E., *Advances in Protein Chem.* **2**, 75 (1946).
46. See Herriott, R. M., *Advances in Protein Chem.* **3**, 169 (1947); Putnam, F. W., *in* "The Proteins" (H. Neurath and K. Bailey, eds.), Vol. 1, Part B, pp. 893–972. Academic Press, New York, 1953.
47. Sanger, F., *Advances in Protein Chem.* **7**, 2 (1952); *Biochem. J.* **39**, 507 (1945); Sanger, F., and Tuppy, H., *ibid.* **49**, 463, 481 (1951).
48. Edman, P., *Acta Chem. Scand.* **4**, 283 (1950).
49. Fraenkel-Conrat, H., and Fraenkel-Conrat, J., *Acta Chem. Scand.* **5**, 1409 (1951).
50. Grassmann, W., and Hörmann, H., *Z. physiol. Chem.* **292**, 24 (1953); Grassmann, W., Hörmann, H., and Endres, H., *Chem. Ber.* **86**, 1477 (1953); **88**, 102 (1955).
51. Chibnall, A. C., and Rees, M. W., *Biochem. J.* **48**, xlvii 1951; see Sanger, F., *Advances in Protein Chem.* **7**, 2 (1952).
52. Lens, J., *Biochim. et Biophys. Acta* **3**, 367 (1949).

53. Bowes, J. H., and Moss, J. A., *Nature* **168,** 514 (1951).
54. Bowes, J. H., and Moss, J. A., *Biochem. J.* **55,** 735 (1953).
55. Porter, R. R., *Biochem. J.* **46,** 473 (1950).
56. Chibnall, A. C., Rees, M. W., and Williams, E. F., *Biochem. J.* **37,** 354 (1953); Tristram, G. R., in "The Proteins" (H. Neurath and K. Bailey, eds.) Vol. 1, Part A, pp. 181–233. Academic Press, New York, 1953.
57. Kuhn, W., *Kolloid-Z.* **68,** 2 (1934); *Experientia* **1,** 6 (1954); Katchalsky, A., Künzle, O., and Kuhn, W., *J. Polymer Sci.* **5,** 283 (1950).
58. Kuhn, W., and Katchalsky, A., *Helv. Chim. Acta* **31,** 1994 (1948).
59. Stainsby, G., *Nature* **169,** 662 (1952).
60. Kuhn, W., Hargitay, B., Katchalsky, A., and Eisenberg, H., *Nature* **165,** 514 (1950).
61. Meyer, K. H., *Biochem. Z.* **217,** 433 (1930),
62. Haurowitz, F., *Kolloid-Z.* **71,** 198 (1935); "Chemistry and Biology of Proteins," p. 104. Academic Press, New York, 1950; *Experientia* **5,** 347 (1949).
63. Pouradier, J., Roman, J., Venet, A., Chateau, H., and Accary, A., *Bull. soc. chim. (France)* **19,** 928 (1952).
64. Ambrose, E. J., and Elliott, A., *Proc. Roy. Soc.* **A205,** 47 (1951).
64a. Bamford, C. H., Brown, L., Elliott, A., Hanby, W. E., and Trotter, I. F., *Proc. Roy. Soc.* **B141,** 49 (1953).
64b. Neale, S. M., *J. Soc. Dyers Colourists* **63,** 368 (1947).
65. Huggins, M. L., *Chem. Revs.* **32,** 195 (1943); *J. Org. Chem.* **1,** 407 (1936).
66. Corey, R. B., *Chem. Revs.* **26,** 277 (1940); *Advances in Protein Chem.* **4,** 385 (1948); Corey, R. B., and Donohue, J., *J. Am. Chem. Soc.* **72,** 2899 (1950).
67. Pauling, L., "The Nature of the Chemical Bond," Cornell University Press, Ithaca, N. Y., 1942.
68. Sutherland, G., *Advances in Protein Chem.* **7,** 291 (1952).
69. Wirtz, K., *Z. Naturforsch.* **26,** 94 (1947).
70. Pauling, L., Corey, R. B., and Branson, H. R., *Proc. Natl. Acad. Sci. U. S.* **37,** 205 (1951).
71. Gustavson, K. H., *Acta Chem. Scand.* **8,** 1298 (1954); *Nature* **175,** 70 (1955).
72. Putnam, F. W., in "The Proteins" (H. Neurath, and K. Bailey, eds.) Vol. 1. Part B, pp. 807–892. Academic Press, New York, 1953; Anson, M. L., *Advances in Protein Chem.* **2,** 361 (1945); Neurath, H., Greenstein, J. P., Putnam, F. W., and Erickson, J. O., *Chem. Revs.* **34,** 157 (1944).
72a. Alexander, P., private communication; see also Alexander, P., and Stacey, K. A., *Proc. Roy. Soc.* **A212,** 274 (1952).
73. Cohn, E. J., and Edsall, J. T., "Proteins, Amino Acids, and Peptides." Reinhold, New York, 1943.
74. Stiasny, E., and Scotti, H., *Ber.* **63,** 2977 (1930); *cf.* Zief, M., and Edsall, J. T., *J. Am. Chem. Soc.* **59,** 2245 (1937).
75. Vickerstaff, T., "Physical Chemistry of Dyeing," p. 288. Oliver and Boyd, London, 1950.
76. Gortner, R. A., Jr., and Gortner, W. A., "Outlines of Biochemistry," 3rd ed., pp. 251–312. Wiley, New York, 1949; *Trans. Faraday Soc.* **26,** 678 (1930).
77. Pauling, L., "The Nature of the Chemical Bond," p. 71. Cornell University Press, Ithaca, N. Y., 1940.
78. Weber, H. H., *Biochem. Z.*, **218,** 1 (1930).
79. Harkins, W., *Science* **102,** 294 (1945); Dole, M., and McLaren, A., *J. Am. Chem. Soc.* **69,** 651 (1947); Davis, S., and McLaren, A., *J. Polymer Sci.* **3,** 16 (1948).

80. Bull, H. B., *J. Am. Chem. Soc.* **66,** 1499 (1944).
81. Fricke, R., and Lüke, J., *Z. Elektrochem.* **36,** 309 (1930).
82. Pauling, L., *J. Am. Chem. Soc.* **67,** 555 (1945).
83. Mellon, E. F., Korn, A. H., and Hoover, S. R., *J. Am. Chem. Soc.* **73,** 1870 (1951).
84. Braybooks, W. E., McCandlish, D., and Atkin, W. R., *J. Intern. Soc. Leather Trades Chem.* **23,** 111 (1939); see also Holland, H. C., *ibid.* **27,** 207 (1943).
84a. Huggins, M. L., *Ann. Rev. Biochem.* **11,** 27 (1942).
85. Gorter, E., *Ann. Rev. Biochem.* **10,** 619 (1941); Bull. H. B., *Advances in Protein Chem.* **3,** 95 (1947); Adam, N. K., "Physics and Chemistry of Surfaces," Oxford University Press, New York, 1941.
86. Gorter, E., and Grendel, A., *Trans. Faraday Soc.* **22,** 477 (1926); Guastalla, J., *Compt. rend.* **208,** 781 (1939); Seastone, C. V., *J. Gen. Physiol.* **21,** 621 (1938); Bull. H. B., *J. Chem. Am. Soc.* **67,** 4 (1945).
87. Ellis, S. C., and Pankhurst, K. G. A., *Nature* **163,** 600 (1949); *Trans. Faraday Soc.* **50,** 82 (1954).
88. Guastella, J., *Compt. rend.* **208,** 781 (1939).
89. Schulman, J. H., and Rideal, E., *Proc. Roy. Soc.* **B122,** 29 46 (1937).
90. Cockbain, E. G., and Schulman, J. H., *Trans. Faraday Soc.* **35,** 716, 1266 (1939).
91. Gorter, E., and Blokker, A., *Proc. Koninkl. Ned. Akad. Wetenschap.* **45,** 288, 335 (1942).
92. Ellis, S. C., and Pankhurst, K. G. A., *Discussions Faraday Soc.* **No. 16,** 170 (1954).
93. Schulman, J. H., and Dogan, M. Z., *Discussions Faraday Soc.* **No. 16,** 158 (1954).
94. Ellis, S. C., and Pankhurst, K. G. A., *Trans. Faraday Soc.* **50,** 82 (1954).
95. Bowes, J. H., and Moss, J. A., *Biochem. J.* **55,** 735 (1953).

CHAPTER 2

The Structure of Skin and the Chemistry of Collagen

From the special point of view of tanning, collagen, the main constituent of the skin, will obviously occupy a predominant position. The solid matter of the corium of the hides and skins which are most important economically consists of 90 to 95 % collagen. As the major constituent of skin, tendon, and connective tissues, collagen is one of the most prevalent and widely distributed proteins of the animal kingdom, comprising about one-third of the total mass of proteins in the body. The tissue from older animals usually contains more collagen than that from young specimens. The degree of orientation of the collagen structures tends also to increase with age.

Apart from its importance as a raw material for leather, collagen serves as the source for glue and gelatin, which are its degradation products. The name collagen is derived from the Greek word for glue, κόλλα, meaning "forming glue," as is also the word colloid, which means "gluelike." Hence, collagen may be considered to be the true parent colloid. In recent years, the collagenous tissues have attracted the attention of the medical specialist, particularly in regard to rheumatic diseases and many disorders of joints and connective tissues. Certain types of disease are believed to be caused by destructive changes of collagen and have been named collagenous diseases. The aging of the body may also involve structural alterations in the tendons and connective tissues. The impaired flexibility of tendons on aging and in certain bodily disorders may well be caused by disturbances in some enzymatic chain, resulting in the enrichment of substances of tanning potency, which in normal systems are destroyed by special enzymes. The importance of collagen for the healing of wounds, as well as the impairment of healing due to the disturbance of the process of collagen formation by a deficiency in ascorbic acid and other vitamins, is another interesting example of the role played by collagen in the normal functioning of the body. In the connective tissues collagen is intimately bound up with elastin in the so-called ground substance, composed mainly of these proteins, mucopolysaccharides, and cellular elements.

1. THE MICROSTRUCTURE OF SKIN

a. General aspects

Since animal skin is the basis of leather, some knowledge of its microstructure is essential for an understanding of the complicated reactions taking place in the fiber weave during the tanning processes. Only the elements of the microstructure of bovine skin will be outlined in this book. Reference is given to the books of Wilson and Küntzel (1, 2).

The microstructure of skin has a decided influence on the properties of leather. A knowledge of the functions of the skin will therefore be helpful for the understanding of the reactions of skin in its conversion into leather by the tanning process. The skin has a number of important functions in the organism. It is an organ for sense, secretion, and excretion, as well as for protection of the body against bacterial infection. It acts also as a buffer against shocks and blows. In strong sunlight it develops color filters for protection of the underlying tissues from the destructive action of the ultraviolet rays of the sun. One of the most important functions of the skin is to keep the body temperature constant. This is done by a delicate mechanism in the upper part of the true skin, which has been called the "thermostat layer." The escape of heat from the body is retarded by the excretion of an oily material to the surface of the skin (sebum). Acceleration of the heat losses of the body is obtained by evaporation of water (perspiration).

The skin is divided sharply into three distinct layers: (*1*) a relatively thin, outer layer of epithelial tissue, the *epidermis*; (*2*) a much thicker layer of connective and other tissues, which constitute the true leather-forming derma or *corium*; and (*3*) *subcutaneous tissue*, consisting of adipose and areolar tissues, known to the tanner as "flesh," by which stratum the skin is attached to the main body. In the preparation of skin for tanning, the epidermis and the adipose tissues must be removed, leaving the purified corium to be converted into leather. This remaining part consists mainly of bundles of collagen fibers, interwoven in all directions.

Figure 6 shows a photomicrograph of a cross section of a calfskin from which the subcutaneous layer has been removed. The sample was taken from the most compact part of the skin, the butt. The picture demonstrates the general structure of skin. The epidermis is shown as a thin, dark line which forms the upper boundary of the skin. The epidermal layer measures only about 1 % of the total thickness of the skin. It consists of cellular strata originating from the ectoderm, which is the outer layer of the young embryo. The corium is derived from the mesoderm, the middle layer of the embryo. These two strata grow independently throughout life. They also show distinctly different chemical and physical properties. The epidermis is built up from keratin, whereas the main constituent of corium is collagen.

Our chief interest will be directed toward the corium. The top of the corium, about one-fifth of its thickness, differs structurally from the main part. It is named the *thermostat* layer, indicating its primary function (Wilson, 1). The chief portion is the *reticular* layer, the name being derived from its

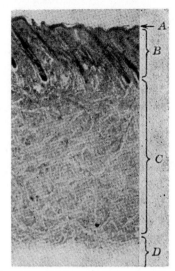

FIG. 6. Vertical section of calfskin, magnification 30 diameters: *A*, epidermis; *B*, thermostat layer; *C*, reticular layer; *D*, subcutaneous tissue.

main feature, the netlike appearance of the fibers of connective tissue. The structure of the thermostat layer is adapted to the physiological function of the skin and determines its appearance in the form of leather, which has a characteristic "grain" depending on the structure of the skin of the animal from which it is derived.

Since the solutions of the generally used tanning agents contain compounds of various degress of dispersity (polydisperse systems), the problem of the degree of accessibility of the reactive groups of collagen makes studies of tanning systems very difficult. The rate of diffusion of the tanning agents into the hide structure, and concomitantly the penetration of smaller molecules into the interior of fibrils and the retardation and even prevention of the diffusion of larger particles of the tanning agent into the smaller interstices of fibrillar units of the skin, presents problems of great difficulty. It is also probably that in many instances the distribution of the tanning agents fixed by collagen is not uniform throughout the interior of the skin or within the various structural elements. These complications of obstructed penetration of tanning agents through the macrostructure may be partly avoided or eliminated in laboratory studies by using skin substrates of a high degree of subdivision, such as hide powder or single-fiber bundles. The latter are preferably applied in studies of theoretical problems by means of physicochemical and mechanical methods, since the macroweave structure is thus eliminated. In any event, the implication of the two-phase systems with the accompanying difficulty of attaining true equilibrium must always be borne in mind.

b. Fiber elements

The major structural elements found in the corium of skin and their dimensions are illustrated in Fig. 7, which gives an indication of the correspondence between these elements and the methods applied for their resolution (3). At the microscopic level with linear magnifications up to 1000, the picture at the top shows a *fiber* of collagen. It is built up from parallelly aligned *primitive* fibers. The fiber has a cross section of 20 to 40 microns, and the diameter of the constituting primitive fiber is of the order of 2 to 5 microns. The ultramicroscopic level shows a primitive fiber split up by mild mechanical treatment (ultrasonics) into its unit, the *fibril*, with an average diameter of some tenths of a micron. By means of the electron microscope the electron-optical level is reached which is required for adequate resolution of the fibril. The fibril with its components, the *filaments*, is depicted at that level. The cross sections of the filaments, the fine structure of which is studied by means of the electron microscope, are of the order of several hundred Ångström units. The possibilities for longitudinal cleavage do not stop with the fibril. The final and highest resolution is reached by means of the diffraction diagram obtained in the small-angle X-ray analysis. The hypothetical thinnest unit of the filament is the protofibril, following the nomenclature of Bear (3) and Schmitt (4). The protofibril carries the essential chemical and configurational structure of collagen, the molecule of which would be equal to or smaller than the protofibril. According to Bear (3), the ultimate structural element of the protofibril is no wider than a very few peptide chains and probably consists most often of *one* polypeptide chain with a diameter of 12 to 17 Å. It is interesting to inquire about the distances between the various structural elements, since the capillaries and channels in the skin structure are expected to determine the possibility for, and the rate of diffusion of, the various reacting substances in systems of tanning processes, such as in vegetable tanning with a polydisperse solution of vegetable tannins. Exact figures of these dimensions are not known, and apparently the dimensions of the cross sections of the interfibrillar spaces vary greatly according to the physical state of the skin, for instance, its degree of swelling. The distance between fibers is probably of the order of a few tenths of a micron, the space between fibrils appears to measure in fractions of a micron, and that between filaments probably involves distances of about a hundred Ångström units.

2. Some Aspects of Structural Organization

Before entering on a discussion of the present conception of the structure of collagen derived from studies using the electron-optical and X-ray diffraction methods, an outline of the general status of organization of

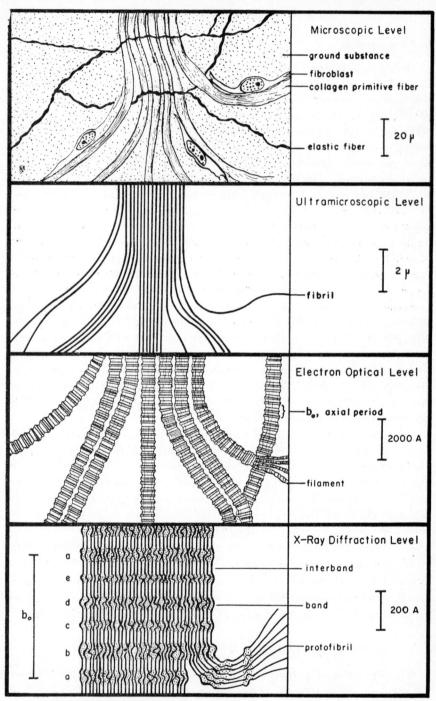

FIG. 7. Structural elements of the collagen fiber, in steps of increasing magnification. From R. S. Bear, *Advances in Protein Chem.* **7,** 72 (1952), Fig. 1.

fibrous proteins and the chemical composition of collagen seems desirable for didactic reasons.

As mentioned in Chapter 1, the classification of the proteins into two main groups, the *globular* and the *fibrous*, is made on the basis of the arrangement of the protein chains, the peptide chains of the fiber proteins being more or less extended in parallel, whereas the molecules of the globular proteins are folded, no preferred direction of orientation being evident. In view of the new ideas of protein structure based on the helical structural principle, originally advanced by Huggins (5), further modified and extended in a more specific form by Pauling and Corey (6), and also promulgated by Bear (3), by Bragg *et al.* (7), by Randall and his school (8), by Ambrose and Elliott (9), and recently by Huggins (9a) from different angles of approach, the dividing line between the globular and the fibrous proteins is somewhat vague. For some time, it has been known that the globular proteins with their compact and fairly rigid molecules may be conceived as potentially fibrous, since their molecules can be opened up and uncoiled by treatment with certain lyotropic agents, such as concentrated solutions of urea, followed by the application of mechanical stress to the modified protein. This was discovered by Astbury and his school (10) and confirmed by the remarkable researches of Lundgren (11). Conversely, it has even been suggested that the molecules of the fibrous proteins, such as keratin and collagen, particularly procollagens, may be built up of globular units forming strings of beads. However, there is still enough difference in general structure between the two main groups to justify adherence to the classification given.

The fibrous proteins and the high-molecular polypeptides are currently classified according to their X-ray diffraction diagrams and their infrared absorption spectra (Ambrose and Elliott, 9; Astbury, 10) into three groups: *(1)* α proteins, with folded polypeptide chains, keratin being the best-known member; *(2)* β proteins, with fully extended chains, silk fibroin being the classic example; *(3)* the collagens, which have as a common characteristic a main axial period at 640 Å. in the small-angle X-ray diffraction diagram and in electron micrographs. The collagen family is subdivided into *(1)* cross-striated structures, represented by collagens from the vertebrates, particularly the mammals, and *(2)* non-cross-striated structures, which are present in collagens of the invertebrates, such as in the earthworm cuticle. This group is also named secreted collagens (Fauré-Frémiet). Both groups give the regular wide-angle X-ray diagram.

The infrared optics, particularly the dichroism of the keto-imide group (stretching and deformation of the C=O and N—H bonds), introduced by the Courtauld research group (9) is particularly valuable because of the classification it gives of the configuration of the polypeptide chains. The method estimates the type of hydrogen bonds in the structure. It has been shown that intramolecular hydrogen bonds are characteristic of the α configuration (lying parallel to the chain) and intermolecular hydrogen bonds of the β configuration (lying perpendicular to the main direction of the chain). The most important feature of this elegant method is that the determination of the type of bond present applies to the *whole* structure, independent of the relative proportion of the band ("amorphous") and interband ("crystalline") regions of the proteins. Hence, the polarized infrared technique does not have the limitations of the X-ray method, which in the form of the wide-angle diagram surveys only the interband regions. In the small-angle modification and from the electron micrographs only the gross structure of the protein chains is obtained. No information as to the presence of mixtures of the α and β configurations is obtained by the earlier methods. Such information is supplied by the infrared examination of polypeptides and proteins.

The properties and reactivity of fibrous proteins are governed primarily by their chemical composition, with due regard to the organization of the protein structures. This fact is clearly brought out by comparing collagen and its secondary product, gelatin, which differ markedly with respect to their physical properties, although their chemical composition is practically identical. The different degrees of organization of the peptide chains and the higher units account for the differences between collagen and gelatin (see Table 3). The collagen units are arranged in parallel and stabilized by valency forces between adjacent peptide chains and micelles (crosslinks). In the conversion of collagen into gelatin, some of these crosslinks are broken, resulting in shortening and disorganization of the protein chains.

The importance of organization of proteins was early recognized by Lloyd (12). Attention was called to the interrelationship of chemical composition, the degree of stabilization of the units, and the physicochemical reactivity of proteins, particularly the degree of swelling (water imbibition),

TABLE 3

ORGANIZATION OF PROTEINS AND DEGREE OF WATER IMBIBITION (SWELLING)

| Protein | Relative Amounts of | | Mg. Equiv. HCl Fixed per g. Protein | Degree of Swelling, % Water Taken up at | |
	Total bases	Total dicarboxylic acids		pH 5	pH 1
Silk fibroin	1	—	0.15	20	22
Keratin	11	15	0.8	30	35
Collagen	15	17	0.9	260	490
Gelatin	15	17	0.9	1300	6500
Muscle protein	17	20	1.0	300	1400

at the pH of maximum swelling and at the pH of minimum swelling (isoelectric range). The data in Table 3 (12) illustrate this point for some typical fibrous proteins (silk fibroin, keratin, collagen, and muscle protein). The acid-binding capacities of the proteins mentioned are included in order to show that the degree of swelling by acids is not a simple function of the amount of acid-binding protein groups. It is evident that fibrous proteins, built up mainly from amino acids with nonpolar groups, possess low affinity for water, whereas proteins containing numerous polar groups take up water readily. However, collagen and keratin, with practically the same degree of polarity and acid-binding capacity, show great differences in water uptake and degree of swelling. The different internal organization of these proteins explains their behavior. Keratin contains the covalent cystine bridge, which resists the action of acids, maintaining the rigid structure in spite of the electrostatic repulsion of those protein groups which are positively charged in acid solutions. In collagen, on the other hand, the negatively charged R groups, to a large extent internally compensated by electropositive R groups, forming saltlike crosslinks, are discharged and the crosslinks broken. By this disorganization of the chains, some of the second type of cohesive forces of the collagen structure, the coordinate crosslinks on the peptide groups (hydrogen bonds), are probably ruptured. Water is added to the protein by polar forces and by association on the coordinate loci of the peptide groups set free by the contraction of the main chains. The effective stabilization of keratin is due to the disulfide bridges and hydrogen bonds. This is evident from the fact that, on breaking of the covalent bridge, the resulting products, the keratoses, swell in acid solution to a degree comparable to the degree of swelling of collagen.

3. The Chemistry of Collagen

a. Amino acid composition

The amino acid composition of gelatin has been extensively studied since the first investigations of Emil Fischer (13), more than fifty years ago, followed by Dakin's important contributions (14). Scant attention has been paid to the precursor of gelatin, the better defined, more uniform, and more easily purified collagen, until recently. The figures on amino acid composition of collagen usually cited in the literature up to the 1940's pertain in fact to gelatin, on the assumption that the compositions of the two proteins were identical. Most of these analyses were carried out by methods which are now obsolete and even considered unsatisfactory, an outstanding exception being the fundamental investigations of Max Bergmann and his associates. Furthermore, the list of amino acid residues in the older literature was derived from a large number of investigations, mainly on one amino acid on different samples of gelatin. As to the analytical work on collagen, most of the data were obtained from analysis of collagens which had been treated in alkaline solutions for unhairing or which had been enzymatically treated in order to remove elastic fibers, accessory proteins of the globular type, and reticular tissue. The alkaline treatment modifies the collagen. It particularly affects the total nitrogen content, since deamidation occurs readily at the high degree of alkalinity corresponding to pH 12 to 13, which is usually employed in the liming process.

By the outstanding work of Chibnall and his school and by the application of the separation techniques of Moore and Stein, great advances have been made in analysis of proteins with reference to their amino acid make-up. These researches have also made feasible an accurate determination of the amino acid composition of native collagen, the only questionable value being that of hydroxyproline, for which there is no reliable method of estimation. The lack of an exact and convenient technique for the estimation of hydroxyproline is especially regrettable, since this particular, and, for collagen, unique, amino acid seems to be the most characteristic one for different types of collagens, which show widely differing values of their hydroxyproline content. Thus, the hydroxyproline figure for mammalian collagen is 14 % (15), whereas only 4 % has been reported for collagen of hake swim bladder (ichthyocol) (16). The teleostean skin collagen contains from 6 to 11 % (15, 17). These figures are in grams of hydroxyproline per 100 g. of protein.

Bowes and Kenton (18) have prepared a sample of collagen with a minimum of chemical treatment. It was considered that any smaller quantities of accessory proteins in the middle of corium would lead to less error in composition of the native collagen than the drastic treatments which are needed for their removal by conventional methods. The mode of preparation is given in detail, a standard procedure being of the utmost importance. The back area, the butt, of a freshly flayed oxhide was cut in pieces of the size 18 × 12 inches. The pieces were drummed, first in water and then in a 10 % solution of sodium chloride for half an hour. They were left stationary overnight in a fresh salt solution of 10 % strength, then drummed further for half an hour the next morning, followed by extensive washing in several changes of distilled water. The grain layer containing the epidermal structures, muscles, and elastin fibers was split off, as was also the adipose layer on the flesh side of the hide specimen. The remaining reticular layer of the corium was cut into 1-cm. cubes which were degreased with three changes of petroleum ether at room temperature for 6 days. The extracted cubes were washed with successive changes of distilled water and finally dehydrated with acetone. The purified collagen contained 0.03 % ash, 23 % moisture, and less than 0.1 % fat.

TABLE 4
AMINO ACID COMPOSITION OF NATIVE UNLIMED COLLAGEN

Amino Acid	N as % Protein N	Gram Residues per 100 g.	Milli-moles per Gram	Assumed Number of Resi-dues	Apparent Minimum Molecular Weight
Amino nitrogen	2.5	—	0.33	—	—
Glycine	26.3	19.9	3.50	136	38.880
Alanine	8.0	7.6	1.06	41	38.580
Leucine ⎱ Isoleucine⎰	3.2	4.8	0.42	17	39.950
Valine	2.2	2.9	0.29	11	37.620
Phenylalanine	1.9	3.7	0.25	10	39.600
Tyrosine	0.6	1.3	0.08	3	37.620
Tryptophan	0.0	0.0	0.00	—	—
Serine	2.5	2.7	0.33	13	39.130
Threonine	1.5	2.0	0.20	8	40.160
Cystine	0.0	0.0	0.00	—	—
Methionine	0.4	0.7	0.05	2	37.640
Proline	9.9	12.7	1.32	51	38.760
Hydroxyproline	8.0[a]	12.1	1.07	41	38.580
Lysine	4.7	4.0	0.31	12	38.400
Hydroxylysine	1.2	1.1	0.08	3	37.680
Arginine	15.3	7.9	0.51	20	39.380
Histidine	1.2	0.7	0.05	2	37.640
Aspartic acid	3.6	5.5	0.47	19	39.750
Glutamic acid	5.8	10.0	0.77	30	38.910
Amide nitrogen	3.5	—	0.47	18	38.740
Total found	99.8	99.6[b]	10.76[b]	419	38.730 (mean)

[a] Determined on gelatin.
[b] Excluding amide nitrogen.

The preparation of the collagen described was analyzed by Chibnall and his co-workers for contents of basic amino acids and aliphatic hydroxy-amino acids, alanine, leucines, valine, phenylalanine, and proline. The contents of glutamic and aspartic acids were estimated by Bowes and Kenten. In Table 4 the final results are tabulated. The total nitrogen content of the native collagen was 18.6%. The mean residue weight of the amino acids is 92.6, a value identical with that of Chibnall (19), calculated from the nitrogen distribution.

In adding up cationic and anionic groups separately, native collagen with its isoelectric point at pH 7.5 to 8.0 will contain 0.95 mg. equiv. of cationic groups and 0.77 mg. equiv. of anionic groups (1.24 − 0.47) per gram of collagen. The location of the isoelectric point in a slightly alkaline medium corresponds then to a slight excess of cationic groups, or 0.18 mg. equiv. per gram of collagen, which is as would be expected.

Using the same figures for alkali-processed gelatin with an average content of amide nitrogen of 0.1 to 0.2 mg. equiv. per gram of gelatin, the cationic groups are equal to 0.95 mg. equiv., and the anionic groups to 1.04 to 1.14 mg. equiv. (1.24 − 0.1 or 0.2). The excess of anionic groups of 0.09 to 0.19 mg. equiv. corresponds to an isoelectric point of 4.8 for this type of gelatin. The composition of native collagen and alkali-processed gelatin thus conforms logically to the location of the pH values corresponding to the isoelectric point of these proteins.

b. Total nitrogen content

With reference to the figures of the table, the total nitrogen and amide contents of this purified sample of native collagen are higher than those previously reported and usually employed. In view of the marked deamidation of collagen taking place in the ordinary liming process, these figures of the nitrogen content should not be used on regular pelt (neutral limed hide) in calculating the factor for conversion of nitrogen into hide substance. The total nitrogen contents of the standard hide powder preparations and of short-limed pelt are generally 18.0 %, in the ash- and fat-free dry substance. Instead of the standard value of 17.8 %, with the conversion factor of 5.62 for nitrogen into collagen, the figure of 18.0 %, and hence a conversion factor of 5.56 (for nitrogen into collagen), seems better to fit the modern practice of short liming, under which considerably less deamidation takes place. This particular aspect of the calculation of hide substances from the nitrogen content of leather has been discussed by Bowes and Kenten (20).

The collagen of sheepskin contains only 17.0 % nitrogen. Since sheepskin contains large amounts of fat, it is possible that the reason for the low nitrogen content is the presence of fatty matter in combination with collagen not extractable with ordinary solvents.

c. General comments on composition

The amino acid figures for glycine and hydroxyproline in Table 4 were selected from the literature. The figure for hydroxyproline is probably the least reliable. In spite of these uncertainties, over 99 % of the total nitrogen of collagen is accounted for by these figures, and the data on the amino acid composition of collagen appear to be virtually complete. In comparing these data with the older values, the main differences are found in the contents of glutamic and aspartic acids, which are nearly twice as large as the earlier values. This will radically affect the proportion of basic (cationic) to acidic (anionic) groups, changing the ratio from 1.5:1 to 1:1.3. The adjusted figures of the dicarboxylic acids, and the resulting ratio of basic to acidic groups, with due consideration of the deamidation of collagen taking place in the alkali treatment, remove the paradox that gelatin and limed collagen are isoelectric in the acid pH range, although according to the old values they should contain a large excess of cationic groups. On the other hand, the new data make the discrepancy between the figures obtained for the base-binding capacity of collagen and its content of free carboxyl groups still wider.

From the data given in the table, it is evident that collagen contains a well-balanced proportion of positively and negatively charged ionic groups, securing a fair degree of ionic reactivity. This reactivity is particularly important for the behavior of collagen in the preliminary processes prior to tanning and in the tanning processes proper. Characteristic for the collagen group of proteins is the large content of nonpolar amino acids, particularly glycine and alanine, which compose about a third of the total amino acid residues. Above all, the prominence of proline and hydroxyproline as well as the paucity of aromatic residues is a unique trait of the collagen molecule. Because of the presence of a large number of residues of the prolines built into the peptide chains, about every fourth or fifth of the regular connecting links of the backbone will appear in the form of —CO—N= links. This will introduce a regular interruption of the regular —CO·NH— links formed by the remainder of the amino acid residues. Since the latter bond is generally considered to be the main site for crosslinking of adjacent peptide chains by hydrogen bonding of proteins, the introduction of the —CO—N= link with an imino group not capable of forming a hydrogen bond will mean fewer sites for the crosslinking of the collagen chains by means of hydrogen bridges.

However, the problem of intermolecular linking is further complicated by the presence of hydroxyproline in the chains. The function of the hydroxy group of aliphatic amino acids as a potential site of crosslinking by interaction with carboxyl ions of an adjacent chain in globular proteins has been suggested by Klotz (21). His basic assumption is that the —OH side chains form hydrogen bonds with other side chains containing —COO⁻ or =NH⁺— groups, the link between the carboxyl and hydroxy groups being preferentially formed. This interaction will increase the rigidity of the protein lattice. Another effect will be the decreased reactivity of the carboxyl ions with an increasing number of hydroxyamino acid residues. Klotz (21) has presented experimental evidence indicating that the reactivity of the carboxyl ion of various globular proteins decreases with increased content of hydroxyamino acids. This behavior is conceived as being due to the inactivation of the charged carboxyl groups by means of neighboring hydroxy groups by a hydrogen-bonding mechanism. The possible bearing of the varying content of hydroxyproline in different types of collagen on their degree of stability will be discussed further on.

It is also interesting to note that hydroxyl groups, contributed by hydroxyproline, serine, hydroxylysine, and threonine, form nearly one-half the total number of polar groups. The possible function of these groups, particularly the primary alcoholic group of the aliphatic amino acids, containing residual negative charge on oxygen (22), in the reaction of tanning agents with collagen has not yet been seriously considered, although suggested by Green (23). The importance of the hydroxy groups in binding of heavy metals by hydroxy acids has been amply demonstrated in Klotz' work, and its participation in the uptake of bivalent cations by proteins has been proved (22). Recent investigations of the reaction of O-acetylated collagen to tanning agents indicate that the hydroxy group participates in the binding of nonionic chromium complexes (sulfito) by collagen (23a).

The minimum molecular weight of collagen calculated from the amino acid distribution (Table 4) is 39,000. In the determinations of the terminal groups of collagen by the Sanger dinitrofluorobenzene (DNFB) method, carried out by Bowes and Moss (24), no terminal amino groups could be detected. Provided that unforeseen complications do not enter, this finding would indicate that the *real* molecular weight must be of the order of millions. If the repeating period of 640 Å., with about 700 residues, in the helical structure is considered to represent the minimum "molecular weight," this will be of the order of 65,000. This value is the minimum molecular weight of "procollagen." As mentioned earlier, the concept of molecular weight as an entity loses its meaning when applied to macromolecules of the type represented by collagen (25). Thus, the molecular weight of acid-extracted skin collagen, estimated by light scattering, is about 10 million (26), the macromolecule being highly coiled, with dimensions 12 × 150,000 Å.

d. Sulfur content

The total organic sulfur content of purified hide, in the form of hide powder and pelt, determined by means of the Grote-Krekeler method, is in the range of 0.3 to 0.5 % for mammalian collagen, and 1.0 to 1.2 % for fishskin collagen, based on the fat- and ash-free dry substance (27). Since the only sulfur-containing amino acid of the collagen molecule is methionine, amounting to 0.7 to 0.8 % in bovine collagen, its sulfur content should correspond to 0.15 to 0.2 %. In some instances, the high sulfur content may be due to impurities in the hide, such as the presence of hair rests in the grain layer. However, even the middle layer of the corium, which is practically free from such debris, contains about 0.3 % sulfur. A plausible explanation is the presence of chondroitin sulfuric acid in combination with collagen, which has been suggested as a cementing substance for the macromolecules of cartilage by Partridge (28), and for tendon by Jackson (29), a possibility also discussed by Bowes and Kenten (30), who considered its effect on the alkaline swelling of hide. However, determinations of the content of chondroitin sulfate (ester sulfur) in bovine hides and skins of various previous history and treatment show only very slight amounts, which are practically unaffected by alkaline pretreatment (liming). The values are of the order of 0.02 to 0.05 % sulfur. Hence, the difference between the total content of organic sulfur and the methionine sulfur, amounting to 0.1 to 0.2 %, is not accounted for by the ester-sulfur present.

Fishskin collagen (*Gadus*) contains more than twice the amount of organic sulfur found in bovine hide, about 1.0 % based on the weight of collagen (31). This is accounted for by the higher content of methionine (2.3 % against 0.9 % for bovine hide) and by the small amount of cystine present (0.12 %). These amounts correspond to 0.5 % sulfur, leaving an equal amount not accounted for.

e. Teleostean còllagen

The collagen of the skin of cold-water fish (Teleostei) differs considerably from mammalian collagen in coordinate reactivity and in physical properties, particularly with regard to the degree of hydrothermal stability and resistance toward proteinases (31). These are markedly lower for fishskin collagen, the shrinkage temperatures being of the order of 60 to 70°C. for mammalian skin (isoelectric pelt) against values of 38 to 45°C for cold-water fishes, and 50 to 56°C for warm-water fishes (17). The experimental findings of the inferior stability of the collagens of the skin of *Gadus*, with shrinkage temperatures of 40 to 43°C. compared to values of 63 to 68°C. for bovine skin collagen, were interpreted to indicate a paucity of crosslinks of the hydrogen-bridge type on adjacent keto-imide groups in fish collagen, in comparison with the mammalian collagen with strongly hydrogen-bonded polypeptide chains (31). At the time of these investigations in the early 1940's, no reliable data on the amino acids were available. Since then, figures on the composition of fishskin collagen (halibut) have been published by Neuman (32) and by Neuman and Logan (15). Table 5 gives the figures of the content (in grams per 100 g. of protein) of the amino acids which differ most markedly in the two types of collagen. Neuman (32) found that collagens from different tissues and from different sources of mammalians were similar in amino acid composition. The main differences in amino acid composition between fishskin collagen and mammalian collagen are the greater amounts (50 to 100 %) of serine, threonine, and methionine in fishskin collagen, and above all the much lower content of hydroxyproline in

TABLE 5

CONTENT OF AMINO ACIDS SHOWING LARGE DIFFERENCES IN BOVINE AND FISHSKIN COLLAGEN (15, 32)

Type	% N	Serine	Threo-nine	Proline	Hydro-xyproline	Methio-nine
Native oxhide	18.1	2.8	2.2	16.5	13.3	0.9
Native fishskin (halibut)	18.4	5.9	3.5	13.7	9.1	2.3

teleostean collagen. Beveridge and Lucas (16) found the same differences between ichthyocol (isinglass from hake swim bladder) and mammalian collagen, their hydroxyproline figure being as low as 4%, probably owing to shortcomings of the method then available.

Takahashi (33), who in collaboration with Tanaka (34) independently discovered the different degrees of hydrothermal stability (T_s) in the skin of cold-water and warm-water fishes mentioned earlier, has determined the T_s and hydroxyproline content of a great number of species of fish. A direct correlation was established, in agreement with the findings of the present author (17). Takahashi reports the hydroxyproline content of skins of cold-water fishes, with T_s values of 33 to 43°C., to be 7.0 to 8.6%. The corresponding values for warm-water fishes, with T_s values of 50 to 56°C., are 9.7 to 11.0%, whereas mammalian skin collagen contains 12.5 to 14%. The values for hydroxyproline listed in the literature and those estimated by Takahashi were obtained by the method of Neuman and Logan (15). The accuracy and reproducibility of this method are not as great as could be desired, since indirect values only are obtained. Hence, a direct estimation of the hydroxyproline content of teleostean and bovine skin collagen are imperative for the problem of the function of hydroxyproline in collagen.

By a combination of the chromatographic procedures of Moore and Stein, the hydroxyproline and proline fractions of the hydrolyzates from collagens of native bovine skin and native skins of codfish and pike have been isolated and these imino acids determined. Table 6 presents the results (17, 35). The directly determined hydroxyproline content of the skin of the codfish, a typical cold-water fish, is appreciably lower than the figure of 9.1% reported for the skin of halibut (with a T_s of 40°C.), indirectly obtained (15). However, the lowest figure found by Takahashi (33) is 7.0% for the skin of the rockfish (*Sebastodes*), which also has the lowest T_s ever recorded for collagens, 33 to 34°C. The sum of the pyrrolidine residues for codskin collagen is hardly more than half the accepted value of bovine collagen. The great variations in the content of these imino acids in various collagens cannot be dismissed when establishing structural models of collagen. Approximately every third amino acid residue of collagen is generally

TABLE 6

CONTENTS OF PROLINES OF VARIOUS SKIN COLLAGENS

Type of Skin	T_s, °C.	Total N, %	Hydroxyproline		Proline		Hydroxyproline + Proline	
			% on protein	% of total N	% on protein	% of total N	% on protein	% of total N
Cod (Gadus morrhua)	40	18.3	5.8	3.4	10.8	7.2	16.6	10.6
Pike (Esox lucius)	55	18.4	7.9	4.6	13.3	8.8	21.2	13.4
Calf (Bos taurus)	65	18.3	12.7	7.4	14.1	9.5	26.8	16.9

considered to be pyrrolidine residue. This proportion has played an integral part in recent structures of collagen, from Astbury's classical model up to the helical structures of Pauling and his school.

The effect of the hydroxyproline content of collagen on its stability and reactivity was first examined in the light of the Klotz concept (21), according to which the hydroxy groups of the residues of aliphatic amino acids in globular proteins form hydrogen bonds of the type —OH---O⁻CO—. This linking should lower the reactivity of the carboxyl ion. The reactions of bovine collagen and codskin collagen with the cupric ion, nonionic complex compounds of chromium, and dyestuffs were studied in the isoelectric range of collagen. The results could not readily be reconciled by an extension of the Klotz concept to the collagens (35). Moreover, according to Bear (3), the electron-optical evidence suggests the presence of the prolines in the interbands of the protofibril, whereas the bands should contain the residues of the dicarboxylic amino acids. Hence, the linking of the hydroxy and ionic carboxyl groups appears improbable for steric reasons.

If collagen is stabilized by interchain hydrogen bonds on adjacent keto-imide linkages mainly, the content of pyrrolidine residues should be a factor of importance. The imino acids form the —CO·N= link, thus introducing a regular interruption of the normal —CO·NH— links formed by the remainder of the amino acid residues. Accordingly, it should result in fewer stabilizing crosslinks (hydrogen bonds), and consequently mammalian collagen should possess a lower degree of stability than teleostean collagen. However, the reverse is true. On the other hand, on the supposition that the hydroxy groups enter into interchain hydrogen bonding with some other groups, e.g., the carbonyl oxygen of the keto-imide linkages, the stability of the structure would be expected to increase with the content of hydroxyproline, as is actually found.

A satisfactory explanation of the correlation between the hydroxyproline content of collagen and its hydrothermal stability has been arrived at by investigations of the behavior of exhaustively acetylated bovine collagen (N- and O-acetylated) (35). The blocking of three out of four hydroxy groups lowers the T_s from 66 to 42°C., indicating the rupture of *interchain* crosslinks by the O-acetylation, since N-acetylation alone has no effect on the T_s. By investigating the fixation of mimosa tannins and nonionic complexes of sulfito-chromium sulfate by intact collagen, N-acetylated, and N- and O-acetylated collagen, experimental evidence for the presence of a strong bond of the following type has been forthcoming (35):

In the new helical model of Huggins, such a bond of 2.9. Å is postulated in collagen (9a).

It should be mentioned that the fixation of both types of reactants by collagen is markedly (50 to 75%) increased by its heat denaturation and by lyotropic pretreatment, which increases the hydrogen-bonding faculty of collagen, probably by rupture of hydrogen bonds, in which the —CO·NH— linkage is a partner. The vegetable tannins possess an exceptionally great affinity for the CO·NH— bond of polyamides, whereas the nonionic chromium complexes mentioned are not fixed at all by the polyamides. Accordingly, the large increase in the uptake of the sulfite compounds by denatured collagen cannot be associated with the keto-imide group by freeing it from its compensation. Moreover, the fixation of mimosa tannins is increased 50 to 75% by O-acetylation, whereas the binding of the sulfito-chromium complexes is lowered by some 30%. These findings, with due consideration of numerous other facts, form the basis for the postulated —OH----OC link.

The rupture of such a bond in the heat denaturation of collagen and by lyotropic agents would satisfactorily explain both the increased fixation of vegetable tannins (by the freed —CO·NH— bond) and the nonionic chromium complexes (by the freed OH— bond), as well as the effects of the blocking of the hydroxy group by its acetylation, i.e., the impaired hydroxy coordination of the chromium complexes, and the increased binding of the keto-imide–attached vegetable tannins. The large T_s decrease is also understandable. In view of the marked reactivity of native collagen for the agents mentioned, it is probable that only a few of the hydroxy- and keto-imide groups are able to form this type of interchain bond. Since the T_s values follow the trend of the hydroxyproline content of the various collagens, being lowered with decreasing content of this amino acid, but run reverse to the figures for the aliphatic hydroxyamino acids in the collagens, it appears as if their hydroxy groups cannot be involved to any appreciable extent. Hence, the hydroxyproline residue should mainly supply the hydroxy- group in the link. This residue should play the same governing role for the stability of collagen as the cystine residue does for keratin. The presence of an ester bond appears possible (Alexander, 35a).

f. The sequence of amino acids

As to the sequence of the amino acid residues of any protein, there are three possibilities: (1) completely ordered, (2) completely randomized, and (3) partly ordered. In the first instance, a definite pattern, identical in different polypeptide chains, is imposed on the protein. The complete pattern may be repeated in the same protein chain, or it may not. It is most likely that definite residues are repeated at definite intervals, according to the frequency number of the particular amino acid residue. The second possibility requires no comment. In the partially ordered pattern, any particular residue is not rigidly fixed, and exchange of similar groups may occur, as for instance between the closely related glycine and alanine. This type of pattern should most probably appear for fibrous proteins, such as collagen. There are two main types of the partially ordered sequence: (1) a regular pattern at intervals along the chain with intermediate intervals of random arrangement; (2) one residue or a type of residue located at fixed intervals, interspaced by one or more fixed types of other residues, and with the remaining intervals randomly fixed.

The collagen structure is characterized by a parallel arrangement of polypeptide chains (protofibrils), which are so arranged as to match each other laterally, accounting for the characteristic periodicity of 640 Å., shown in the electron micrograph and in the small-angle X-ray diagram (3). The crossbanding of the fibrils also suggests that repeating units coincide in the aligned polypeptide chains; this implies a certain order of the different types of residues, at least those of different degrees of hydration. From the complete amino acid composition of a protein, the frequency of the constituting amino acids can be calculated. Thus, from the generally accepted data on the amino acid composition of collagen (18), the frequencies of the principal residues are: glycine 2.95, proline 8.2, hydroxyproline 9.6, alanine 10.2, arginine 21.3, and lysine 33.5. (The figure 2.95, for example, means that about one of every three residues is glycine.) The whole-number sequence of Bergmann and Niemann (36) gave, correspondingly: 3, 6, 9, 18, 24, and 36. However, such figures are of little significance for a protein of the size of collagen, which probably consists only of a partially ordered pattern. Some idea of the most important sequences can first be obtained by isolation and chemical analysis of polypeptides from partial hydrolyzates of collagen.

According to Astbury (37), the amino acid sequence of collagen may be represented by the formula:

$$-P-G-R-P-G-R-$$

where P, with the exception of one residue in eighteen, is prolines, G is glycine, and R is one of the remaining residues. Pauling and Corey (6) assume the same pattern in their evaluation of the X-ray diagrams of collagen in terms of the helical structure. Bergmann and Niemann (36) conceived the sequence from the data of the incomplete amino acid analysis of collagen available in 1936 to be

$$-G-R-P-G-R-R-$$

As early as 1936, Grassmann and Riederle (38) isolated the tripeptide lysyl-prolyl-glycine from a partial hydrolyzate of gelatin. This tripeptide has played an important role in the early development of the periodicity concept of protein structure. Heyns et al. (39) have separated a number of peptides from partial hydrolyzates of gelatin employing paper chromatography and the Sanger DNFB technique. Schroeder el al. (40) have studied the chromatographic separation and identification of di- and tripeptides in such hydrolyzates, using the Moore-Stein Dowex column for the preliminary separation, followed by resolution of the fractions obtained on Celite and end-group determination of the polypeptides separated by the DNFB method. Finally, Kroner et al. (41), employing these and similar methods, have investigated the partial hydrolyzate of native hide collagen. It should also be mentioned that in 1943 Gordon et al. (42) obtained evidence for sequences which contained glycine-leucine, proline-alanine, proline-glycine, and proline-alanine-glycine, but the exact sequences were not determined.

According to the accepted convention of naming the peptides (43), the residue with the free NH_2 group is written first. Using the convention of

TABLE 7

PEPTIDES IDENTIFIED IN PARTIAL HYDROLYZATES OF COLLAGEN AND GELATIN

A. Dipeptides
  1. Containing glycine as C-terminal group
  H·Val-Gly·OH; H·Glu-Gly·OH; H·Ala-Gly·OH; H·Threo-Gly·OH; H·Hypro-Gly·OH
  2. Containing glycine as N-terminal group
  H·Gly-Gly·OH; H·Gly-Asp·OH; H·Gly-Glu·OH; H·Gly-Pro·OH; H·Gly-Ala·OH
  3. Containing   alanine,   but   not   glycine
  H·Glu-Ala·OH; H·Leu-Ala·OH; H·Threo-Ala·OH
  4. Others
  H·Glu-Glu·OH
B. Tripeptides
  H·Ala-Ala-Gly·OH; H·Ala-Gly-Ala·OH; H·Lys-Pro-Gly·OH

Erlanger and Brand (43), alanyl-glycine, for instance, is written H·Ala—Gly·OH. Unknown sequences, in which the N-terminal amino acid is known but the order of the other residues is not known, are written in the form H·Gly·(Ala, Leu).

The peptides identified in the above-mentioned researches are tabulated in the Table 7. In discussing these data, Kroner *et al.* point out that, of the twenty or more dipeptides or tripeptides reported present in partial hydrolyzates of collagen and gelatin, only five fit the sequence —P—G—R—P—G—R— suggested by Astbury (37). These are: H·Lys-Pro-Gly·OH; H·Gly-Asp·OH; H·Gly-Glu·OH; H·Gly-Ala·OH; and H·Hypro-Gly·OH. On the other hand, all these peptides except H·Gly-Gly·OH conform to the —G—R—P—G—R—R— sequence of Bergmann and Niemann (36). However, this sequence was based on Bergmann's value of 19.7 % proline in gelatin (44), which is considerably higher than the currently accepted figure of 15 % (45). Schroeder *et al.* (40) emphasize that, in view of the fact that only one-fourth, instead of one-third, of the residues consists of proline and hydroxyproline, only three-fourths of the prolines could have the sequence —R—Pro(or Hypro)—Gly, and the remaining one-fourth would have no predictable sequence. Accordingly, it would be expected to find sequences which do not agree with the over-all structures proposed. Certainly, more quantitative information is essential for a greater part of the content of amino acids before any definite conclusion can be drawn on structural details of the collagen pattern. Zone 1 of the column in the work of Schroeder *et al.* consisted almost entirely of Threo-Gly, which accounted at least for 40 % of the threonine in the gelatin on the basis of Tristram's analysis (45). If corrections are applied, at least 55 % of the threonine may be accounted for in this form. In zone 2, the Hypro-Gly peptide accounted for about 20 % of the hydroxyproline content of gelatin. Further, the serine in Ser-Gly was equal to about one-third of the total serine. It should also be noted that the isolation of Gly-Gly by Kroner and his co-workers makes it likely that other sequences have to be considered in addition to those suggested. In a recent paper of Schroeder et al. (46), on the isolation and estimation of dipeptides from hydrolyzates of gelatin, it is concluded that the analytical data provide some evidence that the sequence —Gly-Pro-Hypro-Gly— may frequently occur in gelatin and collagen.

It has been pointed out by Eastoe (47) that a promising line of approach would be the quantitative amino acid analysis of different members of the collagen family, both the mammalian and the secreted types. The composition of fishskin collagen (halibut, shark, cod), procollagen, and skin-extracted collagens generally, as well as the non-cross-striated collagens, (15, 45), show widely different contents of some of the amino acids considered to be characteristic for collagens, such as the prolines, and also some nontypical residues, such as tyrosine, methionine, the aliphatic hydroxyamino acids, and even glycine. These findings might indicate that some amino acids form a more permanent framework into which other members of different type can be built, according to the biological requirement. Hence, it would be an important step forward if the rough structure of this framework could be established in order to facilitate the evaluation of the data on the peptide structures.

It seems permissible to conclude from the available experimental data, even though they are rather scanty, that the amino acid residues of the mammalian collagen apparently are laid down according to some definite principle. This conclusion is especially supported by the finding that at least 55 % of the threonine can be isolated as H·Threo-Gly·OH. If it is assumed that the gelatin chains have only random sequences, not more than 33 % of the threonine residues would be followed by glycine, at the most. Since it appears rather improbable that the bond would so break in the hydrolysis that the maximum amount of this dipeptide would be recovered, the figure of 55 % is probably the absolute minimum. Moreover, in view of the fact that glycine and alanine, with frequency numbers exceedingly close to 3 and 9, are found in practically all the isolated dipeptides, it seems quite possible that these two related amino acids can replace each other.

Furthermore, as Eastoe (47) notes, insufficient attention has been given to the possibility that, although a given amino acid may occupy a definite position in the molecular pattern, a further nonstoichiometric amount may occupy some of the optional positions of the framework. Such a replacement would obscure the sequence in the interpretation of the analytical data on the amino acid composition of the protein. Hence, a complete picture of the amino acid composition and the data on the polypeptides isolated for a number of cross-striated and non-cross-striated collagens is an outstanding problem of the collagen chemistry of the future.

REFERENCES

1. Wilson, J. A. "The Chemistry of Leather Manufacture." Chemical Catalog Co., New York, 1929.
2. Küntzel, A., in "Handbuch der Gerbereichemie," (W. Grassmann, ed.), Vol. I, Part 1, pp. 183–358. Springer, Vienna, 1944.
3. Bear, R. S., Advances in Protein Chem. 7, 69 (1952); Cohen, C., and Bear, R. S., J. Am. Chem. Soc. 75, 2784 (1953).
4. Schmitt, F. O., Hall, C. E., and Jakus, M. A., J. Cellular Comp. Physiol. 20, 11 (1942).
5. Huggins, M. L., Chem. Revs., 32, 195 (1943).
6. Pauling, L., and Corey, R. B., Proc. Natl. Acad. Sci. U. S. 37, 272 (1951).
7. Bragg, W. L., Kendrew, J. C., and Perutz, M. F., Proc. Roy. Soc. A203, 321 (1950).
8. Randall, J. T., Fraser, R., Jackson, S., Martin, A. K., and North, A. C., Nature 169, 1029 (1952); Randall, J. T., Fraser, R., and North, A. C., Proc. Roy. Soc. B141, 62 (1953).
9. Ambrose, E. J., and Elliott, A., Proc. Roy. Soc. A206, 206 (1951); A208, 75 (1951).
9a. Huggins, M. L., J. Am. Chem. Soc. 76, 4045 (1954).
10. Astbury, W. T., Dickinson, S., and Bailey, K., Biochem. J. 29, 2351 (1935); Astbury, W. T., Advances in Enzymol. 3, 63 (1943).
11. Lundgren, H. P., Advances in Protein Chem. 5, 305 (1949).
12. Lloyd, D. J., and Phillips, H., Trans. Faraday Soc. 29, 132 (1933); Lloyd, D. J., and Shore, A., "The Chemistry of Proteins." Churchill, London, 1938.
13. Fischer, E., Ber. 34, 433 (1901).
14. Dakin, H. D., Biochem. J. 12, 290 (1918); J. Biol. Chem. 44, 499 (1920).
15. Neuman, R. E., and Logan, M. A., J. Biol. Chem. 184, 299 (1950).
16. Beveridge, J. M. R., and Lucas, C. C., J. Biol. Chem. 155, 547 (1944).
17. Gustavson, K. H., Svensk Kem. Tidskr. 65, 70 (1953).
18. Bowes, J. H., and Kenten, R. H., Biochem. J. 43, 358 (1948).
19. Chibnall, A. C., Proc. Roy. Soc. B131, 136 (1942); J. Soc. Leather Trades Chem. 30, 1 (1946).
20. Bowes, J. H., and Kenten, R. H., J. Soc. Leather Trades Chem. 32, 308 (1948).
21. Klotz, I. M., Cold Spring Harbor Symposia Quant. Biol. 14, 97 (1950); Klotz, I. M., and Ayers, J., Discussions Faraday Soc. No. 13, 189 (1953).
22. Smythe, C. V., and Schmidt, C. L. A., J. Biol. Chem. 88, 241 (1930); Schmidt, C. L. A., "Chemistry of Amino Acids and Proteins," pp. 720–778. Thomas, Springfield, Ill., 1938.
23. Green, R. W., Biochem. J. 54, 187 (1953).
23a. Gustavson, K. H., Nature 175, 70 (1955).
24. Bowes, J. H., and Moss, J. A., Nature 168, 514 (1951).
25. See, e.g., Edsall, J. T., in "The Proteins" (H. Neurath and K. Bailey, eds.), Vol. 1, Part B, pp. 552–555. Academic Press, New York, 1953.
26. M'Ewen, M. B., and Pratt, M. I., in "Nature and Structure of Collagen." (J. T. Randall, ed.), p. 158. Butterworths, London, 1953.
27. Gustavson, K. H., Acta Chem. Scand. 4, 1171 (1950).

28. Partridge, S. M., *Biochem. J.* **43**, 387 (1948).
29. Jackson, D. S., *in* "Nature and Structure of Collagen" (J. T. Randall, ed.), p. 177. Butterworths, London, 1953.
30. Bowes, J. H., and Kenten, R. H., *Biochem. J.* **46**, 1 (1950).
31. Gustavson, K. H., *Svensk Kem. Tidskr.* **54**, 74, 249 (1942); *Acta Chem. Scand.* **4**, 1171 (1950); *J. Am. Leather Chem. Assoc.* **45**, 789 (1950); *J. Soc. Leather Trades Chem.* **33**, 332 (1949); *Biochem. Z.* **311**, 347 (1942).
32. Neuman, R. E., *Arch. Biochem.* **24**, 289 (1949).
33. Takahashi, T., private communication.
34. Takahashi, T., and Tanaka, T., *Bull. Japan. Soc. Sci. Fisheries* **19**, 603 (1953).
35. Gustavson, K. H., *Acta Chem. Scand.* **8**, 1299 (1954).
35a. Alexander, P., private communication; see also Grassmann, W., *Z. Naturforsch.* **9b**, 513 (1954).
36. Bergmann, M., and Niemann, C., *J. Biol. Chem.* **115**, 77 (1936).
37. Astbury, W. T., *J. Intern. Soc. Leather Trades Chem.* **24**, 69 (1940).
38. Grassmann, W., and Riederle, K., *Biochem. Z.* **284**, 177 (1936).
39. Heyns, K., Anders, G., and Becker, E., *Z. physiol. Chem.* **287**, 120 (1951).
40. Schroeder, W. A., Honnen, L., and Green, F. C., *Proc. Natl. Acad. Sci. U. S.* **39**, 23 (1953).
41. Kroner, T. D., Tabroff, W., and McGarr, J. J., *J. Am. Chem. Soc.* **75**, 4084 (1953).
42. Gordon, A. H., Martin, A. J. P., and Synge, R. L. M., *Biochem. J.* **37**, 92 (1943).
43. Brand, E., and Edsall, J. T., *Ann. Rev. Biochem.* **16**, 224 (1947); Erlanger, S., and Brand, E., *J. Am. Chem. Soc.* **73**, 3508 (1951).
44. Bergmann, M., *J. Biol. Chem.* **110**, 471 (1935).
45. Tristram, G. R., *Advances in Protein Chem.* **5**, 84 (1949).
46. Schroeder, W. A., Kay, L. M., LeGette, J., Honnen, L., and Green, F. C., *J. Am. Chem. Soc.* **76**, 3556 (1954).
47. Eastoe, J. E., private communication.

CHAPTER 3

The Architecture and Formation of Collagen

1. Introduction

In the middle 1920's, the problem of the configuration of the protein chains and their arrangement in the final protein structure came into the picture. X-Ray diffraction analysis, particularly in the form developed by the Braggs, had already proved its merits in the elucidation of the structural pattern of simple crystalline compounds. Since the fibrous proteins possess an orderly form and a latticelike structure, as was already known from their mechanical properties and optical anisotropy, the simplest of protein fibers, the silk fibroin, was selected as the most promising object in the first attempt of these researches (1). By directing the X-ray beam perpendicular to the preferred direction of the fiber, X-ray diagrams were obtained which showed definite reflections. Although these reflections were not so well defined as those given by crystals, they nevertheless proved a certain regular crystalline arrangement of the atoms (2).

2. The Wide-Angle X-Ray Technique (3)

Only the general principles of wide-angle X-ray analysis will be presented here. If an X-ray beam passes through a material in which the atoms and molecules are arranged in a fixed position with reference to the three dimensions of space, the emergent beam, when allowed to impinge on a photographic plate, will produce a pattern. This pattern will be mathematically related to the atomic structural pattern of the material. All crystalline compounds show a characteristic X-ray diagram, from which the position of the atoms constituting the molecule or the lattice can be determined and interatomic distances calculated. Materials of a high degree of crystallinity give sharp and well-defined pattern, whereas substances having a poorly defined arrangement of the atoms and molecules give a more diffuse pattern of the X-ray diagram. Any regular periodicity will be indicated by the reflections shown in the pattern. A "powder" diagram is obtained by passing an X-ray beam through these oriented crystallites. The diagram presents itself in the form of rings and arcs, as Fig. 8 shows. This X-ray pattern permits the direct determination of the interplanar spacings. It has recently been discovered that, by stretching the fiber or tendon by about 10 % of its length, much sharper diagrams are obtained, and also some of the spacings unexpectedly are changed (3a).

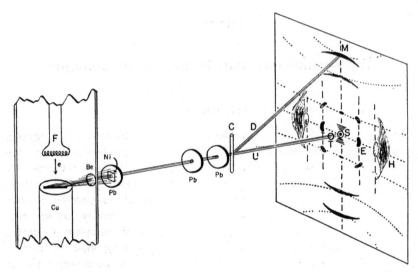

FIG. 8. Schematic illustration of the X-ray diffraction method as applied to collagen fibers. From R. S. Bear, *Advances in Protein Chem.* **7**, 74 (1952), Fig. 2.

There are three groups of spacings which are well defined and characteristic for the fibrous proteins. The first dimension is the spacing between tdentical atomic groupings along the long axis of the fiber, which means ialong the length of the peptide chain. It gives a measure of the length of *the repeating unit* —CO—CH·R—NH. In silk fibroin, which is the most suitable fiber protein for X-ray analysis and the only naturally occurring fibrous protein to show a well-defined and detailed X-ray diagram by reason of its being made up of fully stretched peptide chains, closely and regularly packed in parallel alignment, the repeating unit is 3.5 Å. (2). From the data of interatomic distances, the theoretical figure is 3.65 Å., evidence for some slight contraction, probably due to the presence of some bulky groups (tyrosine) in the silk fibroin lattice. In the fully extended condition the side chains, the R groups, extend alternately from one side and the other of the chain. The distance between two R groups on the same side of such a chain is found to be 7.0 Å., equal to two repeating units. The credit for the interpretation of the diagram belongs to Meyer and Mark (2). The diagram of Fig. 5 gives the interatomic distances and the bond angles in a hypothetical fully extended polypeptide chain (3). Other fibrous proteins—to mention only the two best known and technically most important, the keratin of wool and hair and the collagen of skin—show considerably lower values of the length of the amino acid unit, which is interpreted to signify a coiled or folded state of the protein chains. The type of fibrous proteins which contain more or less contracted polypeptide chains usually possesses the property of long-range elasticity.

The other two characteristic groups of spacings in the X-ray diagram pertain to the distances between sets of planes of the chains running in the direction of the fiber. The first of these two dimensions is practically the same for all proteins and amounts to 4.6 Å. Since the backbones of the chains of proteins are built up from identical structural elements, the —N—C—C— backbone, the spacing of 4.6 Å. is interpreted as the lateral distance between neighboring peptide chains. The constancy of this so-called *backbone spacing* for proteins as a class is significant. The fibrous protein structure is thus indicated and conceived to contain peptide chains arranged in layers. These are parallelly aligned with a distance of 4.6 Å. between the successive chains. The repeating unit of these chains, the —CO—NH— groups, supply valency centers for cohesive forces between adjacent chains, probably by means of hydrogen bridges between the CO— and NH— groups of adjacent chains (4, 5). The formation of a large number of such crosslinks and the occurrence of resonance within the peptide bond should be expected to result in a marked stabilization of the chains (4).

The second lateral group of spacings shows some variation in dimension in the different proteins, and moreover this distance depends on the degree of hydration of the protein. In the case of collagen, dry specimens show an interlayer distance of approximately 10 Å., and moist specimens in the fully hydrated state give values up to 16 Å. This distance is conceived to be the distance between the layers of peptide chains, the space into which the side chains or R groups protrude. It is named the *side-chain spacing.* Obviously, the length of this spacing will be a function of the size and bulkiness of the R groups in the protein. The wide-angle diffraction method discloses the architecture of the crystalline region of the protein. In the fundamental interpretation of the various diagrams of protein fibers, the promulgation of concepts regarding the form of the chains, and the interplay of forms at different extension, thereby creating a science of fiber structure, the name and the school of Astbury (5) are outstanding.

The diffraction pattern of collagen consists of layer lines (vertical dashed lines) and row lines (horizontal dotted lines) of spots [Fig. 8 (6)]. Prominent features of the collagen wide-angle pattern are indicated by M, the important 2.86-Å. arc on the meridian; E, the 10- to 16-Å. equatorial spot; and H, the diffuse "half-halo" of 4.6 Å.

As mentioned earlier, the wide-angle diffraction supplies spatial information on the repeating units of the protein, up to 20 Å. By means of small diffraction angles, the fibrillar and subfibrillar features of the structure can be ascertained (7, 8). This new technique indicates the presence of structures with periods of several hundred Ångström units in length along the fibril axis. These diffraction lines were first resolved and explained by Bear (9), who found that they represent a fibrillar period of 640 Å. This was verified the very same year by Schmitt and his group by an independent method, the electron-microscopic technique (10). This new development and the subsequent researches of Bear and his group on the fine structure of collagen fibrils have been of decidedly greater importance than the wide-angle diffraction studies of collagen, from the point of view of the changes collagen undergoes in the tanning processes. The contribution of the wide-angle technique to our knowledge of the nature of the combination of tanning agents with collagen was very disappointing, since no, or only slight, changes in the diffraction pattern could be ascertained by the incorporation of tanning agents. The alteration in the side-chain spacing on hydration of collagen, already mentioned, was practically the only quantitative finding of importance. By means of the small-angle diffraction method, important contributions bearing on the mechanism of tanning have been made by the Bear group, in close collaboration with the electron-microscopic investigations of the Schmitt school.

Some fundamental structural differences among the three principal fiber proteins—collagen, silk, and keratin—were established by the classical X-ray researches. It was a happy coincidence that silk fibroin came to be the first object for this work, since it contains almost fully extended peptide chains, and further since the chains can be closely packed because of the dominance of glycine and alanine residues, the R groups of which are small and nonpolar. With regard to the crystalline part of the fibers of silk formed by these residues mainly, the structural similarity to cellulose fibers is obvious. In fact, the X-ray work of Dore and Sponsler in 1926 (11) prepared the way for the interpretation of the silk fibroin diagram. Astbury has pointed out that this protein is the only one for which X-ray evidence suggests a periodicity of 3.5 Å. along the fiber axis, a periodicity which corresponds nearly to the calculated length of the repeating unit, $\cdot N \cdot C \cdot C \cdot$, which is contributed to the polypeptide backbone by each amino acid residue. The scarcity of charged side chains, such as diamino and dicarboxylic acids, is probably responsible for the complete extension of the protein chains.

It was soon found, however, that X-ray diagrams of hair (keratin) and collagen were much more complicated and did not yield to this simple analysis. The main features of all structures of fibrous proteins are probably analogous, since they are all based on long-chain molecules with parallel or spiral alignment. However, differences of configuration were soon found from investigations of other protein fibers, especially the various forms of keratin, such as in hair and feathers, as evidenced by the fundamental pioneering work of Astbury (5, 12). Astbury and his co-workers (5, 12, 13), showed that an intramolecular transformation of keratin occurs when hair is stretched. It has long been known that hair can be reversibly stretched if moistened. This property is made use of in the hair hygrometer, which measures the change in length of the hair with changing relative humidity of the air. The increase in length was shown by changes in the X-ray diagram, which was interpreted to indicate a reversible intramolecular transformation. By application of heat, the natural keratin fiber is further contracted, the supercontracted state being reached. Astbury gave the name α-keratin to the normal state of hair and wool, which contains folded chains forming a series of loops, shown in the diagram of the α–β transformation in Fig. 9. The keratin with extended chains with a backbone spacing approximating that of silk fibroin represents the β modification, which term implies the presence of nearly fully extended protein chains. The nomenclature of α and β types of proteins and polypeptides generally used is derived from the keratin types of Astbury. Astbury's daring intuitive interpretation of his researches, particularly the concept that the elasticity of hair is due to intramolecular alterations and is that of a molecular spring, has had profound consequences in the study of the movement of biological structures in general. Thus, the α–β transformation of the molecular grid of myosin and

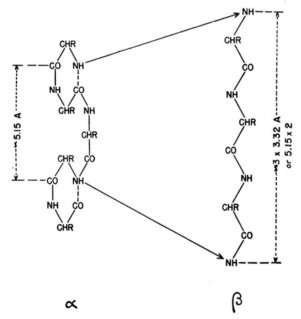

FIG. 9. The α–β keratin transformation. The α fold contains three residues per 5.1-Å. period. From B. W. Low, in the "The Proteins" (H. Neurath and K. Bailey, eds.), Vol. 1, Part A, p. 255, Fig. 11. Academic Press, New York, 1953.

of the muscle itself has been demonstrated experimentally, showing the myosin molecule normally to be in the folded α configuration and hence endowed with inherent long-range elasticity (Astbury et al., 14). It is to be noted, however, that radical modification of our concepts of the architecture of keratin and collagen fibers is inevitable in the light of the helix concept of Pauling and Corey (15–17), which will be discussed later.

It has been mentioned that the keratin molecule is an exceedingly rigid structure because of the strong lateral cohesion between chains (18). Keratin contains a moderate amount of strongly polar groups, cationic ones in the form of arginine and lysine, and anionic ones due to glutamic and aspartic acids. Its acid-binding capacity, for instance, is comparable to that of collagen (0.8 mg. equiv. of H^+ per gram of keratin). Still more important for its structural stability is the large amount of cystine it contains. The very strong lateral, covalent bridge formed by the interchain incorporation of the cystine yielding the—$CH_2 \cdot S \cdot S \cdot CH_2$— bridge puts its mark on the properties and behavior of keratin. In the natural form, the α modification, the looping of the chains facilitates the formation of numerous strong intramolecular hydrogen bonds. The results of recent work point to the governing importance of such crosslinks for the elastic properties of keratin (wool) (18), particularly for the transformation of the natural keratin into the supercontracted state, a type of denaturation similar to the hydrothermal shrinkage of collagen fibers. By concentrated solutions of strongly hydrogen-bonding agents, such as phenol, the contraction of the α form is markedly promoted. In the pioneering investigations of Speakman and his school (19), it was suggested that the ionic groups of keratin are involved in the intermolecular linking through their mutual attraction, the saltlike links being the result. Speakman considers the saltlike links to be important for the processes of relaxation and the set of keratin fibers.

Whatever will be the final fate of the α and β models of Astbury, it must be admitted that the concept of the α–β transformation and its experimental background furnishes a wealth of information of lasting significance for the knowledge of the structure of protein fibers.

Astbury (20) has classified the native fibrous proteins into two distinct families according to their diffraction patterns: the *collagen* class, and the *k-m-e-f* class, i.e., the keratin-myosin-epidermin-fibrinogen family. The validity of this diffraction classification of the fibrous proteins appears to be independent of the particular models of the corresponding peptide chain configurations, since the diffraction patterns may be regarded as furnishing empirical criteria for the structural similarities and dissimilarities of the protein fibers. However, the classification of Ambrose and Elliott, based on the α–β configuration, seems to have wider and more general applicability, since the infrared dichroism is independent of the degree of crystallinity (band and interbands) of the protein fibers, measuring directly the proportion of the α and β forms of the polypeptide chains in any protein. The original concept is also significant for the large body of globular proteins which on denaturation are transformed into fiberlike structures, as was first demonstrated by Astbury and his co-workers (14).

The history of the interpretation of the X-ray diagram of the structural unit of collagen reveals the difficulties in evaluating fiber diagrams. As already stated, the main spacings are the meridional arc of 2.86 Å., the diffuse halo of 4.6 Å., and the side-chain spacing which is a function of the water content of the structure. Of these spacings, the dimension of 2.86 Å., believed to represent the mean length of one residue in the direction of the chain, presented a real puzzle. It was not until the X-ray diagrams from the α–β transformation of keratin fibers were interpreted by Astbury that it became possible to make any significant advance. The indications suggested that the 2.86-Å. spacing corresponded to the 3.5-Å. distance in a fully extended polypeptide chain of silk fibroin and the 3.3-Å. diffraction of β-keratin, i.e., to the length of an amino acid residue incorporated in the chains. The lower value of the collagen diffraction suggested that the collagen chains were folded as in α-keratin, although to a much smaller degree. This should imply the possibility of stretching collagen fibers into a fully extended form similar to the α–β transformation. As Astbury aptly remarked, that has never been found possible. In the electron-optical work on collagen fibrils by the Schmitt-Bear group, such an extensibility has been demonstrated; but it has nothing to do with any α–β transformation, as will be evident from a subsequent discussion of this issue. Although the final explanation arrived at by Astbury (21) some fifteen years ago is no longer valid, the ideas involved are of sufficient general interest, and may even apply in part to the new helical models of collagen, to be briefly discussed.

The main question to be answered was why the average length of an amino acid residue of collagen is so much shorter than it is in the β-proteins, in spite of the fact that the collagen fiber appears to be practically inextensible. In the explanation suggested by Astbury (21), it was first postulated for probable reasons that the backbone of the collagen chain assumes an alternating *cis-trans* form and that the ultimate reason for the shortening of the chain was the unique chemical composition of collagen, primarily its high content of proline and hydroxyproline. These bulky residues form about one-fourth of the side chains of collagen. Astbury was led to believe that the preponderance of these large pyrrolidine residues, which together with the insignificant hydrogen of the glycine residue occupy one side, the remaining side chains being located on the opposite side of the chain, should restrict the backbone of the collagen structure. Astbury even attempted to verify his concept by data on the chemical composition and by the X-ray diagrams available at that time for gelatin. By inserting the newer values of the side-chain and backbone spacings of collagen, 10.4 and 4.6 Å., respectively, and assuming the residue to be inclined at an angle β, the length of one residue in the direction of the main chain can be calculated. With a density of 1.35 and a mean residue weight of 93, the figure will be 2.4 sin β Å., or 2.86 Å. The Astbury model of collagen was the crowning effort of the classical X-ray analysis of collagen by means of the wide-angle technique.

3. The Modern Interpretation of the X-Ray Diagram

Several general objections to the Astbury model have been raised. In 1943, Huggins (22) in his now classical paper, "The Structure of Fibrous Proteins," pointed out some weaknesses of the Astbury model. He introduced the important concept of resonance of the peptide bond and assumed the most probable configuration of these proteins to be the spiral one. Huggins made the following two general points about the symmetry of a stable protein chain configuration: First, polypeptide chains must each have a screw axis of symmetry. The unbalanced forces on opposite sides of a chain which has no screw axis, and that applies to the collagen model just discussed, would tend to bend the chain continously in the same direction. This criterion has been accepted by Bragg, Kendrew, and Perutz (23) in their account of the polypeptide chain configurations in crystalline globular proteins. The second requirement of a stable structure is that corresponding atoms along the main chain should be surrounded with similar configurations of atoms, which the Astbury model does not show. The high content of pyrrolidine side groups of collagen may invalidate the second objection. Ambrose and Elliott (24) have modified the original model, and recently Huggins has suggested a helical model to be described below.

In the collagen models discussed, the interpretation of the main spacings in the wide-angle reflection pattern is essentially the same, the main difference being the explanation of the contraction of the chains, i.e., the meaning of the 2.86-Å. reflection. In his lucid analysis of this problem, Bear (6) stressed the point that the interpretation of this spacing as corresponding to *one* residue has been so firmly fixed in the minds of investigators of the molecular chains of collagen that it has delayed the advancement of other models which might better account for the *actual* extensibility of the collagen protofibril as demonstrated by the electron microscope (Schmitt and his school).

4. THE LOW-ANGLE X-RAY PATTERN

As the basis for the current view of the structure of collagen, additional information has been gathered from interpretations of the low-angle diffraction pattern of collagen and from electron-optical investigations. The results of these innovations will be summarized, as simply as possible, in order to present the essentials of a highly specialized and complicated subject which at the present time is in a state of flux. This discussion is derived primarily from the illuminating exposition on "The Structure of Collagen Fibrils" by Bear (6).

Mammalian tendon (kangaroo tail), which possesses the highest degree of fibrillar orientation of any collagen structure, is the most suitable object for X-ray diffraction. Although it provides good *fibrillar* orientation, the intrafibrillar elements, the protofibrils, showing up in the wide-angle diffraction, are not as well oriented as the larger units. The result is faint and diffuse reflections and inability to recognize hazy lines. Herzog and Gonnel (25), two pioneers in the X-ray analysis of collagen, pointed out more than twenty years ago that a period of approximately 20 Å. would satisfactorily account for the collagen wide-angle lines. The lines of 19.1 and 20 Å., which form pseudoperiods, have been long ignored, probably because of their diffuse appearance. At one time Bear (6) considered the 20-Å. pseudoperiod to be significant for the spiral structure of collagen. His present model is based on a 28.6-Å. period (private communication).

The diffraction patterns of collagen (Fig. 10) obtained by the low-angle diffraction method show a set of axially oriented diffractions related to a single fundamental fibril period of approximately 640 Å. in air-dry specimens. This large characteristic spacing is present in each diagram of Fig. 10, as represented by a series of equally spaced layer lines. Figure 10a shows how the moist specimen of tendon forms short lines closely applied to the axis of the diagram which is interpreted to imply a strong coherence of the entire fibrillar structure. This fibril may be described as a smooth cylinder. The constant diameter of the cylindrical structure is reflected in the constant width of the diffraction lines, transversally measured. From Fig. 10c it is obvious that the drying of the fibril results in lengthening of the lines, the increase being accentuated with increasing distance from the center of the diagram. This is believed to indicate intrafibrillar distortions and diminished coherence of the structural units.

The findings indicate that the fundamental units, the protofibrils, are arranged in parallel so that parts of corresponding chemical structures are matched transversely to the fibril axis. The periodic pattern of the proto-fibril is approximately 640 Å. Since the matching varies somewhat, *bands* of distorted structure alternate with *interbands* that appear to be more

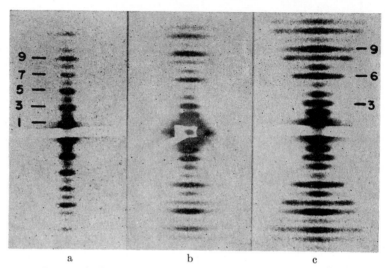

a   b   c

FIG. 10. Low-angle X-ray diffraction patterns of kangaroo tail tendon: *a*, after extensive soaking in water and drying under tension; *b*, after complete hydration and drying under tension; *c*, after brief exposure and drying under tension. Layer-line indices are indicated. From R. S. Bear, *J. Am. Leather Chem. Assoc.* **46**, 110 (1951), Fig. 2.

nearly perfect. This matching of the collagen molecule in pattern of bands and interbands, clearly shown in the electron micrographs, may be due to a regular sequence of amino acid residues along individual polypeptide chains of the collagen molecule. However, the data available give no definite evidence as to the chemical make-up of the bands and the interbands, although certain indications point to the accumulation of amino acid residues with large polar side chains, such as those of the diamino and dicarboxylic acids, in the bands with distorted protofibrillar organization. The interbands would then contain the hydroxy acid side chains preferably. The nonpolar groups would be expected to be evenly distributed along the chains, since they form the great majority of residues (hydrogen and methyl groups). Some support is given to the assumption that the ionic protein groups, particularly the cationic ones, are predominantly localized at the bands by the low-angle X-ray diffraction pattern of collagen and also of collagen which has been treated with stains, such as phosphotungstic acid, and which has combined irreversibly with certain agents, such as polymetaphosphates and basic chromic salts (26). Since the anions of the two polyacids mentioned appear to be attached to the cationic protein groups, and since the cationic chromium complexes are known to interact with the anionic groups of collagen, the main fixation of these agents taking place in the band would indicate a preferential accumulation of the strongly electrovalent side chains in the bands. Some significance may be attached to the fact that those substances which are recognized as tanning agents, for instance the basic chromium salts and polyacids, possess the unique property of forming intrafibrillar crosslinks through the anionic and cationic side chains of the protofibrils. The ionic R groups would be most easily accessible if present in the bands. However, in their interpretation of their electron micrographs and the density curves of collagen, to be discussed below, Grassmann et al. (35) take a view diametrically opposed to that of Bear.

An interesting technique for the differentiation and estimation of the crystalline and noncrystalline regions (interbands and bands) of keratin (wool) has been devised by Hailwood and Horrobin (26a). It is to be noted that the crystalline regions of keratin appear to be inert and inaccessible, even to small molecules like those in water vapor. Since reactions with keratin and collagen are usually carried out in aqueous media, the fraction of the protein which is accessible to water molecules is of primary importance, whether or not it can be identified strictly with the amorphous region (bands). According to Hailwood and Horrobin (26a), the water adsorption isotherm of fibers is given by the equation:

$$\frac{M \cdot r}{1800} = \frac{\alpha \cdot h}{1 - \alpha h} + \frac{\alpha \cdot \beta \cdot h}{1 + \alpha \beta h}$$

where α and β are constants, h is the relative humidity, and M is the molecular weight of the unit which can combine with 1 g. mole of water. The regain, r, is given in g. of water absorbed per 100 g. of dry fibers. If the whole of the wool fiber were accessible to the water molecules, M would have a value of the mean residue weight of keratin, 122. Much higher values are found, however. The part of the keratin molecule which is inaccessible to water molecules is obtained from the expression $(M - 122)/M$. The crystalline fraction of wool is about 0.4, according to this method. Collagen shows no crystalline regions.

Speakman and his co-workers (26b) have introduced a direct method of estimating the amorphous (band) portions of wool keratin. It is based on the determination of the gain in dry weight of the wool after it has been exposed repeatedly to saturated vapor of heavy water, deuterium oxide (D_2O). If all the labile hydrogen atoms of the keratin molecule were replaced by deuterium, the gain in dry weight would be 1.61%. Speakman (26b) found gains of 1.13 to 1.21% only, which implies that 30 and 25% of the keratin molecule were inaccessible to D_2O. It appears probable that these methods would yield values of little significance for collagen because of its more open structure, and consequently the easy penetration of water vapor. These techniques are nevertheless unique and worthy of mention.

The concept of Bear, with a preferential distribution of certain types of amino acid residues in the regions of bands and interbands, has recently received substantial experimental support by the results of the investigations of the Zahn school (see p. 237). The difluorodinitrodibenzene-sulfone-treated tendon collagen contained, after hydrolysis, the sulfone bislysine and the sulfone bishydroxylysine compounds, in addition to a compound with the two amino acids crosslinked, indicating the presence of the ε-amino groups of lysine, and the hydroxyamino group of hydroxylysine within a distance of less than 20 Å. on adjacent polypeptide chains.

5. THE HELICAL CONCEPT

A turning point in our knowledge of the architecture of the proteins will in the future most likely be attributed to the authoritative concept of Pauling and Corey (15, 16), advanced in 1951. These workers established a broad basis for the structural theory of proteins by means of their conception of the helical configuration as the general form for protein chains. The structure of the fibrous proteins of the collagen-gelatin group is included. Pauling and Corey are of the opinion that it is possible to narrow down the conceivable coiled configurations to a very few types, in which the bond distances and angles conform rigorously to those of amino acids and peptides. The first determination of the interatomic distances and of the bond angles of glycine and diketopiperazine was carried out by Corey, as mentioned earlier. Pauling and Corey have used this information to arrive at configurations of the chains of various proteins compatible with these data, the wide-angle X-ray pattern of collagen, and the nature of the —CO—NH— bond. The Pauling-Corey model is based on the supposition that the 2.86-Å. spacing represents the projection of one residue length on the fiber axis, that the prolines represent one-third of the total residues, that the collagen structure is essentially inextensible, and that the keto-imide group should be planar. The only configurations of the chains compatible with these requirements are helical models. It is further assumed, with due

consideration of the resonance in the

$$-\overset{\displaystyle |}{\underset{\displaystyle |}{C}}-\overset{\displaystyle O}{\overset{\displaystyle \|}{C}}-\overset{\displaystyle H}{\underset{\displaystyle |}{N}}-\overset{\displaystyle |}{\underset{\displaystyle |}{C}}-$$

bond, that the

configuration of the keto-imide link is planar. The final conclusion is that there are only two possibilities of hydrogen-bonded helical structures for the polypeptide chain, one the α helix with 3.7 residues per turn, and the other the γ helix with 5.1 residues per turn. It is believed that the former model represents the structure of synthetic polypeptides, α-keratin, and myosin, and that it also constitutes an important structural feature in some globular proteins, particularly in hemoglobin. The 5.1-residue helix is conceived to be laid down in supercontracted keratin and possibly also in collagen, according to Bear (6). Pauling and Corey themselves originally considered the molecule of collagen to be cylindrical in shape, consisting of three polypeptide chains with 3 residues, the projection of each residue being 2.86 Å. Because their proposed model did not adequately explain the collagen X-ray wide-angle diagram, Pauling (17) abandoned the three-chain helical structure for collagen, and instead he suggested a single-chain helix with seven turns per 29 Å. of axial projection. The original Pauling-Corey model of collagen has been revised recently (16). The present discussion of the collagen lattice will follow the lines of Bear's interpretation (6) (Fig. 11).

The Pauling-Corey models have the attractive feature that the position of the $>$ NH groups toward the $>$ CO groups leaves ample opportunity for stabilization of the structure by hydrogen bonding. Bear (6) considers the model with 5.1 residues per turn to be applicable to collagen after some minor adjustments. With a projection of each residue equal to 0.95 Å., it would require 21 residues for the 20-Å. pseudoperiod of collagen in four coils of 5.25 residues per each turn. Such a coil should satisfy the bond and angle distances of the simple units established by Corey. Figure 11 shows an outline of such a coil. Consideration of space accommodation should eliminate all but the models with four to five turns per pseudoperiod. In a paper by Cohen and Bear (27), preference is given to a helix with seven equivalent groups of 3 residues each that make two turns per 20 Å. However, this model has already become obsolete.

Bear's most recent model is based on a left-handed helix with 28.6 Å. period which would contain 10 equivalent scattering groups, arranged in three turns of a discontinuous helix. Consideration of the density of collagen (1.41), together with other facts suggest that there may be four residues per equivalent scattering group, instead of three as in his earlier models (personal communication (1954)).

In Huggins' (28) model, which he claims is in agreement with all experimental facts, the sequence of residues is $X \cdot X \cdot P$, where P represents the prolines and X the other residues. The chain is coiled in a left-handed helix. Huggins further bases his model on the following assumptions: (1) 30 residues per three turns and per 28.6 Å; (2) Pauling-Corey bond angles and lengths in the polypeptide chain; (3) rectilinear N—H $\cdots$ OC $<$ hydrogen bonds; (4) planar C—CO—NH—C groups. The computed —NH $\cdots$ CO hydrogen bond is 2.83 Å. The hydroxyl oxygen of the hydroxy-proline residue is 2.9 Å. from a carbonyl oxygen in the next turn of the helix, indicating OH————O=C $<$ hydrogen bonding. Such an *interchain* bond has

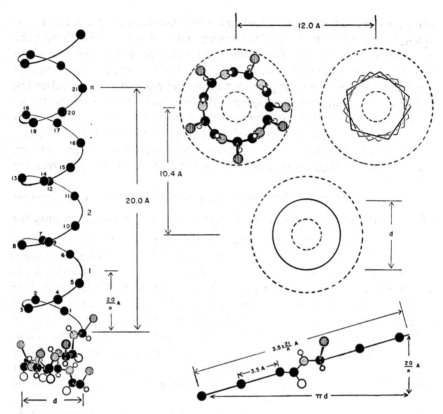

FIG. 11. Helical models for the collagen polypeptide chain (protofibril). On the left is the skeleton of the helix, with the location of atoms filled in for the bottom turn. The numbered carbon (solid black) atoms of the skeleton represent the twenty-one places (α-carbon atoms) at which residue side chains are attached in one full period of the helix. The number of turns per period illustrated is 4, indicated in general as n. The diameter of the helix is d. The upper right part of the drawing indicates cross-sectional plans for three helices and their mode of packing in the collagen fibril. In one helix the atoms of a single turn are shown; in another, lines directly joining the α-carbon atoms of the residues are given for a full period; and in the third, their general circular locus of projection is indicated. Dotted lines show rough domains within which penetration of side chains from outside each helix is largely prohibited by van der Waals repulsions of the helix skeleton. At the lower right is shown one unrolled coil, with one residue indicated in detail. Stippled circles represent nitrogen atoms; small open circles are hydrogen; large open circles are oxygen; and shaded circles show the general direction for emergence of R groups (side chains). From R. S. Bear, *Advances in Protein Chem.* **7**, 131 (1952), Fig. 31.

been postulated by the present author as a result of chemical studies (29). However, Huggins' corresponding link is an *intrachain* bond. There are no large holes within the helix, although about one water molecule can be accommodated per three residues by hydrogen bonding. With a mean residue weight of 93 and closely packed helices 12 Å. apart, the computed density of collagen with one H_2O per 3 residues is 1.38, in good agreement with the value of 1.41 for dry collagen (30).

Bear (6) sounds a note of caution in translating optical properties of fibers into characteristics of subfibrillar structures because of the marked anisotropy of the fibers, and furthermore in view of the fact that the models are constructed merely for the interbands. The general concept of the helical configuration of protein structures is acceptable chemically and physically. Thus, the helix structure of collagen is consistent with certain evidence obtained by M'Even and Pratt (30a) in estimation of the molecular weight of acid-extracted collagen by means of the light-scattering method. It was indicated that collagen exists in the form of highly coiled threadlike macromolecules formed from a single polypeptide chain of about 150,000 Å. in length and a width of 12 Å. (molecular weight $\sim$ 10 million).

6. Electron-Microscopic Findings

The contributions of electron-microscopic investigations will now be briefly reviewed. Of all direct-imaging optical instruments, the electron microscope has the greatest resolving power, the theoretical lower limit lying at about 10 Å., i.e., about the width of an average polypeptide chain. In practice, 20 Å. is about the highest resolution of biological materials. The optical principles of the electron microscope are essentially the same as those of the common microscope (31). The illuminating radiation in the form of a high-velocity, monochromatic beam of electrons is focused by magnetic lenses in high vacuum. The image is viewed on a fluorescent screen for selection of fields to be photographed. Magnifications ranging from 1000 to 20,000 are obtained, which are subsequently enlarged to micrographs up to 200,000 ×. The material is usually completely desiccated and of thickness of 0.01 to 0.5 micron to make it possible for the electron beam to penetrate and to obtain a sufficient degree of resolution of fine details. The specimens are fragmented by teasing, blending, homogenizing, and particularly by the use of ultrasonics. Important preparatory procedures are metal shadowing (31), staining, and making of replicas in plastics (31).

Collagen has proved to be an ideal material for electron-microscopic studies. It is readily obtained, and it is easily manipulated because of its resistance. Further, it possesses a highly developed structural unit in the form of fibrils which show a regular axial repeating period of approximately

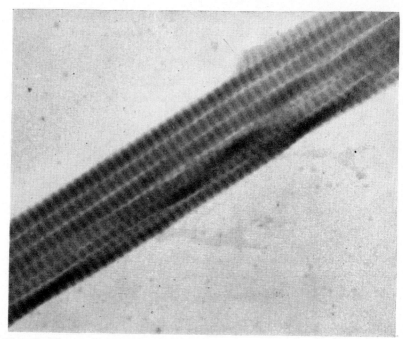

FIG. 12. Electron micrograph of cowhide collagen stained with phosphotungstic acid, magnification 29,000X. Reproduced through the kindness of Dr. R. Borasky.

640 Å. Finally, it shows a distinct intraperiod fine structure. It is remarkable how closely the characteristics of the low-angle X-ray diagrams check with the pictures of the electron microscope.

Figure 12 shows an electron microphotograph of bundles of collagen fibrils from corium. The interlacing of bundles is characteristic for skin tissue. Collagen fibrils are many microns in length, with the width in the range of 200 to 2000 Å. All forms of vertebrate collagen known are characterized by an axial repeating period of extreme regularity, manifested by alternating dark and light bands which make the fibrils look something like the flexible metal tubes used in bathroom equipment.

The axial repeating period close to 640 Å. was discovered by Bear in 1942. Shortly after this discovery electron-microscopic investigations of collagen fibrils by the Massachusetts Institute of Technology group headed by Schmitt (32), the pioneer investigator of biological materials by electron-microscopic methods, also showed collagen fibrils to have a banded, cross-striated structure with an average distance between like bands of about 640 Å. Independently, Wolpers (33) had found similar cross-striations. Variations of the periods from 500 to 800 Å. were found, probably caused

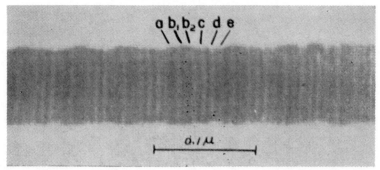

F<small>IG</small>. 13. Six intraperiod bands in fibril of chrome-tanned calfskin stained with phosphotungstic acid, magnification 274,000X. From F. O. Schmitt and J. Gross, *J. Am. Leather Chem. Assoc.* **43**, 661 (1948), Fig. 2.

by the mechanical distortion in manipulation, with an average close to 640 Å. By extreme stretching of the fibrils, periods as large as 4000 Å. have been observed occasionally. These findings are extremely important, since they require the assumption that the collagen *protofibril*, unlike the native macrofiber, is highly extensible. The extensibility of the collagen protofibril is a strong argument for the spiral structure of the polypeptide chains as postulated by Bear (6) and is incompatible with the orthodox model of Astbury (21). It is interesting to note that both the Pauling and the Astbury groups have based their models on the assumption of a non-extensible structure.

In the later work of the Schmitt group, in which the name of Gross is prominent, collagen fibrils stained by phosphotungstic acid were studied. A pattern with six intraperiod bands was found. Each band has a characteristic position and density. The pattern is asymmetric in the axial direction, which is of importance from the point of view of crystallography. Similar findings were independently reported by Nutting and Borasky (34) in an important study. Figure 13 shows these intraperiod bands of calfskin collagen. They are designated a, b_1, b_2, c, d, and e. Probably more will be found as the technique improves. Thus, Grassmann has discovered ten bands (35), each with 15-Å. extension, and measured their intensities. The main part of these bands is also present in unstained native collagen. Further, their existence is indicated in Bear's X-ray diagrams (see Fig. 44).

Dry specimens show that the dense bands are wider. In the moist fibril a smooth contour devoid of bands is shown. Hence, it appears that the form of the collagen fibril in its native environment, fully hydrated, is a smooth cylinder. The distribution of water in the ordered and disordered regions (interband and band) is probably different, depending on the nature

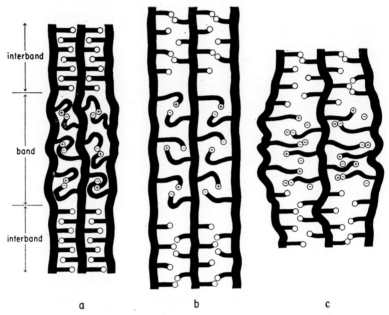

a   b   c

FIG. 14. Diagrammatic representation of the swelling of the collagen fibril at bands and interbands, showing the difference between *a*, a dry fibril; *b*, a fibril swelling in water at neutrality; and *c*, the result of acid swelling. Only polar side chains are shown, with open-circled heads representing uncharged side chains, + and − signs designating correspondingly charged heads or ions, and H indicating hydrogen ions. The long charged side chains at the bands normally distort the vertical main-chain helices from a straight course. Neutral water (not shown) penetrates the bands and interbands, separating the main chains to an extent limited by the hydrogen bonds between the polar heads at the interbands, and simultaneously more room becomes available for the charged side chains at the bands, which now permit straightening of the main chains. Addition of acid discharges the negative side chains by means of hydrogen ions, and the equal number of free negative ions required to remain at the bands produce local osmotic swelling, which contracts the structure axially. From R. S. Bear, *Advances in Protein Chem.* **7**, 149 (1952), Fig. 32.

of the side chains in these regions and probably also on the interaction of the main chains with each other laterally. From Bear's investigations (6), it appears that the interband regions should possess the highest degree of parallel alignment of protofibrils, whereas the bands apparently are disordered structures. Since removal of water leads to the appearance of a banded structure, the different degrees of hydration of the two regions probably enter as a factor. The bands show a very much greater affinity for the heteropolyacids than the interbands do. This applies also to the fixation of basic chromium complexes, which treatment, however, also markedly accentuates the interband structure. Figure 14 presents a schematic picture of the changes in the band and interband regions of collagen on swelling (Bear, 6).

The continuous cross-striations of the collagen fibril shows that the protofibrils are aligned according to the chemical features of the regions, forming a transverse matching. As to the lateral structure of the collagen fibrils, significant differences in the strength of this bonding are found for different types of collagens. Fibrils from fishskin and rat tail tendon fray rather easily, whereas bovine collagen does not show this tendency at all. Rat tail tendon, fishskin, and ichthyocol (from fish swim bladder) dissolve easily in dilute acids. On the other hand, skin collagen only swells but is not dissolved in dilute acid solutions, the probable reason being its weave structure. The relative strength of the lateral cohesion and the degree of bonding of protofibrils of collagen from different sources are probably connected with the presence of cementing substances (mucoids and chondroitin sulfate), factors involving steric environment and differences in chemical constitution, until now a field barely studied.

7. BIREFRINGENCE

The rather easily demonstrated classical evidence for the lattice structure of collagen fibers, their birefringence (double refraction) (36), should not entirely be overlooked in these days of X-ray diffraction and electron-microscopic impacts on the structural make-up of collagen. The histological structural features of collagen fibers and fiber bundles, revealed by microscopic methods, particularly the informative dark-field technique, and polarization optics, laid the foundation for better understanding of the macrostructure of skin, since they supplied knowledge of the fibrils, permitted estimates of their dimensions, orientation, and weave, and also gave some idea of the changes they undergo during swelling, contraction, and tanning. Researches on the chemical level of collagen structure were also an early development. At the time of the introduction of X-ray diffraction and the electron microscope, there existed a large gap in our knowledge of the dimensions (in the range of millimicrons), which has been left unexplored. As a result of the investigations of the past decade, this gap is gradually being filled by means of new techniques.

The studies of the anisotropy of collagen fibers by means of double refraction have shown that normally the double refraction is positive in the direction of the fiber axis (36), which is an indication of the presence of rodlets or chains aligned parallelly in this direction. Thus, the intrinsic double refraction is due to the anisotropic property of the aligned units, for instance the fibrils. The sign and extent of the birefringence of collagen fibers may be varied through introduction of various substances, e.g., tanning agents within the structure (37). One of the pioneers in this field, von Ebner (38), observed some sixty years ago that certain phenols and aromatic aldehydes reversed the sign of the double refraction of collagen, making it negative. By the incorporation of certain vegetable tannins into the structure, the same shift occurs (37). Such tannins include those of gambier, myrobalans, sumac, and mimosa. Others, such as the tannins of oak bark, quebracho, and chestnut wood, do not alter the optical sign of the fibers (37).

It is a remarkable fact that all leather fibers show positive refraction when wet, irrespective of the sign of the refraction when dry. The original character is restored on drying, provided that the solubles of the leather are not removed by extending washing. If however the water solubles are removed, then the fibers on drying always possess positive values of the refringence. This fact points to the orientation of the uncombined matter in a crystalline order within the leather structure; accordingly, the reversal is probably caused by this impregnation and has nothing to do with the property of the collagen in irreversible combination with tannins. Marriott's (39) finding of a certain correlation between the sign and extent of the birefringence of vegetable-tanned sole leathers and their resistance to abrasion is interesting. It appears that leather containing isotropic fibers should have a lower degree of resistance to abrasion than leathers of strongly negative, or with definitely positive, values of the birefringence.

Küntzel (37) asserted that it is possible from the study of the birefringence of tanned fibers to prove the occurrence of intra- or inter-micellar types of combination of tanning agents with collagen. Thus, this investigator concluded, from the inversion in the sign of the birefringence of collagen noted in leathers tanned with certain types of vegetable tannins, chiefly belonging to the pyrogallic class, that the tannins are incorporated intra-micellarly, which in the new vocabulary of submicroscopic dimensions would mean intrafibrillarly. In view of the marked effect of uncombined vegetable tanning matter on the optical behavior of leather fibers just referred to, Küntzel's conclusion does not seem convincing. Certainly additional work is required to elucidate this point and the meaning of the birefringence phenomena for collagen and leathers generally. Further, agents which should be able to penetrate into the fibril and filaments, such as formaldehyde, simple basic chromic salts which, as the low-angle diffraction studies just reviewed indicate, do so, show no tendency of reversing the sign of the refraction, although some of these reagents reduce the positive values.

To conclude, the normal positive sign of the birefringence of collagen fibers may be interpreted to indicate the parallel orientation of intrafibrillar molecular chains in the direction of the fiber axis. The effect of tanning agents on this property may involve intramicellar penetration of these agents, or oriented absorption, or even reactions of a chemical nature, changing the collagen lattice.

8. Reconstituted Collagen

In this connection some remarks on the problems of the reconstitution and formation of collagen are opportune. The collagen fibrils formed from dilute acid dispersions of collagen, in which no fibrils can be detected, are known as reconstituted collagens.

The early work of Nageotte (40) and of Fauré-Frémiet (41) showed that by extraction of some forms of connective tissue, such as the tail tendon of rat and the swim bladder (tunic) of fish (carp), with dilute organic acids such as 0.01 N acetic or formic acid, a considerable part of the collagen was solubilized. The dissolved collagen was reprecipitated from the filtered solution by the addition of salt or by neutralization. The reprecipitated protein was characterized as collagen by chemical and microscopic examination. It was later found that the fibrils formed may show cross-striation if certain conditions of the precipitating bath are fulfilled, particularly a certain ionic strength of the solution.

Schmitt and his co-workers (42) have been able to reconstitute fibrils precipitated from an acid solution. The reconstituted fibrils possess identity periods and the fine structure characteristics of native collagen. In view of the evidence of an extracellular formation of collagen fibrils, it seems probable that the cell secretes a precursor, a procollagen, possibly in the form of simple polypeptide chains, which on alteration of the physicochemical environment aggregate in a manner similar to the acid-dissolved collagen. Porter and Vanamee (43) reported on their electron-microscopic investigation of the synthesis of collagen in fibroblast tissue cultures. In addition to the typical fibrils, small nodular filaments were found. According to their view, the small filaments of collagen consist of chains of globular protein molecules.

In 1948, Orekhovich and his associates (44) reported the preparation of a so-called procollagen, obtained by extraction of skins with citrate buffers of pH 3 to 4. The extract is a viscous solution. On dialysis against tap water, fibrils are obtained which chemically are essentially identical with native collagen (45). The Russian group considers this material to be the biochemical precursor of collagen. It is to be noted that collagen dissolved in weak solutions of acetic and formic acids yields only transparent gels on dialysis against water: by adjustment of the ionic strength of the added electrolyte (salt), cross-striated fibrils are formed.

The electron-microscopic study of the reconstituted fibrils of Orekhovich carried out by Highberger, Gross, and Schmitt (45) revealed two types of fibrils: the ordinary cross-striated type of collagen fibrils with an axial period of 640 Å., and a new type of fibril with an axial period in the range 2000 to 3000 Å. These "fibrous long-spaced" (FLS) fibrils are most easily obtained from citrate-buffered extracts of the skin of the rat, calf, and steer, rat tail tendon, and fish swim bladder. There are no indications that this new fibrous form of collagen pre-exists in the tissues. It appears to be artificially produced from the precursors present in the extract. As to the important researches of the Randall group, reference is given to his symposium publication (46).

The M.I.T. group made the important discovery that collagen prepared by the method of Bergmann and Stein (47), involving repeated extractions with 10 % solution of sodium chloride, followed by extraction with solutions of sodium diphosphate, yielded hardly any long-spaced fibrils. This might mean that the precursor is removed from collagen in the extraction with these agents. The material extracted by means of phosphate gave on dialysis against water a flocculent precipitate, which electron-microscopic examination showed to be amorphous. However, on extraction with citrate buffer of pH 3.8, ionic strength 0.2, and dialysis against water, the typical long-spaced fibrils were obtained. These exceedingly interesting findings focused the attention of Gross, Highberger, and Schmitt (48) on the nature of the material which is extracted from collagen by phosphate and subsequently transformed into the long-spaced form of collagen.

In view of the close association of mucoproteins with collagen in connective tissue and in consideration of the solvent action of phosphate solution, it was suspected that the mucoprotein may play some part in the formation of the anomalously spaced collagen fibrils (48). In order to test this working hypothesis, one part of the mucoprotein preparation, which was obtained from connective tissue and calfskin was added to a filtered acetic acid solution of rat tail collagen (10 parts) which had been pre-extracted with phoshate in order to remove the precursor. The fibrous precipitate obtained on dialysis of this mixture consisted almost entirely of long-spaced fibrils. A purified monodisperse glycoprotein from plasma, described by Schmid (49), behaved identically. As the authors point out, however, it seems safe to conclude, after careful control experiments, that the mucoprotein, or some of its components, combines with the highly solvated collagen in acid solution to produce the long-spaced fibrils. It was found that no long-spaced fibrils were formed by addition of mucoproteins to intact native collagen fibrils. The findings of Gross et al. (48) suggested that mucoproteins may be instrumental in the formation of collagen fibrils. With low ratios of mucoprotein to collagen (1:1000), the normal type of fibrils is preferentially formed; intermediate ratios yield mixtures of the two types of fibrils; and high ratios (1:10) result chiefly in the long-spaced fibrils *in vitro*.

The FLS collagen formed by dialysis of solutions of acid-extracted skin and other tissue, or by the addition of glycoprotein to solutions of ichthyocol, show a characteristic intraperiod fine structure, consisting of at least fourteen bands. This intraperiod banding differs from that of ordinary collagen fibrils not only in the relative positions of the bands but particularly in the symmetry of the pattern and the lack of polarization. It was found that besides glyco-protein several other substances are able to initiate the formation of cross-striated fibrils, although glycoprotein is far more effective. Thus, phosphatase and heparin are active and may play some role in the formation of collagen (50), as are also chondroitin sulfate, gum arabic, and many other substances ill-defined chemically (51). The results from the researches of Highberger *et al.* (45) indicated that the components necessary for the formation of cross-striated fibrils are present in the collagen extracted from connective tissue.

Schmitt, Gross, and Highberger (52) have investigated the extract obtained from connective tissue by phosphate buffer at 0.15 M ionic strength at pH 8. In an earlier work (48), it was found that such extracts contain everything required for the formation of cross-striated fibrils, although they yield only amorphous precipitates on dialysis against water. By extraction of these precipitates with the citric acid buffer, however, fibrils of ordinary and of FLS collagens were obtained. The Boston team found that, when the phosphate-extracted connective tissue was dialyzed against the citric acid buffer, precipitates were formed which contained considerable amounts of an entirely new form of collagen. On electron-microscopic examination this new type of collagen appeared as broad, flat segments of characteristic fine structure, with a length of about 2000 A., and with as many as eighteen intraperiodic bands. The pattern is polarized. Segment long spacing (SLS) is the name given this new form of cross-striated collagen.

Gross, Highberger and Schmitt (52a) have recently presented evidence in support of the view that the three structural forms of collagen may be derived from a parent collagen (protofibrillar particles of 2,000–3,000 Å. lengths). Normal collagen, FLS and SLS should represent different states of aggregation of this unit particle, called *tropocollagen*. They consider it possible that, in the biogenesis of collagen, tropocollagen is synthesized by the cells, subsequently being converted into the characteristic fibrous form in the ground substance. Boedtker and Doty (52a) found this tropocollagen to consist of rod-shaped particles of 14 Å. diameter and 2,900 Å. length, with molecular weight about 300,000, from measurements of light scattering, osmotic pressure, sedimentation constant, intrinsic viscosity, and flow birefringence. All these methods gave values of the same order of magnitude. They conclude that this particle, which evidently is an extended single polypeptide chain (protofibril) appears to embody the essential characteristics of the tropocollagen postulated by the Schmitt group. Their discovery will likely have fargoing consequences on our knowledge of the biogenesis and nature of the collagens.

In his highly informative paper (53) on the new developments in this field, Highberger states that extracts from which SLS collagen is produced show a strong ultraviolet absorption in the region of 2600 A. This indicates the presence of nucleic acids or nucleotides. This suggestion received some support from the finding that, by the addition of ATP (adenosine triphosphoric acid) to ichthyocol solution, the SLS form is directly produced. The fibrils formed show the amino acid characteristics of collagen and the typical wide-angle X-ray diagram of ordinary collagen. An important advance was the demonstration of the complete interconversion of the various forms, i.e., the ordinary fibrils and the FLS and SLS fibrils, one into another. The important contributions of the British laboratories to the study of reconstituted collagens, particularly the amino acid composition of various acid-extracted skin collagens (ES) are comprehensively discussed in Randall's book (46).

Of great interest also are the data on the amino acid composition of the ES collagens. From comparative analyses of rat tail tendon and ES collagen, Brown, Kelley, and Watson (54) found that the amino acid compositions are very similar. The chief differences are that the contents of glutamic acid and hydroxyproline in native collagen are less than those in ES collagen; on the other hand, the tyrosine and proline contents of the tendon collagen are both higher than those for ES collagen. The ES collagen consists of banded segments of about 2400-Å. length, together with fine filaments. The finding of similar segments, the SLS fibrils, is also of current interest. Randall (46) believes that the chemical differences between native and ES collagens are similar to those observed for albumin and plakalbumin, the latter being a secondary protein formed from the native one by hydrolysis and splitting off of some simple polypeptides.

The research of Bowes et al. (55) on the chemical composition of citrate-extracted calfskin indicates that the conversion of the procollagen (acid-extracted skin) to ordinary collagen would require the addition of a protein fraction relatively rich in tyrosine, histidine, lysine, proline, and amide nitrogen, and relatively low in alanine, serine, and hydroxyproline. An interesting and probably important difference is the lower hexosamine content of the ES collagen, which may be due to the splitting off of a mucopolysaccharide. Treatment of native skin collagen in solutions of alkali of pH 13 for 14 days produces changes similar to those caused by acid extraction, particularly marked losses in tyrosine and hexosamine, and gains in hydroxyproline. Hence, it is indicated that in the solubilization of skin collagen a fraction low in hydroxyproline and rich in tyrosine and hexosamine is split off. On the basis of the data reviewed, Bowes *et al.* point to the possibility that fiber formation may involve the association of the soluble protein (ES) with a mucopolysaccharide, which may function as a cementing substance. N-Terminal groups are not present in native collagen. However, ES collagen contains aspartic acid and alanine as N-terminal groups. It is possible that the amino group of aspartic acid in some way participates in the attachment of the mucopolysaccharide to the collagen molecule. Jackson and Randall (51) consider it significant that all precipitants or initiators of the formation of long-spaced fibrils which were tried in his survey contained polysaccharide. Moreover, Randall points out that the effective chondroitin sulfate and the gum arabic contain end groups of 2,3,4-trimethylglucuronic acid.

The work of the Schmitt and the Randall schools has indicated that mucoproteins and hyaluronic acid are involved in the development of fibrils. Thus, the tail tendon of the young rat shows a higher proportion of mucopolysaccharide content than that of the adult rat. The embryonic and young collagen fibrils are argyrophilic. Hence, the reticulin may be collagen in association with mucopolysaccharides. According to the investigation of Little and Kramer (56), reticulin has a membrane structure consisting of minute, randomly oriented collagen-type fibrils embedded in a structureless matrix, which is probably a glucoprotein. In connective tissue there is a continuous series of structures, from this appearance to the familiar collagen fibrils. A gradual transition of the fibrils into aggregates of bundles seems to take place at the expense of the amorphous matrix. These observations are in line with the view of reticulin as a muco-collagen association product.

From the point of view of the genesis of collagen and the possible role of polysaccharides, it is of interest to note that collagen of skin contains on the average 0.65 % polysaccharide, based on its dry weight. Grassmann and Schleich (57) found that carbohydrate to consist of galactose and glucose. Beek (58) found about 0.5 % of carbohydrate residues, consisting of glucose and galactose, the latter either bound by means of a difficultly hydrolyzable linkage to the protein or composed of a mixture of the L forms (not fermentable by a galactose-active yeast).

9. SOME BIOCHEMICAL AND MEDICAL ASPECTS OF THE FORMATION OF COLLAGEN

The formation of collagen and connective tissue in healing wounds is disturbed by a deficiency of vitamin C, as was first noticed by Höjer in

1924 (59) and subsequently confirmed by a great number of medical specialists. In the absence of ascorbic acid, abnormal swollen collagen fibrils are deposited, associated with large amounts of polysaccharides. According to Robertson (60), ascorbic acid (vitamin C) may be of importance for the formation of the prolines of collagen. Robertson and his co-workers assayed collagen in tissues with various degrees of scurvy and found a fairly constant value. However, in studies of the collagen required to fill in wounds in guinea pigs, i.e., replacement collagen, it was found that this material was deposited in up to 60 days and was satisfactory only when the diet included ascorbic acid. For instance, on an ascorbic acid-free diet collagen is not deposited until after 14 days. On the other hand, a tissue with only 2 % of collagen, due to vitamin C deficiency, will show an increase to 11 % in 3 days when ascorbic acid is introduced. Evidence for the presence of a collagen precursor in tissue from deficient animals was not conclusive. However, the results of Robertson and his co-workers show that, if a precursor is present, it does not contain hydroxyproline. It is suggested, therefore, that ascorbic acid may be necessary for the production of hydroxyproline.

It appears that the abnormal collagenous tissue formed in rheumatoid arthritis is low in hydroproline. This degenerated collagen is also more soluble in alkali than the ordinary collagen. Robertson and Schwartz (60) also found that precollagen (collagen in tissue from deficient animals) contains less hydroxyproline than does normal collagen. Apparently ascorbic acid is needed for replacement of the collagen destroyed by wear and tear but not for the maintenance of organ collagen.

Further investigations have shown that vitamin A plays some role in the healing of wounds, vitamin E even more so, as the clinical findings of Burgess and Pritchard show (61). In cases of necrobiosis, characterized by swelling of collagen, the necrobiotic processes disappeared, and normal collagen fibrils were formed when vitamin E was administered. A rehabilitation of the collagenous system together with its ground substance was probably fundamental in this change induced by vitamin E injection. This finding was of particular interest in World War II, the term "diffuse collagen diseases" having been introduced at that time by the pathologist Klemperer (62). He came to the conclusion that the collagen fibers are markedly altered during certain pathological conditions of the body, as in the case of *lupus erythematodes*. He submitted the thesis that alteration of the collagenous system is the basic anatomic manifestation of disseminated lupus and also of the case of scleroderma and muscle rheumatism. The changes taking place in the collagens of tendons in certain diseases and on aging, investigated by Stucke (63), and some interesting suggestions by

Bjorksten (64) on aging and collagen will be considered in Chapter 10 in "The Chemistry of Tanning Processes."

10. Some Accessory Proteins of Skin

Some proteins more or less related to the biochemical aspects of collagen will be briefly surveyed in this section.

Reticulin. Reticulin is the protein of the fine network surrounding the collagen fiber bundles and more abundantly present in the grain surface, its characterization being mainly histological (argyrophilic). At least four different views can be mentioned: (*1*) Reticulin and collagen are two distinct proteins, with no chemical relationship whatsoever. (*2*) Reticulin represents an early stage of development of collagen; it is a "procollagen." (*3*) The two proteins are chemically identical, the difference being in degree of subdivision, reticulin forming very much finer fibrils than collagen, (*4*) Reticulin tissue is a complex between collagen and mucoproteins or polysaccharides.

Considering the apparently conflicting ideas, the concept of reticulin as a collagen type of protein modified by association with polysaccharides seems to be the most acceptable. The amount of reticulin of the reticular layer of corium is less than 0.4 % of the dry weight of corium.

Elastin. Next to collagen, the elastin of the elastic fibers is the most important protein of the connective tissue. They appear as branched fibers, of varying length and width, yellow colored in the native state. They are resistant to boiling water and also to dilute acids and alkalis, which properties are helpful in separation of elastin from its normal associate in tissues, the collagenous fibers, since the latter are gelatinized and go into solution in the treatments mentioned. Unlike native collagen, elastin is susceptible to tryptic digestion. As the name implies, elastic fibers possess rubberlike elasticity. Since dry fibers are not elastic, this property must be bound to the hydrated form of the elastin molecule.

Whereas collagen and reticular fibers can be regenerated throughout life, elastic fibers cannot be replaced to any extent in the adult human. A consequence is that scars contain an abundance of collagen but not of elastin (65). Nothing is known of any specific factor inducing the formation of either elastin or collagen.

Force extension and thermoelastic studies of elastic fibers indicate a mechanical behavior very similar to that of rubber. Our knowledge of the amino acid composition of elastin is still fragmentary. Its hydroproline content is about 1.5 %. However, the large content of nonpolar residues is characteristic for this protein, and the elastic property has been ascribed to their presence in the elastin molecule. It is generally considered that the polypeptide chains are disordered, forming a tangled mass of long, mainly apolar chains. Elastin is optically isotropic in the unstretched condition. By stretching, birefringence of the fibers is induced. Astbury's X-ray studies (66) showed no indication of ordered structures. Hence, the properties of elastin are in accord with the concept of a structure composed of extensively folded chains which on stretching become more or less unfolded but tend to return to the original state of disorder.

Elastin is commonly prepared from the neck ligament of cattle, the *ligamentum nuchae*. The finely divided ligament is extracted with dilute sodium chloride solution, washed, and then extracted repeatedly with boiling water in order to gelatinize and solubilize the collagen, which forms about 15 % of the ligament. Extraction with a 1 % solution of potassium hydroxide is followed by washing in water and in a dilute solution of acetic acid. In the final stage, the stock is left in cold 5 % hydrochloric acid solution and washed thoroughly. A final extraction with boiling water then follows, after which treatments with hot alcohol and ether are applied before the final air-drying. This drastic mode of preparation will probably result in partial denaturation and degradation of the elastin. A preparation which avoids these alterations, although a less complete removal of collagen is effected, is obtained by pretreatment of the chopped ligaments in saturated lime solution for 2 to 3 weeks, followed by extraction in 60°C. water for 1 to 2 days, and washing and dehydration with acetone. The corium of skin contains only small amounts of elastin, less than 1 % of the weight of collagen, located mainly in the grain layer and the layer of the adipose tissue. Since elastin swells considerably less than collagen fibers, the presence of elastic fibers in the grain layer of the corium will impart less desirable properties to the grain during the processing of skins into leather, which involves conditions requiring swelling. A wrinkled and drawn grain is such a defect. The breaking up of the elastic fibers of the grain layer by means of the action of proteinases, mainly tryptic enzymes, is therefore attempted and considered by some people to be accomplished in the bating process. However, it has recently been demonstrated by Banga and Baló (67) that animal pancreas, used in bating, show elastolytic activity, which is attributed to a special enzyme, elastase. It has been suggested that the degeneration of human elastic tissue in arteriosclerosis is caused by elastase. Elastase liberates carbohydrates, glucosamine, and even sulfuric acid, from elastic tissue (68). The elastase problem is complicated by the presence of an inhibitor.

In the bating process, the lime solution retained in the interstices of the hide is removed by washing. The limed skins are then treated in a bate solution which contains an extract of pancreatin and large amounts of ammonium salts which interact with and remove the fixed calcium oxide of the skin and simultaneously function as an effective buffer, establishing a pH environment suitable for the tryptic degradation of elastin (pH 8 to 9). The partial removal or dislocation and breaking up of the elastic fibers in the bating process counteracts the strain in the grain membrane set up by the inelastic elastin fibers which will show up particularly in the chromed state. The difference in extensibility and other mechanical properties of chrome-tanned collagen and chrome-tanned elastin fibers is very marked, and hence the deaggregation and, if possible, the removal of the native elastic fibers of the skin before chrome tannage is desirable for the attainment of a smooth grain surface of the final chrome leather.

As to the reactivity of elastin, the acid-binding capacity is about 0.3 mg. equiv. of hydrogen ion (0.1 N HCl) per gram of elastin (69). Its affinity for basic chromium sulfates is about one-fourth of that of collagen (69). On the other hand, its degree of fixation of vegetable tannins nearly equals the values recorded for collagen (70). It is interesting to note that heat denaturation of "native" elastin has no noticeable effect on its binding capacity for vegetable tannins (70), whereas heat shrinkage of collagen, in the form of hide powder, connotes a marked increase in the fixation of vegetable tannins. Chrome-tanned elastin is inelastic and brittle, its appearance being an excellent argument for its removal by bating in the production of chrome upper leather.

11. The Glycoproteins of Skin

Although skin contains only small amounts of glycoproteins, their presence is interesting from the physiological point of view, particularly with regard to the genesis of the collagenous structure. If purified corium (salt-extracted and washed) is extracted in a cold solution of half-saturated calcium hydroxide solution and the filtered solution neutralized with acetic acid, a cream-colored bulky precipitate is formed which on drying turns into a dark-brown, brittle mass. The amount of the dry substance thus obtained is usually about 0.5 % of the weight of the collagen. Analysis of this mucoid shows a nitrogen content of about 12 % and 2.4 % of sulfur in the ester-bound form, which is present as sulfate (7.3 % sulfuric acid). Although a strong Molisch reaction for carbohydrate is obtained, no reducing sugars are present. This is proved by the fact that Fehling's solution is first reduced by the carbohydrate after its hydrolysis with acid. Grassmann (71) found 7.7 % galactose and glucose and 1.5 % hexosamine. It seems probable that this interfibrillar or cementing substance, which may function as a lubricating agent for the collagen bundles, contains chondroitin sulfuric acid, as one of its components, mucopolysaccharides, and related compounds, which are attached to the protein moiety through salt formation. The content of ester sulfate (chondroitin sulfate) of corium is rather low (about 0.02 to 0.04% sulfur) as already mentioned. Since the chrondroitin sulfate and similar sulfur compounds are prominent constituents of the ground substance in association with hyaluronic acid, mucoproteins, collagen, and elastin, their presence in corium is of biochemical interest. Discussion of the numerous minor constituents of skin, such as globular proteins, lipids, phospholipids, cholesterol, and mineral constituents, which have no direct bearing on the problems to be considered is outside the scope of this book.

12. CLASSIFICATION OF COLLAGENS

Since there are many members in the collagen class of proteins, some means of characterization of the class as a whole are desirable, and even necessary. Classification by a set of properties is indeed very difficult. The collagen present in mammalian tissues is economically the most important and hence the most thoroughly investigated and best-known type. These collagens of various species are apparently basically similar, although the collagen of mammalian corium differs in many properties from the collagen of tendons of the identical species, e.g., the skin and the tail of the rat. As mentioned earlier, the collagen of sheepskin has markedly lower nitrogen content than that of calfskin, and differences in hydrothermal stability of the two skins are noted, as evidenced by the shrinkage temperatures being about 60 and 67°C., respectively. The properties of cat and dog skins resemble those of sheepskin. In the Teleostomi (bone fishes), the collagens of the skin show varying stability, depending on the habitat of the species, ranging from 38 to 56°C. As a class, the fishskin collagens differ also in many other respects from the bovine type, in chemical composition, physical properties, and physicochemical behavior (72).

Turning our attention to some uncommon collagens, such as the elastoidin present in shark fins, and to the ichthyocol (73) of swim bladders of fishes, they appear superficially not to have much in common with bovine skin collagen, if physical properties and chemical reactivity are the main criteria. Thus, ichthyocol is readily turned into a soluble gelatinized form at blood heat, whereas bovine skin first shrinks in water at temperatures of about 65 to 70°C. The latter requires extensive acid or alkaline pretreatment and application of heat for gelatinization. On the other extreme, elastoidin shrinks in the range 60–66°C. This shrinkage is reversible, similar to that of formaldehyde-tanned collagen which also shows the Ewald reaction (73), i.e., a spontaneous re-extension of the heat-shortened fiber to about its original length on cooling. The presence of crosslinks of the type supplied by the fixed formaldehyde seems to be a requisite for this reversal. Since elastoidin contains rather large amounts of sulfur, the presence of cystine interchain links may well explain the unique behavior of elastoidin.

The causes for these differences among collagens of various organs and species may be assigned to differences in the amino acid pattern, varying degrees of cohesion, and intermolecular linking, i.e., a problem of the steric conditions, kind and degree of micro and macro-orientation of the units, such as fibers and fiber bundles, degree of hydration, and general histological differences.

By considering a group of properties, it should be possible to establish some sort of classification. Apart from the chemical characteristics, such as the high hydroxyproline content of collagen, such general properties of collagens are: insolubility in cold water, ability to swell in acid and alkaline solutions, considerable shortening of the fibers in water at certain temperatures, and transformation into gelatin on prolonged boiling of collagen which has undergone swelling pretreatment. Further, native collagen possesses marked resistance toward the action of proteinases of the type of trypsin and papain. However, collagen swollen in solutions of strong acids and alkalis, or by lyotropic agents, and mechanically defective collagen (fibers damaged or cut) are attacked by these proteinases, as is fishskin collagen. Moreover, the immunological inertness of collagen is characteristic, as is the practically complete inextensibility of the collagen fiber bundles; the fibrils possess great extensibility, on the other hand. The only methods which give clean-cut information for isolating and identifying collagens, are those based on physical criteria, such as the low-angle X-ray diffraction pattern and electron-microscopic photographs. However, these criteria may not always specifically denote collagens, since even proteins lacking in hydroxyproline and with low content of proline may show the typical low-angle X-ray diffraction diagram of collagen. It has been found, however, that collagens of widely different origin can be identified and classified by the wide-angle X-ray diagram (21). Also the electron micrographs give promise of being able to record the long spacings and the band-interband intraperiods which are the common features of collagens.

In the investigations of Robertson and Schwartz on ascorbic acid and the formation of collagen (74), the difficulties encountered in the quantitative assay of collagen in tissue are excellently exemplified. Robertson and Schwartz employed the two main methods available: first, a method (75) which depends on the precipitability by tannic acid of gelatin formed on the hydrolysis of collagen, after removal of other proteins by heat coagulation; second, the method of Neuman and Logan (76), which is based on the determination of the hydroxyproline content of the tissue, alloting a figure of 13.5 % of hydroxyproline to mammalian collagen. The values obtained with these two techniques varied considerably, as is shown by the figures of 18.6 % and 16.5 %, respectively; an even lower value of 9.0 % was obtained by the alkali-extraction method (77). In view of the wide variations of the hydroxyproline content of different collagens, for instance, that of *Teleostei*, the Neumann-Logan method should be restricted to the assay of mammalian collagen. Apparently the tannic acid method is not sufficiently specific for collagens, since most globular proteins form precipitates with tannic acid.

REFERENCES

1. Herzog, R. O., and Jancke, W., *Ber.* **53,** 2162 (1920); Brill, R., *Ann.* **434,** 204 (1923).
2. Meyer, K. H., and Mark, H., *Ber.* **61,** 1932 (1928).
3. See Low, B. W., *in* "The Proteins" (H. Neurath and K. Bailey, eds.), Vol. 1, Part A. Academic Press, New York, 1953; see also ref. 5.
3a. Cowan, P. M., North, A., and Randall, J. T., *in* "Nature and Structure of Collagen" (J. T. Randall, ed.), pp. 241–249. Butterworths, London, 1953.
4. Mirsky, A. E., and Pauling, L., *Proc. Natl. Acad. Sci. U. S.* **22,** 439 (1936); Pauling, L., and Niemann, C., *J. Am. Chem. Soc.* **61,** 1866 (1939); Huggins, M. L., *J. Org. Chem.* **1,** 407 (1936).
5. Astbury, W. T., "Fundamentals of Fibre Structure." Oxford University Press, London, 1933.
6. Bear, R. S., *Advances in Protein Chem.* **7,** 69 (1952).
7. Clark, G. L., Parker, E. A., Schaad, J. A., and Warren, W. J., *J. Am. Chem. Soc.* **57,** 1509 (1935).
8. Wyckoff, R. W. G., Corey, R. B., and Biscoe, J., *Science* **82,** 175 (1935); Wyckoff, R. W. G., and Corey, R. B., *Proc. Soc. Exptl. Biol. Med.* **34,** 285 (1936).
9. Bear, R. S., *J. Am. Chem. Soc.* **64,** 727 (1942); **66,** 1297 (1944).
10. Schmitt, F. O., Hall, C. E., and Jakus, M. A., *J. Am. Chem. Soc.* **64,** 1234 (1942); *J. Cellular Comp. Physiol.* **20,** 11 (1942).
11. Dore, W. H., and Sponsler, O. L., *Colloid Chem. Monograph* **4,** 174 (1926).
12. Astbury, W. T., and Street, A., *Phil. Trans. Roy. Soc.* **A230,** 75 (1933).
13. Astbury, W. T., and Woods, H. J., *Phil. Trans. Roy. Soc.* **A232,** 333 (1933).
14. Astbury, W. T., Dickinson, S., and Bailey, K., *Biochem. J.* **29,** 235 (1935).
15. Pauling, L., and Corey, R. B., *Proc. Natl. Acad. Sci. U. S.* **37,** 272 (1951).
16. Pauling, L., and Corey, R. B., *Proc. Roy. Soc.* **B141,** 31 (1953).
17. See Edsall, J. T., *Science* **119,** 302 (1954).
18. Lundgren, H. P., *Advances in Protein Chem.* **5,** 305 (1949).
19. Speakman, J. B., and Hirst, M. C., *Trans. Faraday Soc.* **29,** 148 (1933); Speakman, J. B., and Stott, E., *ibid.* **30,** 539 (1934); Speakman, J. B., and Townend, F., *ibid.* **32,** 897 (1936).
20. Astbury, W. T., *Compt. rend. trav. lab. Carlsberg* **22,** 45 (1938); *Trans. Faraday Soc.* **34,** 378 (1938).
21. Astbury, W. T., *J. Intern. Soc. Leather Trades Chem.* **24,** 69 (1940).
22. Huggins, M. L., *Chem. Revs.* **32,** 195 (1943).
23. Bragg, W. L., Kendrew, J. C., and Perutz, M. F., *Proc. Roy. Soc.* **A203,** 321 (1950).
24. Ambrose, E. J., and Elliott, A., *Proc. Roy. Soc.* **A208,** 75 (1951).
25. Herzog, R. O., and Gonnel, H. W., *Ber.* **58,** 2228 (1925); Herzog, R. O., and Jancke, W., *ibid.* **59,** 2487 (1926).
26. Bear, R. S., Bolduan, O. E. A., and Salo, T. P., *J. Am. Leather Chem. Assoc.* **46,** 107 (1951).
26a. Hailwood, A., and Horrobin, S., *Trans. Faraday Soc.* **42B,** 84 (1946).

26b. Speakman, J. B., *J. Soc. Leather Trades Chem.* **37,** 37 (1953).

27. Cohen, C., and Bear, R. S., *J. Am. Chem. Soc.* **75,** 2784 (1953).

28. Huggins, M. L., *J. Am. Chem. Soc.* **76,** 4046 (1954).

29. Gustavson, K. H., *Acta Chem. Scand.* **8,** 1299 (1954).

30. Pomeroy, C. D., and Mitton, R. G., *J. Soc. Leather Trades Chem.* **35,** 360 (1951).

30a. M'Even, M. B., and Pratt, M. I., *in* "Nature and Structure of Collagen" (J. T. Randall, ed.), p. 158. Butterworths, London, 1953.

31. Wyckoff, R. W. G., "Electron Microscopy," Interscience, New York, 1949; *Advances in Protein Chem.* **6,** 1 (1951).

32. Schmitt, F. O., *Advances in Protein Chem.* **1,** 25 (1944); Schmitt, F. O., and Gross, J., *J. Am. Leather Chem. Assoc.* **43,** 659 (1948).

33. Wolpers, C., *Naturwissenschaften* **28,** 461 (1941); particularly *Das Leder* **1,** 3 (1950).

34. Nutting, G. C., and Borasky, R., *J. Am. Leather Chem. Assoc.* **43,** 96 (1948); Borasky, R., and Rogers, J. S., *ibid.* **47,** 312 (1952).

35. Grassmann, W., Hofmann, V., and Nemetschek, T., *Z. Naturforsch.* **7b,** 509 (1952).

36. Schmidt, W. J., "Die Bausteine des Tierkörpers in polarisiertem Licht." Cohen, Bonn, 1924.

37. Küntzel, A., *Collegium* **1925,** 63; Küntzel, A., and Schwank, M., *ibid.* **1940,** 489.

38. von Ebner, V., *Sitzber. Akad. Wiss. Wien, Math.-naturw. Kl.* **103,** 162 (1894).

39. Marriott, R. H., *J. Intern. Soc. Leather Trades Chem.* **19,** 133, 169, 246 (1935).

40. Nageotte, J., and Guyon, L., *Arch. biol.* (Liége) **41,** 1 (1930); *Am. J. Pathol.* **6,** 631 (1930); Nageotte, J., *Compt. rend. soc. biol.* **98,** 15 (1928).

41. Fauré-Frémiet, E., and Garrault, H., *Arch. anat. microscop.* **33,** 81 (1937); Fauré-Frémiet, E., and Baudouy, C., *Bull. soc. chim., biol.,* **19,** 1134 (1937); Fauré-Frémiet, E., and Cougny, A., *Bull. muséum natl. hist. nat. (Paris)* **9,** 188 (1937).

42. Schmitt, F. O., Hall, C. E., and Jakus, M. A., *J. Cellular Comp. Physiol.* **20,** 11 (1942).

43. Porter, K. R., and Vanamee, P., *J. Exptl. Med.* **94,** 255 (1951).

44. Orekhovich, V. N., *Biokhimiya* **13,** 55 (1948); *Communs. 2e congr. intern. biochim.,* Paris (1952).

45. Highberger, J. H., Gross, J., and Schmitt, F. O., *Proc. Natl. Acad. Sci. U. S.* **37,** 286 (1951).

46. Randall, J. T., ed., "Nature and Structure of Collagen." Butterworths, London, 1953.

47. Bergmann, M., and Stein, W. H., *J. Biol. Chem.* **128,** 217 (1939).

48. Gross, J., Highberger, J. H., and Schmitt, F. O., *Proc. Soc. Exptl. Biol. Med.* **80,** 462 (1952).

49. Schmid, K. J., *J. Am. Chem. Soc.* **72,** 2816 (1950).

50. Morrione, T. G., *J. Exptl. Med.* **96,** 107 (1952); Gold, N. K., and Gould, B. S., *Arch. Biochem. and Biophys.* **33,** 155 (1951).

51. Jackson, S. F., and Randall, J. T., *in* "Nature and Structure of Collagen" (J. T. Randall, ed.), p. 181. Butterworths, London, 1953.

52. Schmitt, F. O., Gross, J., and Highberger, J. H., *Proc. Natl. Acad. Sci. U. S.* **39,** 459 (1953).

52a. Gross, J., Highberger, J. H., and Schmitt, F. O., *Proc. Natl. Acad. Sci. U. S.* **40,** 679 (1954); **41,** 1 (1955); Boedtker, H., and Doty, P., *J. Am. Chem. Soc.* **77,** 248 (1955).

53. Highberger, J. H., *J. Am. Leather Chem. Assoc.* **48,** 704 (1953).

54. Brown, G. L., Kelly, F. C., and Watson, M., in "Nature and Structure of Collagen" (J. T. Randall, ed.), p. 117. Butterworths, London, 1953.
55. Bowes, J. H., Elliott, R. G., and Moss, J. A., in "Nature and Structure of Collagen" (J. T. Randall, ed.), p. 199. Butterworths, London, 1953.
56. Little, K., and Kramer, H., Nature 170, 499 (1952); "Nature and Structure of Collagen" (J. T. Randall, ed.), pp. 33–43. Butterworths, London, 1953.
57. Grassmann, W., and Schleich, H., Biochem. Z. 277, 320 (1935); Schneider, F., Collegium 1940, 97.
58. Beek, J., Jr., J. Am. Leather Chem. Assoc. 36, 696 (1941).
59. Höjer, J. A., Acta Paediat. 3, 1 (1924); see also Wohlbach, S. B., Am. J. Pathol. 9, 689 (1933); Danielli, J. F., Fell, H. B., and Kodicek, E., Brit. J. Exptl. Pathol. 26, 367 (1945); Bradfield, J., and Kodicek, E., Biochem. J. 49, xvii (1951).
60. Robertson, W. van B., J. Biol. Chem. 197, 495 (1952); Communs. 2e congr. intern. biochim., Paris (1952); Robertson, W. van B., and Schwartz, B., J. Biol. Chem. 201, 689 (1953).
61. Burgess, J. F., and Pritchard, J. E., Arch. Dermatol. and Syphilol. 57, 953 (1948); Burgess, J. F., Lancet 265, 215 (1948).
62. Klemperer, P., Pollack, A. D., and Baehr, G., Arch. Pathol. 32, 569 (1941); J. Am. Med. Assoc. 119, 331 (1942); Klemperer, P., Bull. N. Y. Acad. Med. 23, 581 (1947); Am. J. Pathol. 26, 505 (1950).
63. Stucke, K., Langenbecks Arch. klin. Chir. 265, 579 (1950).
64. Bjorksten, J., J. Am. Chem. Soc. 64, 868 (1942).
65. Jacobson, W., in "Nature and Structure of Collagen" (J. T. Randall, ed.), p. 6. Butterworths, London, 1953.
66. Astbury, W. T., Trans. Faraday Soc. 34, 377 (1938); J. Intern. Soc. Leather Trades Chem. 24, 69 (1940); Kolpak, H., Kolloid-Z. 73, 129 (1935).
67. Banga, I., and Baló, J., Nature 164, 49 (1949); 171, 44 (1953).
68. Hall, D. A., Reed, R., and Tunbridge, R. E., Nature 170, 264 (1952).
69. Gustavson, K. H., unpublished investigation.
70. Gustavson, K. H., Biochem. Z. 311, 347 (1942).
71. Grassmann, W., Janicki, J., Klenk, L., and Schneider, F., Biochem. Z. 294, 95 (1937).
72. Gustavson, K. H., Svensk Kem. Tidskr. 65, 70 (1953).
73. Fauré-Frémiet, E., and Woelffin, R., J. chim. phys. 33, 801 (1936).
74. Robertson, W. van B., and Schwartz, B., J. Biol. Chem. 201, 689 (1953).
75. Spencer, H. C., Morgulis, S., and Wilder, V. M., J. Biol. Chem. 120, 257 (1937).
76. Neuman, R. E., and Logan, M. A., J. Biol. Chem. 186, 549 (1950).
77. Lowry, O. H., Gilligan, D. R., and Katersky, E. M., J. Biol. Chem. 139, 794 (1941); Robertson, W. van B., ibid. 187, 673 (1950); 196, 403 (1952).

CHAPTER 4

The Isoelectric Points of Collagen

1. INTRODUCTION

By definition, the isoelectric point of a protein is that pH value of its solution or suspension at which it does not migrate in an electric field. The concept of the isoelectric point had its origin in Hardy's (1) experiments on the migration of suspensions of egg albumin in an electric field. For the proteins, this important point, expressed as the pH value of its location, also connotes some distinct properties, such as the minima of swelling and solubility, osmotic pressure, membrane potential and viscosity, further minimum ionization, and accordingly the minimum in acid- and alkali-binding properties. In gels, the isoelectric state also denotes the maximum light-scattering power (Tyndall effect) and gel strength (relative resistance to shear). When the values of these properties are plotted as functions of the pH value, the curves show a sharp drop, or incline, at or near the iso-electric point. Although the first determinations of the isoelectric point of globular proteins were carried out by electrophoresis, by noting the pH of the medium at which the migration of the protein reversed its direction, most investigations of the isoelectric state of collagen have made use of the abrupt changes in various physical properties and in the chemical reactivity of the protein taking place at the pH of this point.

2. METHODS OF DETERMINATION

Determinations by such techniques are relatively easy to perform. However, only approximate values of the location of the isoelectric point are obtained by taking physical properties, such as the minimum degree of swelling of skin, as the criteria. The first systematic studies of Wilson (2) were carried out by this method on gelatin and skin, the former substrate yielding a very much sharper minimum than the solid skin (see Fig. 28). Another method is based on the fact that collagen, or any protein, will not alter the pH of an unbuffered solution when its value is identical with that of the isoelectric point of the protein (3).

a. The dyestuff technique

A third method is the dyestuff-staining procedure, extensively used by Loeb in his lucid researches on gelatin (4) and later introduced by Thomas and Kelly for the study of the reactivity of collagen and for the estimation of the isoelectric point of collagen (hide powder) (5). The basis for this method is the fact that acid dyestuffs, i.e., anions of aromatic sulfonic acids, will combine with collagen only on the acid side of its isoelectric point, whereas basic dyestuffs (cations of dyestuff salts) possess affinity for collagen on the alkaline side only. If two simple dyestuffs are considered, such as Martius yellow and fuchsin, originally used by Thomas and Kelly (5), it will be found that the specimens treated with the yellow acid dye will stain the hide substrate at pH values below 5, whereas the red coloring of the basic dye will appear only on hide powder equilibrated at pH values greater than 5. The isoelectric point of hide powder (limed and subsequently delimed collagen) is thus fixed at pH values in the vicinity of 5. The dyestuffs selected for such tests should preferably be rather simple compounds which for their irreversible combination with the hide protein rely on simple ionic groups in the dyestuff molecule. Dyestuffs of more complicated constitution, containing coordination-active groups, are less selective for the ionic reactions, which are the basic functions of the protein, since secondary reactions, feasible through coordination on nonionic protein groups, will partially mask the primary electrovalent reaction. Some dyestuffs carry both positively and negatively charged functional groups, the ampho-ionic class. These cannot be used, because they dye the substrate in its isoelectric state. Even such a simple dyestuff as α-naphthol orange shows this tendency, reacting in its dipolar form,

$$SO_3^- \langle \bigcirc \rangle N\overset{+}{H}{=}\overset{+}{N}H \langle \bigcirc \rangle O^-$$

as investigations of Kuhn (6), have shown. In the more complicated and larger molecules of polyazo dyestuffs, this tendency is further developed (Otto, 7). The application of the dyestuff technique for determination of the shift of the isoelectric point of collagen resulting from its combination with tanning agents will be discussed under the appropriate headings of the various tannages in "The Chemistry of Tanning Processes."

b. Titration curves

A method combining simplicity with precision for determination of the isoelectric point is based on the construction of the titration curve of collagen (see Fig. 18). In this method, which will be discussed later, the intersection of the titration curve with the abscissa denoting the pH values gives the value of the isoelectric point, when the amounts of hydrogen and hydroxyl ions removed from the solution by collagen are plotted as a function of the equilibrium pH of the system. In the case of fibrous proteins, for instance silk fibroin, the titration curve obtained in a salt-free solution may show an isoelectric zone instead of a sharp point. Of course, only nonswelling proteins or those showing only a slight swelling, such as silk and keratin (hair), may be titrated in salt-free systems. For collagen, on the other hand, because of its marked tendency to swell, and because of the accompanying complications of Donnan effects and phases of different concentrations of hydrogen ions, addition of neutral salt, preferably having a common anion with that of the acid used, will be an absolute requisite for elimination of these difficulties. Even with insoluble proteins which are relatively resistant to swelling, the effect of the addition of salt to the titrated system is shown by the form of the curve obtained. Its intersection with the pH axis is sharply defined, and an isoelectric point instead of a zone is obtained. In the system hydrochloric acid–sodium chloride, complicating secondary effects do not occur.

c. Electrophoresis

The method of electrophoresis, particularly in its modern, highly developed form, is the logical technique for the determination of the isoelectric point by virtue of the definition of this property. For insoluble proteins, such as collagen in the form of hide powder, a suspension of the material is used. It must possess a sufficient degree of subdivision in order to hold the particles in suspension during the time necessary to carry out the experiment. The microcell method is the most convenient. For collagen in combination with such tanning agents which themselves react with the added acid and alkali, plotting of the acid- and base-binding curves is not feasible. This applies to chrome-tanned hide powder and chrome leather for which methods based on changes in electrical migration or potential of the tanned collagen are practically the only ones available.

In microelectrophoresis, the motion of individual particles of the substrate in an electrical field is observed and determined by means of a microscope or an ultramicroscope. In order to minimize the error introduced by the Brownian movement, the mean of many observations has to be taken. A variety of cells have been devised for this type of electrophoresis. The Abramson cell (8) is representative and generally used. Reversible electrodes (Cu in saturated $CuSO_4$ solution, or Ag in NaCl solution) are inserted in the electrode vessels which are fused to the cell. Agar-agar plugs prevent streaming of the solution from the electrode system into the system being measured.

This microtechnique and the standard moving-boundary method (9) gave identical values of the mobilities of serum albumin in comparative experiments. In the following paragraphs, some typical results from investigations on collagen will illustrate the salient points of the electrophoretic technique. The mobility is usually given in microns per second per volt per centimeter. The curve thus obtained for positive and negative migration values will intersect the pH axis. The intersection gives the value of the isoelectric point of the substrate tested (see Fig. 15).

d. The electrokinetic technique

When a stream of a dilute solution of an electrolyte is forced through a plug of fibers, an electric current is produced. This method has been applied by Neale and Peters (10) and by Neale (11), to the determination of the isoelectric point of wool, nylon, silk, and collagen. It is based on the fact that the surface potential varies with the hydrogen ion concentration and is zero at the isoelectric point.

Finally, measurement of the dialysis potential has been used by Staverman (12) to determine the isoelectric point of membranes prepared from lupin proteins or hide powder by pressing, or applied in the form of a split (middle layer) of skin. The simple apparatus is shown in Fig. 16. The dialysis potential is the potential measured between two KCl solutions of 0.1 and 0.01 M strength. In the cell, the membrane m, in the form of a split of skin, separates the two KCl solutions. Nitrogen is bubbled through the cell in order to ensure homogeneity of the two phases and to avoid the polarization of the solution in the immediate neighborhood of the membrane. The potential difference between the two half-cells is measured by means of two identical calomel electrodes with saturated KCl bridges, e. For deter-

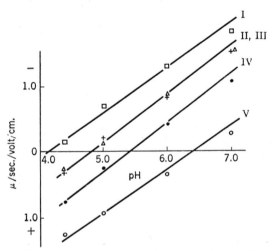

FIG. 15. pH-mobility curve of chrome-tanned powder: I, cationic chromed hide powder (No. 1) in acetate buffer; V, in borate buffer; II, anionic chromed hide powder (No. 5) in acetate buffer; III, in borate buffer; IV, untreated hide powder (blank).

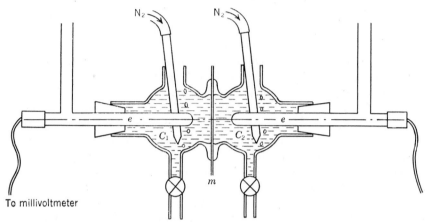

Fig. 16. Cell for measurement of dialysis potentials of membranes (skin), according to Staverman (12): m, membrane; C_1, glass compartment with 0.1 M KCl solution; C_2, with 0.01 M KCl solution; e, calomel electrodes.

mination of the isoelectric point of the membrane, for instance chrome leather in the form of the middle layer of skin, the cell is filled with the appropriate buffer solution of a given pH value and the voltage is measured in millivolts. By selecting buffers of pH values located on both sides of the probable isoelectric point of the membrane, not to far from this point, a curve intersecting the pH axis will be obtained. The results of a series of determinations on delimed (isoelectric) splits of sheepskin as such (pelt) and after oil tanning of the pelt (unfixed oil removed) are graphically represented in Fig. 17. This method has been found very useful for the study of the potential of various leathers.

3. The Isoelectric State of Collagen

In the early determinations of the isoelectric point of collagen by localization of the swelling minimum, by the dyestuff technique, and by titration curves, standard hide powder was usually the substrate. Hide powder is a fluffy powder of finely divided corium of hide, which has been limed, delimed, dehydrated, and ground into a powder. Hence, it really is a collagen modified by alkaline pretreatment and mechanical treatment. Its use as a standard substrate for tannin analysis and for experiments in tanning, which are the prototypes for technical processes, is justified because of its relatively high uniformity and the feasibility of eliminating, or at least lessening, the topochemical complications inherent in the hide structure as a whole. Although standard commercial hide powder is by no means representative of native collagen, its properties and particularly its isoelectic point

are of the utmost importance in its behavior and use as a universal substrate for a modified collagen, representing the skin after dehairing and
conditioning into a state suitable for tanning. Native collagen is rarely met
with in practice, although sometimes it is found in the fur industry and in
biological systems in physiology and medicine.

The isoelectric point of hide powder has by several independent methods
been established in the neighborhood of pH 5 (2–5), values only slightly
higher than that of gelatin of the normal alkali-processed type (4). As already emphasized, the importance of the isoelectric conditions of limed
(alkali-treated) collagen is obvious, in view of the fact that the hide material
undergoing tanning in practice is always limed.

A simplified expression for the relationship between the hydrogen ion
concentration corresponding to the isoelectric point, expressed as the pH
value, and the values of the contents of cationic and anionic groups of
collagen and their relative strength cannot be derived. However, for simple
amino acids the isoelectric point is defined by the equation:

$$\mathrm{pH}_I = \frac{pK_A + pK_B}{2}$$

The correlation between the value of the isoelectric point of collagen and
the number and strength of the acidic and basic groups of the protein becomes evident. In earlier days this presented an exceedingly puzzling problem, since the data on the amino acid composition of collagen available at
that time showed a large excess of basic groups, whereas the isoelectric

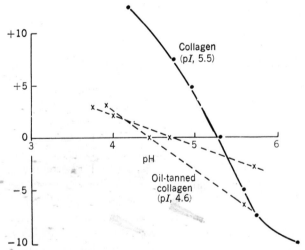

FIG. 17. Determination of the isoelectric point of pelt (skin) and oil-tanned pelt
by Staverman's method of electrodialysis.

point was found in a zone opposite to that expected, i.e., in the acid range, at a pH of about 5. However, in view of the fact that not only the quantity of polar groups but also their strength enter into the equation of the location of the isoelectric point, the possibility that the pK values of the acidic groups are increased, compared to the value of the simple amino acids by the ionic environment of the protein chains, could not be wholly discounted. The proximity and space arrangement of the charged protein groups in an insoluble protein of fixed configuration must not be disregarded. This problem was simplified by the availability of complete quantitative data on the amino acid make-up of collagen and by information on the effect of alkali treatment (liming) on the proportion of cationic to anionic groups in the collagen molecule.

In the early 1920's Wilson and Gallun (13) found two isoelectric points of collagen and gelatin, particularly in systems at room temperature, located by the minima of swelling at pH 5 and pH 7.6. At that time it was taken for granted that the minimum of swelling of collagen and gelatin denoted precisely the isoelectric state. By selection of buffers of different composition, however, the minimum of swelling may be attained at different pH values. The existence of two different isoelectric points in one protein was a remarkable discovery, in many respects quite disturbing. It was, and still is, quite contradictory to our conception of proteins. Since the second isoelectric point was found in the alkaline pH range, the possibility that a rearrangement of the collagen molecule occurs when the ionic environment is changed could not wholly be discounted. Another possible explanation would be the presence of two types of collagen in corium; the early X-ray diffraction patterns were indeed interpreted on the basis of the existence of a crystalline part, responsible for the lattice structure and the diffraction effects. The ordered structure was believed to be embedded in an amorphous constituent. Such two-phase structures of proteins, crystalline and noncrystalline, are also indicated by the infrared spectra of fibrous proteins, particularly in silk and the keratins (14). Since Wilson used phosphate buffers in his swelling experiments, it has also been suggested by Atkin and Douglas (15), and later by Küntzel (16), that the second isoelectric point might be an artifact due to the action of the polyvalent phosphate ions.

The possibility that gelatin is a mixture of two proteins with isoelectric points at pH 5 and 7.8, having double isoelectric points corresponding to their composition, was tested by Kraemer (17) in his work on pigskin gelatin. Kraemer prepared various mixtures of alkali-treated gelatin with an isoelectric point of pH 5, and acid-treated gelatin isoelectric at pH 7.8. He found that the isoelectric point, as determined by the influence of pH on the Tyndall effect, was at a pH intermediate between those of the two components. In general, the component with an isoelectric point near pH 5 was more effective than the other component in determining the pH of the mixture.

It seems safe to conclude that there is no justification for considering the point of minimum swelling to be the isoelectric point of the protein. The problem then may be restated: Two points of minimum swelling of gelatin and collagen are discernible under certain experimental conditions; but this by no means implies two isoelectric points of collagen, since the swelling property is no conclusive criterion of the isoelectric state of the protein. On the other hand, it is perhaps merely a coincidence that the isoelectric point of native collagen is located at about the same pH value as that found by Wilson for the second isoelectric point, whereas the normal isoelectric point of limed (alkali-treated) collagen coincides with the pH of the normal minimum of swelling.

4. LOCATION OF THE ISOELECTRIC POINT

The turning point in our concept of the isoelectric point (1) as a constant value and (2) as a characteristic property of protein was brought about by the findings of Kraemer and Dexter (18) and of Briefer (19). These workers showed that the isoelectric point of gelatin obtained from acid-treated pigskin which has not been limed corresponds to pH values of 7 to 8, whereas alkali-treated (limed) pigskin gives a gelatin with a normal isoelectric point at pH 5. In these investigations the light-scattering capacity of the gelatin, the Tyndall effect, was assumed to have its maximum at the isoelectric point.

A number of investigators later showed that the location of the isoelectric point of hide collagen is a function of its previous history, particularly the degree of alkali treatment (liming). The final experimental proof of this assertion and an explanation of the displacement of the isoelectric point was given by Beek and Sookne (20) in their cataphoretic investigations of collagens subjected to different pretreatment, according to the procedure of Moyer (21), using a microcell. The finely ground collagen powders were suspended in buffer solutions of 0.02 N ionic strength. The results of the electrophoresis of native hide collagen and limed hide collagen were plotted with the mobility of the collagen suspension as a function of the pH value, the intersection of the curves with the pH axis giving the value of the isoelectric point. The pH of the isoelectric point of native hide collagen was found to be 7. By liming of the hide, the isoelectric point of collagen was shifted to about 5.3 on the pH scale. From determination of the amide nitrogen of the two types of collagen, the conclusion was drawn that the decrease in amide nitrogen, as a result of the deamidation taking place in the liming, was accompanied by an increase in the number of free carboxyl groups, which in turn caused an increase in the net negative charge. Thus the isoelectric point of collagen is displaced toward the acid pH range.

Independently, and also by electrophoresis, Highberger (22) found the isoelectric point of native collagen of hide to be at pH 7.8 in buffers of ionic strength 0.005. It was suggested that the normal value of the isoelectric point of limed hide, hide powder, and regular gelatin (alkali-treated) at pH near 5 is due to some structural change in the protein caused by the alkaline treatment given these materials.

New data on the contents of dicarboxylic acids and amide groups (23) in native collagen offer a rational explanation of the location of the isoelectric point of native hide in the slightly alkaline pH range, and that of gelatin and limed collagen generally in the acid pH range, if due regard is paid to the hydrolysis of acid amide groups, with the formation of free carboxylic groups taking place in the regular liming process. Generally, in the regular practice of liming, about half of the amide nitrogen appears to be split off during treatment of the hide for a few days in saturated lime solutions containing small amounts of a depilatory (sodium sulfide) (24). Thus, limed collagen contains about 1.0 mg. equiv. of *free* carboxylic groups (total anionic groups, 1.24 − amide groups, 0.2 to 0.3) and 0.87 mg. equiv. of cationic groups, or a surplus of anionic groups of about 0.1 to 0.2 mg. equiv. per gram of collagen (23). The new data also satisfactorily account for the location of the isoelectric point of native (*not* alkaline-treated) collagen in the pH range of 7 to 8, since the amount of *free* carboxylic groups is 0.77 mg. equiv. (total anionic groups, 1.24 − amide groups, 0.47), whereas the content of basic groups is 0.87 mg. equiv., or a surplus of 0.1 mg. equiv. of cationic groups per gram of collagen (23).

According to Cassel and McKenna (25), the amide groups of native steer hide collagen (Highberger) amount to 0.43 mg. equiv. of nitrogen per gram of collagen. Limed hide (hide powder) was found to contain 0.27 mg. equiv. and common gelatin 0.14 mg. equiv. of amide nitrogen per gram of collagen. The main source of the amide nitrogen in collagen is indicated to be asparagine. By comparing the rate of hydrolysis of the amide group in N sulfuric acid at 100°C., on the one hand, and in a phosphate-borax buffer of pH 6.5, on the other, it is possible to ascertain whether the residue of glutamic or aspartic acid is deamidized, since in the first instance all the amide groups are liberated, whereas in the second case, (at pH 6.5) complete hydrolysis of glutamine is accomplished, with practically no hydrolysis of asparagine (26). Comparative experiments with collagen in sulfuric acid and in the buffer solution indicated the ratio of asparagine to glutamine to be about 4:1.

It is evident that the shift of the isoelectric point of native collagen toward the acid side by the alkali treatment may also be due to partial destruction or weakening of cationic protein groups by the action of alkali alone, in addition to the principal reaction, production of new anionic groups by means of the deamidation process. In any alteration of the basic groups by the alkali, the guanidyl group of the arginine residue should be expected to be most susceptible. It is known that arginine is decomposed into urea and ornithine by the action of alkali, and hence the arginine residue of collagen may react with alkali according to the equation:

$$
\begin{array}{c}
| \\
CO \\
| \\
H\overset{|}{C}(CH_2)_3 \cdot NH \cdot C \cdot (NH) \cdot NH_2 + H_2O \rightarrow \\
| \\
NH \\
|
\end{array}
$$

$$
\begin{array}{c}
| \\
CO \\
| \\
CO(NH_2)_2 + H\overset{|}{C} \cdot (CH_2)_3 \cdot NH_2 \\
| \\
NH \\
|
\end{array}
$$

The reaction of splitting off ammonia with formation of citrulline is practically absent. The ornithine residue contains a basic group in the side chain, but this group is much less strongly basic than the original guanidyl group. Highberger and Stecker (27), investigating the chemical action of saturated lime solutions containing added sodium hydroxide on native collagen of steer hide, found that urea is definitely formed in the processing. However, the destruction of the guanidyl group is insignificant in ordinary liming i.e., during periods of a few days. These workers found the major factor in the shift of the isoelectric point of limed collagen to be hydrolysis of the acid amide groups with the formation of ammonia and new carboxylic groups. The work of Bowes (24) has fully confirmed this conclusion. Highberger and Stecker (27) further report that apparently all the acid amide groups are completely hydrolyzed in 4 days at ordinary temperature at pH values about 13 (saturated lime solution containing 1.0 % w/v NaOH), 0.25 mg. equiv. of NH_3 per gram collagen being set free. However, this figure is only slightly more than half the value given by Bowes and Kenten (23) for the total amide content of native hide collagen, 0.47 mg. equiv. per gram of collagen. In ordinary liming for 3 days with sharpened limes at pH 13.7, about two-thirds of the amide groups is removed (24).

In regard to the formation of ornithine residues from the arginine residues of collagen, which takes place under intensive pretreatment of collagen in its transformation into gelatin, the following incident is of interest. Berg-ström and Lindstedt (28), in estimating the content of hydroxylysine in gelatine, found that some constituent of the completely acid-hydrolyzed high-grade gelatins interfered with this determination. The trouble was traced to small amounts of ornithine, which was found to be a regular constituent of the gelatins. By direct hydrolytic breakdown of native fish-skin by hydrochloric acid, this complication was avoided. Thus, evidence for the formation of ornithine in alkali-treated collagen was obtained.

Theis and Jacoby (29) have also studied the effect of the degree of liming on the isoelectric state of hide collagen. Their results show the same trend as those obtained in the pioneering investigations of Beek and Sookne and of Highberger, although Theis and Jacoby apparently failed to realize the theoretical significance of the earlier investigations. Theis and Jacoby consider *deaminization* or a change in amino acid content of collagen to be the main reason for the shift of the isoelectric point, emphasizing that histidine and lysine are most drastically affected. Thus the loss in basic groups should be responsible for the lowered pH of the isoelectric point. Further, they state that the changed amino acid content is shown in the formaldehyde and chrome fixation of the various limed specimens of col-lagen. There are doubts about the correctness of the experimental data—for instance the finding that the arginine group is more resistant to alkali than the ϵ-lysine residue—and under no circumstances are the conclusions drawn from the data presented justified. Theis and Jacoby also claim to have pre-pared collagens with isoelectric points at pH 4.25 on 15 days' liming in a straight saturated solution of lime at room temperature, the isoelectric point being localized by means of microelectrophoresis. This exceedingly low value of the isoelectric point of moderately limed collagen at pH 4.25 is without a parallel and is probably due to insufficient familiarity with the electrophoretic technique, since the lowest pH value of the isoelectric point recorded for gelatin after months of liming is 4.5 (30). According to modern, more precise methods, the isoelectric point of gelatin cannot be brought to a pH value lower than 4.7.

5. The Effect of Alkali

It was once believed—or guessed, since experimental foundation for the statement was lacking—that on prolonged alkali treatment of collagen, as in the conditioning of limed stock for the making of gelatin, hydrolysis of peptide links may occur to a considerable extent. Since about every fourth linking of the amino acid residues in the backbone of bovine collagen contains the —CO—N= group, formed by the linking of proline and hy-droxyproline, the effect of the opening up of such links on the isoelectric reaction of collagen may be an important factor. By hydrolysis of the regular —CO—NH— group, *equal* amounts of strong carboxylic and amino groups are formed, whereas the cleavage of the —CO—N= group results in the formation of one strong carboxylic group and one weakly basic group, the =NH. Hence, in the latter instance the hydrolytic breaking of the keto-imide groups formed by the residues of the prolines (the —CO·N= groups), would be expected to increase the net negative charge of collagen, i.e., to shift the isoelectric point toward lower pH values. This type of reaction appears to be relatively rare, to judge from modern work on gelatin and the distribution of the molecular weights of its constituents.

The problem suggested involves many important questions which are no longer outside the reach of the investigator, such as the relative stability of the various —CO—NH— and —CO—N= bonds present in collagen to H and OH ions, and its dependence on the type of adjacent side chains and on the general ionic environment of the lattice. If only a few links of the regular peptide links are hydrolyzed in the liming process, they should contribute very little, or in an amount hardly measurable, to the potential of acidic and basic groups. The reason is that the small number of liberated groups which are added to the large number of ionic groups already present in the original molecule of collagen with a molecular weight of the order of a few millions would cause a very small change in the total number of ionic groups already present in the intact protein molecule (31). Provided the proline residue is not an end group of collagen and making use of a method of the same specificity and degree of accuracy as the Sanger dinitrofluoro-benzene method for determination of N-terminal residues in the estimation of the C-terminal groups, the carboxylic groups, it should be possible to determine both N- and C-terminal groups of collagens that have been subjected to various treatments in acids and alkalis. Thus unequivocal information could obtained as to the degree and art of splitting of the backbone links of collagen, and the occurrence of any preferential splitting of the —CO·N= bond over that of the —CO—NH— bond. Such an investigation will be discussed.

The main results of the investigations by Bowes *et al.* (24, 32, 33) on the effect of alkaline solutions (pH 12 to 14) on collagen indicate:

1. Hydrolysis of amide groups, by which the amount of free carboxyl groups is increased, and nitrogen is lost in the form of ammonia.
2. Modification of the guanidine groups (the arginine residue).
3. Minor destruction of aliphatic hydroxy acids (serine and threonine).
4. Some hydrolysis of keto-imide groups of the backbone of the collagen chains.

Specimens of native hide collagen were treated for 14 days in solutions of calcium and sodium hydroxides of final pH 13 at 20°C. The treated collagen and the solutions were analyzed. Apart from the marked decrease in amide nitrogen, and a slight lowering of the arginine content, Bowes *et al.* found that amino nitrogen had increased from 0.33 to 0.36 mg. equiv. per gram of collagen, which is accounted for by the ornithine formed. Furthermore, the total basic groups increased by 0.06 mg. equiv., which probably was due to the slight hydrolysis of the $CO \cdot N=$ link formed by proline and hydroxyproline (24).

About 5 % of the collagen was dissolved, and the amount of total nitrogen solubilized was largely in excess of the ammonia formed by deamidation and the urea due to the ornithine formation. The high value of the amino nitrogen found by Bowes *et al.* suggests that it represents amino acids or small peptides. An additional important point was the lower content of dicarboxylic acids of the alkali-treated collagen as compared to that of the native collagen. This may be due to a preferential release of aspartic acid, glutamic acid, or peptides rich in these amino acids. It is interesting to note that Partridge and Davis (34) found a preferential release of dicarboxylic acids on acid hydrolysis of several globular proteins also, which may indicate that the keto-imide groups which these acids form are more easily split than the major part of the $CO \cdot NH$— links of the protein backbone.

In a subsequent paper Bowes *et al.* (33) submit further data on the composition of the breakdown products of collagen on alkali treatment. About one-fourth of the dissolved matter was precipitable with acetone. Amino nitrogen determination indicated that the precipitated fraction consists of large polypeptides, and the soluble fraction contains small peptides or amino acids mostly. Less tyrosine and hexosamine and more hydroxyproline were found in the alkali-treated collagen than in the original native collagen. The paper chromatogram of the acetone-precipitated fraction was similar to that of collagen, except that the hydroxyproline spot was weaker and the tyrosine spot more marked than is usual with collagen. The more soluble fraction gave a paper chromatogram without any hydroxyproline and with a very strong tyrosine spot. These results indicate that a fraction of collagen is split off in the alkaline treatment.

Bowes and Moss (32), investigating the reaction of fluorodinitrobenzene with the α- and ϵ-amino groups of native collagen and variously treated collagen, including alkali-treated specimens, detected no α-amino groups (terminal NH_2) in the native collagen. The alkali-treated specimens contained α-amino groups as terminal groups in the form of the following amino acid residues, given in millimoles per 100 g. of collagen: aspartic acid 0.07; glutamic acid 0.17; glycine 0.42; and phenylalanine 0.04. The Sanger reagent was able to react with 55 % of the total amount of ϵ-amino groups of the lysine residues, and the accessibility was not increased by alkali treatment. The end groups formed by the various treatments of collagen are probably derived from hydrolysis of the keto-imide links, with the possible exception of aspartic acid, which, as Bowes and Moss suggest, is either a terminal residue inaccessible to DNFB or the peptide bond involving its α-amino groups is especially labile. Also the possibility that the ends of the collagen chain split off in the form of simple polypeptides, similar to the formation of the plakalbumin by certain proteolytic agents, should be investigated by the new end-group methods (35). This issue is of particular interest for the understanding of the process of bating, in which the presence of polypeptidases may cause a similar hydrolytic breakdown of a specific amino acid or a few amino acids located at the end of the protein chain. This suggestion is prompted by the observation of Harris and Knight (36) that carboxypeptidase splits off about three thousand residues of C-terminal threonine groups per mole of tobacco mosaic virus. This finding stands, however, in marked contrast to the absence of a similar number of detectable N-terminal residues. Probably the threonine or the N-terminal residues are bound through the ω-carboxyl group of aspartic or glutamic acid to the chain, yielding either true α-peptide rings or 6-shaped chain rings containing one ω-linkage and C-terminal threonine, as suggested by Fraenkel-Conrat and Singer (36). Similar structures have been proposed for tropomyosin (Bailey, 37). The existence, formation, and alteration of terminal groups of the collagen molecule, particularly the effect of alkali on collagen in that respect, may not appear to belong to a discussion of the isoelectric point of collagen. However, the formation of new groups and the kind of backbone links split in the alkali treatment are problems intimately bound up with the electro-chemical changes of collagen in liming and the other preparatory processes in the manufacture of leather. The location of the isoelectric point of collagen in combination with tanning agents is important for the theory of tanning and leather formation and will be considered in connection with the various tannages in "The Chemistry of Tanning Processes."

REFERENCES

1. Hardy, W. B., *J. Physiol.* **24**, 285 (1899); **33**, 251 (1905).
2. Wilson, J. A., "The Chemistry of Leather Manufacture," Vol. 1, pp. 148–156. Chemical Catalog Co., New York, 1928.
3. Michaelis, L., *Biochem. Z.* **47**, 250 (1912); Meunier, L., Chambard, P., and Jamet, A., *J. Intern. Soc. Leather Trades Chem.* **9**, 200 (1925).
4. Loeb, J., "Proteins and the Theory of Colloidal Behavior." McGraw-Hill, New York, 1922.
5. Thomas, A. W., and Kelly, M. W., *J. Am. Chem. Soc.* **44**, 194 (1922); Gustavson, K. H., *Collegium* **1926**, 437.
6. Kuhn, R., *Naturwissenschaften* **20**, 618 (1932).
7. Otto, G., *Collegium* **1938**, 509; *Kolloid-Z.* **83**, 120 (1938).

8. Abramson, H. A., Moyer, L. S., and Gorin, M. H., "Electrophoresis of Proteins," pp. 44–46 (Fig. 13). Reinhold, New York, 1942.
9. Tiselius, A., *Trans. Faraday Soc.* **33**, 524 (1937).
10. Neale, S. M., and Peters, L., *Trans. Faraday Soc.* **42**, 478 (1946).
11. Neale, S. M., *J. Colloid Sci.* **1**, 371 (1946); *Trans. Faraday Soc.* **42**, 437 (1946).
12. Staverman, A. J., and Petri, E. M., *Discussions Faraday Soc.* **No. 13**, 151 (1953).
13. Wilson, J. A., and Gallun, A. F., *Ind. Eng. Chem.* **15**, 71 (1923); Wilson, J. A., and Kern, E. J., *J. Am. Chem. Soc.* **44**, 2963 (1922); **45**, 3139 (1923).
14. Ambrose, E. J., and Elliott, A., *Proc. Roy. Soc.* **A208**, 75 (1951).
15. Atkin, W. R., and Douglas, F. W., *J. Intern. Soc. Leather Trades Chem.* **8**, 359 (1924); Atkin, W. R., and Campos, J. M., *ibid.* **8**, 406 (1924).
16. Küntzel, A., *Biochem. Z.* **209**, 326 (1929).
17. Kraemer, E. O., *Colloid Symposium Monograph* **4**, 102 (1926).
18. Kraemer, E. O., and Dexter, S. T., *J. Phys. Chem.* **31**, 764 (1927).
19. Briefer, M., *Ind. Eng. Chem.* **21**, 266 (1929).
20. Beek, J., Jr., and Sookne, A. M., *J. Research Natl. Bur. Standards* **23**, 271 (1939); *J. Am. Leather Chem. Assoc.* **34**, 641 (1939).
21. Moyer, L. S., *J. Bacteriol.* **31**, 531 (1936).
22. Highberger, J. H., *J. Am. Chem. Soc.* **61**, 2302 (1939).
23. Bowes, J. H., and Kenten, R. H., *Biochem. J.* **43**, 363 (1948).
24. Bowes, J. H., *J. Soc. Leather Trades Chem.* **33**, 176 (1949).
25. Cassel, M., and McKenna, E., *J. Am. Leather Chem. Assoc.* **48**, 142 (1953).
26. Vickery, H., *Biochem. J.* **29**, 2710 (1935).
27. Highberger, J. H., and Stecker, H. C., *J. Am. Leather Chem. Assoc.* **36**, 368 (1941).
28. Bergström, S., and Lindstedt, S., *Acta Chem. Scand.* **5**, 157 (1951).
29. Theis, E. R., and Jacoby, T. F., *J. Am. Leather Chem. Assoc.* **36**, 375 (1941).
30. Thomas, A. W., "Colloid Chemistry," p. 336. McGraw-Hill, New York, 1934; Küntzel, A., *in* "Handbuch der Gerbereichemie" (W. Grassmann, ed.), Vol. I, Part 1, p. 542. Springer, Vienna, 1944.
31. Bowes, J. H., "Progress in Leather Science," Vol. 1, p. 158. BLMRA, London, 1946.
32. Bowes, J. H., and Moss, J. A., *Nature* **168**, 514 (1951); *Biochem. J.* **55**, 735 (1953).
33. Bowes, J. H., Elliott, R. G., and Moss, J. A., *in* "Nature and Structure of Collagen" (J. T. Randall, ed.), p. 199. Butterworths, London, 1953.
34. Partridge, S. M., and Davis, H. F., *Nature* **165**, 62 (1950).
35. Linderstrøm-Lang, K., and Ottesen, M., *Compt. rend. trav. lab. Carlsberg* **26**, 403 (1949); *Nature* **159**, 807 (1947).
36. Fraenkel-Conrat, H., and Singer, B., *J. Am. Chem. Soc.* **76**, 180 (1954); see also Harris, J. L., and Knight, C. A., *Nature* **170**, 613 (1952).
37. Bailey, K., *Proc. Roy Soc.* **B141**, 45 (1953).

CHAPTER 5

The Interaction of Collagen with Acids and Bases and the Titration Curves of Collagens

A. REVERSIBLE SYSTEMS

1. INTRODUCTION

Collagen contains moderate amounts of positively and negatively charged groups, which are derived from the diamino and dicarboxylic acids built into the collagen molecule. In the isoelectric state and in equilibrium with water in the pH range from 5 to 8, these polar groups are almost completely ionized.

Collagen is an amphoteric ionic structure attaining the highest degree of charge, both positive and negative, in the isoelectric pH range. These charged centers of the protein zwitterion exist in electrostatic balance with each other. It appears that this balance can be disturbed only by some mechanism which is able to suppress either the positive or the negative charge. The two outstanding ions in this respect are the hydrogen and the hydroxyl ions, as would be expected. Hence, the interaction of collagen with aqueous solutions of acids and bases is of fundamental importance for the understanding of the general reactivity of collagen, especially in the tanning processes.

The hydrogen ions are attached to the negatively charged carboxyl groups, the COO⁻ groups, which thereby are discharged and turned into —COOH groups. Since the simplified general structure of isoelectric collagen is of the type COO⁻·R·NH₃⁺, it is evident that by complete discharge of the carboxyl ions the positively charged groups are left intact and free to react. This state is reached for strong mineral acids at equilibrium pH values of about 1.2 to 1.5 on their interaction with collagen.

The hydroxyl ions, supplied by means of dilute solutions of sodium hydroxide for instance, are attracted to the positively charged protein groups. In this reaction the cationic protein groups lose protons and are discharged. The proton is transferred to the hydroxyl ion, the final result being the formation of a molecule of water. At the point of complete discharge of the positively charged protein groups of the collagen molecule, which requires final pH values of the solution of the order of 13, the carboxyl ions are all free and able to react. Accordingly the transference of the proton from one position of binding to another will depend on the pH value of the solution,

102

as the following simplified equations bring out:

$$COO^- \cdot R \cdot NH_3^+ + H^+ \rightarrow COOH \cdot R \cdot NH_3^+ \text{ (in acid solution)}$$

$$COO^- \cdot R \cdot NH_3^+ - H^+ \rightarrow COO^- \cdot R \cdot NH_2 \text{ (in alkaline solution)}$$

Collagen   Proton

Once the dipolar partnership has been broken, opportunities for numerous other ionic reactions are created. All the electrovalent reactions of proteins generally take place either in acid or alkaline solutions. The presence of the ionic groups at a fixed position in a long molecular chain must be of governing importance for enforcing the apparent ionic inertness which collagen shows in the isoelectric range of pH values. The architecture of the molecule influences the function and properties of the positively and negatively charged centers of the dipolar structure in several ways. Thus, the charged sites of the collagen chains do not have the freedom of action found with ions of soluble amphoteric electrolytes. For instance, in contrast to soluble proteins, solid proteins such as collagen bind very small amounts of acid or alkali within a certain limited pH range on both sides of the isoelectric point from solutions devoid of neutral salts. This is probably due to the interaction of cationic and anionic side chains with each other, forming the saltlike crosslinks. A certain minimum potential of hydrogen or hydroxyl ions is probably required within the fiber structure between the polypeptide chains before this link can be broken. However, when a neutral salt containing a common anion of the acid used is added to the acid solution, this zone of inert reactivity, or the noncombining range, is eliminated. This is probably due to the increased concentration of the anion which, apart from the elimination of the Donnan effect, will help to overcome the potential barrier set up against the anions of the strong acid, which is preponderantly electrostatically balanced by, and not combined with, the cationic protein groups. The role played by the affinity of the anion of the acid is shown by the fact that acids containing anions which are irreversibly fixed by collagen do not show this noncombining range, for instance polysulfonic acids of dyestuffs. This problem will be considered later.

2. Titration Curves

The titration curves of the globular proteins are similar in form. The curve for alkali-processed gelatin given by Ames (1) illustrates the general type of curves (Fig. 18). The titration curves for limed and native collagen in the form of hide powder are also shown in Fig. 18.

The titration curves of globular proteins are usually obtained on 1% solutions of the proteins and hence in a homogeneous system. As a rule, the curve for gelatin is obtained in the same manner. In the determination of the titration curve of a heterogeneous system, such as insoluble collagen-acid solution, the experimental conditions may be similar to those for water-soluble proteins, if the object is merely a comparison of the two types of proteins, for instance gelatin with collagen, with respect to their electrochemical behavior. However, this method is not suitable for quantitative determination of the acid and base binding of collagen, for reasons to be presented later.

The conventional method is to titrate a dilute ($\sim$1%) solution of the protein and to plot the pH value observed on one axis against the amount of acid or base added on the other axis. A curve serving as a blank is obtained by adding acid and base to water, within the pH range covered. The amount of acid or base removed by the protein is the difference between the two curves at any given pH. The data so obtained, expressed in milliliters of decinormal acid or base, or milligram equivalents of the same, may finally be plotted against the pH value attained at equilibrium.

From the titration curves, the pK values of the different sections or the various reacting groups of the protein can be ascertained, since the pK of any group is the midpoint of the titration range over which it gains or loses protons. (Table 8 gives the pK values of the principal groups of collagen.)

The titration curve of gelatin forms a sharp intersection with the pH

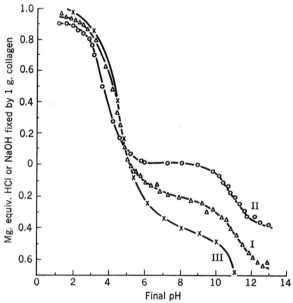

FIG. 18. Titration curves of collagens and gelatin: I, limed collagen (corium); II, native collagen (unlimed corium); III, alkali-processed gelatin.

axis, which is evidence for a well-defined isoelectric point of gelatin, as is the case with water-soluble proteins in general. The maximum binding capacity for hydrogen ions is 0.96 mg. equiv. per gram of protein reached at equilibrium pH of approximately 2, and the alkali binding attains the highest value at pH 12.5, with about 0.9 mg. equiv. of base per gram of gelatin. As subsequent work will show, the final base-binding capacity is not reached even at final pH values of 13; no definite figure can be given for this property of gelatin. Evidently secondary reactions, which may be expected to increase the number of available base-binding groups by the hydrolytic rupture of peptide bonds, introduce complications in systems of such high degree of alkalinity. They make any such attempt appear fruitless and the data derived of doubtful value. The corresponding titration curve of collagen differs in many fundamental respects from that of gelatin. The acid-binding capacity is practically identical. However, in the intermediate pH range from 2 to 5, the proton-accepting capacity of gelatin is markedly higher than that of collagen. The difference is probably intimately connected with the very different structural organization of the two proteins. Gelatin in solution contains simple molecular chains in which the carboxyl ions are free to react, whereas a certain interaction or compensation between electropositive and electronegative groups of the parallelly oriented chains of the rigid collagen structure makes the carboxyl ions less reactive. By the addition of sodium chloride to the solution of hydrochloric acid, for instance making it 0.2 M with respect to chloride ions, the curve of fixation of the acid by collagen will practically coincide with that of gelatin for reasons already stated.

On the alkaline side, very much lower fixation of base by collagen is shown throughout, compared to gelatin. A broad plateau in the pH range 8 to 11 is characteristic of the collagen curve, and no maximum is reached in the uptake of the base, which probably is connected with the fact that the guanidyl ion requires still higher pH values than the highest one applied for complete discharge. An isoelectric zone in the pH range 4.5 to 7, with negligible reactivity of collagen, is also characteristic for this protein. This nonreactive zone may be attributed, partly at least, to the presence of almost an equal number of ionized cationic and anionic groups in internal compensation, and hence a large shift in pH is needed to fix any considerable amounts of added ions. The fact that the base-binding capacity of collagen is much lower than that of gelatin may be due to a more extensive and stable interaction of the negatively charged groups with oppositely charged groups, possible the guanidyl group. The presence of ester crosslinks may also be involved (2). Grabar's researches (2a) on gelatin have indicated that the guanidyl group has an important function for gel formation, and the anomalous chemical inertness of the arginine residue of collagen points in the same direction. Such an internal compensation of groups would be expected to require high concentration of hydroxyl ions for its dislocation and the subsequent discharge of the guanidyl ion, which has been found to be so.

3. The Effect of Neutral Salts

It was early recognized by Atkin (3), who in collaboration with Campos published the first titration curve of collagen (hide powder) in 1924, that it is essential to eliminate the Donnan potential and the concomitant swelling of the protein by the addition of a neutral salt in systems containing an insoluble protein, such as collagen, which is highly susceptible to swelling by acid and alkali. This applies to two-phase systems generally. Accordingly, the solutions to be titrated were all made 0.1 M in potassium chloride. This neutral salt concentration will nearly equalize the internal pH of the solution present in the hide powder with that of the external solution, and hence eliminate the large error in calculation due to variations in acid concentration between the hide substrate and the external solution. Moreover, since the solubilization of hide powder is facilitated by swelling of the substrate, which is very large at extremely low and high pH values, the swelling-depressing action of the neutral salt will make for greater accuracy also. Concentrations of neutral chloride, mostly the sodium salt in solutions of hydrochloric acid, up to 1.0 M NaCl per liter of solution, may be used. That neutral salts, such as sodium chloride, alter the titration curve of proteins was first shown by Speakman and Hirst (4).

Figure 19 shows a collection of titration curves of collagen (hide powder) with hydrochloric acid in the presence of varying amounts of sodium chloride. The effect of increasing the chloride ion concentration of the acid solution is shown by the form of the curves (5). These become steeper, because the salt tends to increase the amount of acid fixed by collagen at any given pH value between the zones of maximum and minimum fixation of hydrogen ions. The concentration of the anion does not appreciably increase the maximum uptake of acid; neither does it induce interaction of acid with collagen at the isoelectric point. There are probably several factors involved in this neutral salt effect. At low concentrations of added salt, the elimination of the differences in the pH values of the two-phase system due to the Donnan effect in the absence of salt—with pH values of the solution held within the solid protein considerably higher than those of the external solution—and the prevention of swelling are probably the main effects of the salt which are responsible for the increased uptake of hydrogen ions in the intermediate pH range. It is noteworthy that the shift of the curves is markedly less with increased salt content beyond 0.1

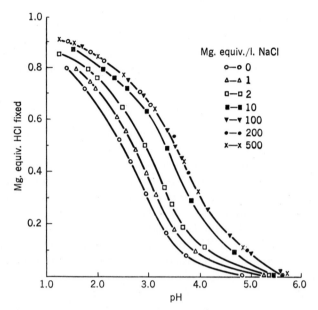

Fig. 19. Titration curves of collagen in the presence of varying amounts of sodium chloride.

M. The augmentation of the acid binding is shown to be considerably less with increasing concentration of chloride ions until the solution is made about 1 M with respect to sodium chloride. This trend is clearly shown in the corresponding curves from the system wool–hydrochloric acid–NaCl, investigated by Steinhardt et al. (6).

The effect of the increased concentration of the chloride ions in the higher molarity range of salt is probably due to the mass action effect of the chloride ions on the equilibrium between the cationic groups of collagen and the anions of the acid electrostatically held at these sites, resulting in a greater number of chloride ions combining with the protein. This should be expected to lead to a lowering of the net positive charge of the protein, which would in turn facilitate the interaction of the protons with the charged carboxyl groups of collagen. Apart from the properties inherent in a two-phase system, the internal compensation of the ionic groups of collagen by the formation of salt links may possibly be a factor contributing to the relative inertness of collagen compared to other proteins at pH values near the isoelectric point, as has been pointed out earlier. In alkaline solution, sodium sulfate should be used as the swelling-depressing agent, and not sodium chloride, since under these conditions neutral sulfates are effective, but not neutral chlorides. Evidently the concept of the Donnan equilibrium fails in alkaline solution, which throws serious doubts on the justification of its application to acid two-phase systems. The interpretations of the salt effect on the titration curves by means of the Donnan concept on one hand, and the Gilbert-Rideal approach on the other, will be discussed subsequently.

4. ERRORS OF THE PRESSING METHOD

It has been maintained by McLaughlin and Adams (7) that the addition of neutral salt to an acid solution tends to decrease the fixation of acid. This statement is at variance with previous findings of a number of workers (8). McLaughlin and Adams (7) base their erroneous claim on an investigation of the effect of sodium sulfate on the uptake of sulfuric acid by pelt (limed collagen). The amount of acid bound by collagen was determined by analysis of the stock after the treated pelt was pressed twice at 5000 p.s.i. in an hydraulic press. The pressed stock was air-dried and analyzed for nitrogen and sulfate. No correction was applied for the sulfur content of collagen since, as the authors state, "the original prepared skin squares showed a negligible sulfate content." However, collagen in the form of pelt shows mean values of 0.3 to 0.5 % sulfur in terms of the weight of the collagen, or amounts of sulfur equal to 1 to 1.5 % in terms of sulfuric acid. The statement may be explained by the fact that nitric acid was used to destroy the organic matter. The organic sulfur of hide protein, exclusive of the small amount of ester sulfate present—mainly the sulfur present in methionine, in this instance—is rather incompletely oxidized to sulfate by nitric acid. Highly variable results are obtained, depending on the experimental conditions and the type of protein, as was shown by the classical investigations of sulfur estimation in proteins by Mörner, some sixty years ago (9).

This oversight however, is not the main cause of the statement of McLaughlin and Adams (7), claiming diminished fixation of sulfuric acid by pelt in the presence of sodium sulfate. The underlying reasons lie in the shortcomings of the pressing technique employed and, further, the fact that the system of plain sulfuric acid was not compared with the system of sulfuric acid–sodium sulfate at the same final pH values. It has been proved experimentally (10) that stock pressed according to the method devised by McLaughlin contains a large percentage of free solution of acid in addition to the water of hydration. Since no corrections for the two kinds of water present in the pressed stock were made, the results may show errors as large as 20 to 30 % of the true values of bound acid. Since the paper cited (7) gives no information as to the amounts of water of hydration and of free solution of the acid-salt solution in the pressed collagen, data on the contents of dry substance and collagen of stock after pressing by the same method, given in papers by McLaughlin *et al.* (7, 11), must be consulted to determine the extent of the error. The water not removed from the skin by application of pressure is composed of: (*1*) *free water*, in the form of the acid-salt solution held in the interstices of the substrate; (*2*) *bound water*, which is associated with the protein and which cannot function as a solvent for the electrolyte. The probable value of the water of hydration is 20 % of the weight of the protein. The amount of the total water in the pressed stock obtained in the experiments of the authors cited averaged 124 %, on a hide substance basis. With correction for 20 % water of hydration, about 100 % water in the form of solution will be left in the pressed skin. From the data of the composition of the straight sulfuric acid solution equilibrated with collagen at pH 1.0 given by McLaughlin and Adams (7), the external solution contained 0.854 % sulfuric acid. Hence, 1 g. of collagen was associated with 8.9 mg. of sulfuric acid, or 0.89 % acid, on the basis of hide substance. The error is about 15 %.

This criticism of the pressing method applies also to the investigations carried out by McLaughlin and his associates on chromium salts (12), vegetable tannins (13), formaldehyde (14), and any tanning agent of which a considerable part is left unfixed in the bath. By this erroneous method, data were obtained which formed the basis for McLaughlin's (7) explanation of the effect of neutral sulfate on the fixation of sulfuric acid and of chromium by collagen from solutions of basic chromium sulfates. It is claimed that the reduced chrome fixation by collagen, resulting from the addition of neutral sulfate to the solution of chromium sulfate, is due to the lowered uptake of sulfuric acid by the hide substrate, which in turn will affect the uptake of chrome and reduce its fixation. Evidently, this concept is invalidated by the false premises.

In the interaction of acids with insoluble proteins, the degree of affinity of the anion of the acid for the cationic protein groups plays a prominent role, as was proved by the important researches of Steinhardt and his coworkers (6). The sulfate ion possesses greater binding tendency than the chloride ion. Accordingly, collagen fixes greater amounts of sulfuric acid than hydrochloric acid in the absence of the corresponding neutral salt. At low pH values, an additional factor favors the uptake of sulfuric acid over that of hydrochloric acid, because at high acidity sulfuric acid will partially function as a monobasic acid.

5. The Effect of Deamination of Collagen on its Titration Curve

By deamination of collagen with nitrous acid, the strongly basic ε-amino group of lysine is removed and replaced by the weakly basic hydroxy group. The effect of the removal of the amino-lysine group on the fixaticn of HCl is illustrated in Fig. 20 (15).

By the removal of the amino group of the lysine side chain, the acid binding is markedly decreased and the isoelectric point of collagen shifted from pH 5.3 to pH 4.6. The most remarkable change is shown in the pH range from the isoelectric point to about 9, the base binding of the deaminated collagen being much greater than that of ordinary collagen. It is interesting to note that Thomas and Foster (16), who were the first scientists to investigate the influence of deamination of collagen on its properties and reactivity, noted very large swelling in that particular pH range, whereas ordinary collagen hardly showed any swelling at all. The titration curve of gelatin has a form similar to that of deaminocollagen. This fact indicates less interaction of oppositely charged carboxyl and amino groups in this type of degraded collagen. The reason for the large swelling and high alkali-binding power of the deaminated protein in this pH range is probably the fact that by removal of the charged amino groups, originally present in internal compensation by carboxyl ions, the latter are set free, since the hydroxy group introduced to replace the ammonium ion is too weak for interaction with the carboxyl ions. The result is the freeing of the carboxyl groups from their compensation. A comparison of the titration curves of collagen, on the one hand, and collagen devoid of its ε-amino group, on the other, shows that the removal or substitution of one particular protein group is not restricted to the specific reactivity of this group. The fact is that the reactivity of other groups are radically changed, in

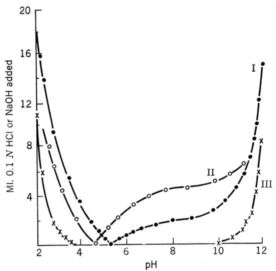

Fig. 20. Titration curves of ordinary and deaminated collagen: I, ordinary hide powder; II, deaminated hide powder; III, correction blank for HCl and KOH.

this instance the reactivity of the carboxyl group. The reciprocity within the protein molecule complicates the interpretation of the changed reactivity of the protein by blocking of an individual group.

For determination of the acid-binding capacity of collagen and of collagen tanned by means of agents which do not interact with mineral acid, the following simple procedure has proved useful, giving reproducible and accurate values (17). Portions of hide substrate equal to 1.00 g. of collagen are intermittently shaken for 4 to 6 hours, according to the degree of subdivision of the stock, in 25.0 ml. of 0.1 N hydrochloric acid, containing 0.5 M sodium chloride per liter. Aliquots of the filtrate are titrated, with methyl red as indicator. Correction is applied for the water introduced with the substrate, allowing 20% of the weight of the substrate (0.2 ml.) as the water of hydration. Thus, if 1.00 g. of collagen holds 2.0 g. of water, the total volume titrated will be 26.8 ml. The amount of acid fixed is obtained as the difference between the acid added and the acid present in the exhaust. For the determination of the acid-binding capacity of collagen, the following points are of interest. In the system HCl-NaCl, with amounts of added salt adequate for complete depression of the swelling of collagen at equilibrium pH values >1.3, the amount of protein nitrogen going into solution is practically negligible in bovine pelt (hide powder) treated for periods of 4 to 8 hours, within which time equilibrium is generally attained. At lower final pH values, some collagen is lost to the solution (17a), which will introduce an error in the values of acid bound by collagen obtained by titration of the residual solution. In acid solutions free from neutral salt, a condition that allows swelling of the collagen to take place freely, the dissolved protein nitrogen reaches fairly large values, even at pH 2. Therefore it cannot be neglected, particularly on prolonged treatment, as Armstrong's data (17b) prove. Lollar and his co-workers (17a) have been critical of the data on the determination of the acid-binding capacity of collagen given in the literature (including those of the present author), because of the error due to hydrolysis products in the final solution. Their critical attitude is not valid, however, since the equilibrium pH values of the systems were in the range of 1.3 to 1.5, and, moreover, the solutions contained at least 2.5% w/v sodium chloride. No such determinations have been undertaken in neutral salt-free acid solution. In the author's series of determinations, mainly with pelt of calfskin, which were carried out according to the method described above, the amount of solubilized collagen was in all instances less than 1% of the weight of the original collagen.

6. TITRATION CURVES OF COLLAGEN

The titration curve of native (unlimed) collagen has been studied by Bowes and Kenten (18). The curve (Fig. 18) was interpreted in terms of

TABLE 8

ANALYSIS OF THE TITRATION CURVE OF NATIVE (UNLIMED) COLLAGEN (18)

Groups Titrating	Method of Calculation	pK from Curve	Amounts Present, mg. Equiv./g. Protein	
			From curve	From analysis of amino acids
(a) Total basic groups	Titration from pH 1.5 to 7.0	—	0.90	0.94
(b) Imidazole + imino + α-amino groups	Titration from pH 4.9 to 9.6	7.5	0.07	—
(c) ε-Amino	Titration from pH 9.6 to 12.5	11.0	0.34	0.39 (0.33 by van Slyke)
(d) Free carboxyl	Titration from pH 1.5 to 4.9	3.5	0.87	0.79
(e) α-Amino + imino	(b) − 0.05 mg. equiv. imidazole	—	0.02	—
(f) Guanidine	(a) − (b) − (c)	14	0.49	0.51
(g) Amide	From analysis	—	—	0.47
(h) Dicarboxylic acids	(d) + (g) − (e)	—	1.32	1.26

titratable groups, and the values obtained were compared with those derived from chemical analysis of the participating groups of amino acid residues in the same specimen. These data have already been given in Table 4. A close agreement between the values derived from the two methods was found, as the data of Table 8 show. The table also gives an idea of which groups titrate in the various pH intervals and the method chosen for calculating the amounts of the various reactive protein groups.

The main differences between the titration curves of native collagen and limed collagen are as follows: The isoelectric point of the native protein was near pH 7.0. The acid-binding capacity was 0.85 to 0.90 mg. equiv. of acid (HCl) per gram of protein, and the maximum base binding showed values of 0.4 to 0.5 mg. equiv. As a rule, the curves of alkali-treated collagen show a considerable removal of hydroxyl ions in the pH range 6 to 8 which is absent in the curve of native collagen. The curve of the latter can roughly be derived from three sections: (1) pH 1.5 to 5.0; (2) pH 5.0 to 9.6; and (3) pH 9.6 to 12.5. With the probable pK values of the various groups known, the data given in Table 8 are obtained. The pK value of the carboxylic group is figured from the titration curve obtained in the presence of 0.5 M NaCl. At this concentration, the pH inside the collagen probably is identical with the pH measured in the external solution.

An important point brought out by these data is that the guanidyl group is not titrating in the pH range covered, i.e., up to pH 12.5. The pK value of this strongly basic group is indicated to be greater than 14. This is also indicated in the titration curve of gelatin (19).

7. THE EFFECT OF THE CHARGE OF THE PROTEIN ON ITS pK VALUES

The apparent pK values of soluble proteins are generally not very far from those of the corresponding groups in the free amino acids. This is not the case with insoluble protein. Thus, for instance, the pK values of the dicarboxylic amino acids, about 4 in the amino acids themselves, show values of about 3 for the γ-carboxylic groups of collagen.

The pK value of 2.1 for the carboxyl ions of collagen, given by Vicker-staff in his monograph (20), appears to be too low. A figure of 3.0 to 3.5 is more in line with the available data (Bowes and Kenten, 18). Collagen and other fibrous proteins appear to be much stronger acids than the globular proteins, and the latter in their turn seem to possess slightly more developed acidic function than the amino acids. A plausible explanation is the rigid structure of the insoluble proteins and the concomitant distribution of the charged groups. It seems probable that the different behavior noted is connected with the electrical charge carried by the fibrous proteins and the structural restraint of the parallelly aligned chains. A similar, although less marked, trend is also shown by the water-soluble proteins which give titration curves of less slope than the corresponding amino acids.

Cannan (21) has attempted to explain this tendency in terms of the electrical charge of the proteins. In the reaction of a proton with an uncharged protein molecule, the free energy of the system is increased. Hence, the combination of a second proton with the charged protein will be retarded, or even prevented, by the repulsion of the charge possessed by the positively charged protein. The free energy involved in the second reaction will thus be less than that of the first reaction. Accordingly, it becomes increasingly difficult for each successive hydrogen ion to combine with the protein. The slope of the titration curve will be less, and the curve will take on a greater spread. If a spherical form is assumed for the globular proteins, it can be easily shown that the potential of a charged sphere decreases inversely as the radius, but the number of ionizable groups within a sphere of a protein will increase as the cube of the radius. Consequently the potential produced when any given proportion of the ionizable groups in a protein is ionized will increase as the square of the radius of the protein molecule. It has been concluded that, if the size increases from molecular dimensions to macroscopic dimensions of the wool fiber, such a high potential will be set up as to prevent the uptake of additional protons. Then, further combination of protons with the protein which has partly reacted with the acid only will take place, if the positive charge of the protein is diminished. This is effected most simply by the simultaneous attachment of the anion of the acid. The conclusion to be drawn from these findings is that the difference in the pK values of insoluble and soluble proteins is caused by the positive charge of the chainlike molecule of the insoluble protein. The large differences reported (20) in pK values of the carboxyl group are hence only apparent. This view is also held by Speakman (22), who expresses it in terms of the Donnan equilibrium. It has recently been further developed quantitatively by Peters and Speakman (23). From the thermodynamic point of view, Gilbert and Rideal (24) have arrived at the same conclusion.

By increasing the concentration of the anion by the addition of a neutral salt containing an anion in common with the acid—for instance, addition of sodium chloride to hydrochloric acid—the binding of the acid (hydrogen ion) will be promoted by increasing the uptake of the anion, i.e., by decreasing the net positive charge of collagen. This will be a mass action effect. From the point of view of the Donnan equilibrium, the positive effect of neutral salts on the uptake of hydrogen ions is explained as the result of eliminating the difference in pH of the solid phase and the external solution. It is considered that, by making the solution of hydrochloric acid reacting with collagen about 0.5 M with respect to chloride ions, the pH of the outside solution will be identical with the pH of the interior of the substrate. The salt effect and the influence of the affinity of the anion of the acid for the cationic groups of collagen will be discussed in later chapters.

Steinhardt et al. (25) have presented evidence in support of the view that the combination of wool with hydrochloric acid may be resolved into two partial reactions, one with the protons and one with the chloride ions, each reaction being governed by its own equilibrium constant. On the basis of this assumption and by application of the law of mass action to the association of both protons and chloride ions with the protein, it proved possible to account quantitatively for the large effects produced by various concentrations of hydrochloric acid on the curve relating combination of the protein with hydrochloric acid to pH. The existence of such a variation in the position of titration curves would constitute critical evidence in support of the hypothesis of stoichiometric anion association, i.e., the Gilbert-Rideal concept, since an analysis of the salt effect based on the Donnan effect offers no apparent basis for the prediction of such an effect, or for its corollary, combination to unequal extent with each of two or more anions present in mixtures.

Peters and Speakman (23) have criticized the concept of Gilbert and Rideal (24) and that of Steinhardt and his co-workers, claiming that the data of Steinhardt *et al.* (25) satisfy the Donnan theory better than the other two theories. Gilbert and Rideal, as well as Steinhardt, assume that there is no difference in concentration of the solution inside and that outside the fibers and that the amount of acid or base combined with the protein is equal to the difference between the amount originally added and that remaining in the solution. The experimental data forming the basis of these theories were obtained from wool, which is only slightly susceptible to swelling, compared to collagen. For collagen the assumption of the equalization of the acid is apparently not true for systems free from neutral salts. However, Armstrong's data from a recent investigation (17b) of the collagen–hydrochloric acid system indicate that collagen in contact with acid forms a two-phase system and that the results are in harmony with the Donnan theory.

In an important paper on the combination of wool with acids, Olofsson (26) has compared the results calculated on the basis of the Gilbert-Rideal, Donnan, and ion-exchange theories. The essential conclusion drawn from the statistical analysis is that the Gilbert-Rideal theory is applicable, whereas the Donnan theory fails. The probable reason is the specific thermodynamic differences between fiber and solution phases. This effect should be still more prominent in the collagen structure because of its marked tendency to swell and, hence, the application of the Donnan concept to collagen should not be valid. An interesting point deduced from the statistical analysis of the systems is that some sulfate ions are unipointly attached; i.e., every SO_4^{--} ion is attached to only one positive site of the keratin. It is indicated that there is statistical distribution between sulfate ions of uni- and bipointal attachment. It appears that Olofsson's arguments are well-founded and convincing.

8. The Effect of Temperature on the Binding of Acid and Alkali by Collagen

The effect of temperature on the titration curve is an interesting and instructive problem. Since collagen is rather easily broken down in solutions of acids and alkalis at temperatures of about 35°C., it is not a very suitable substrate for investigations of this type. On the other hand, wool is exceedingly stable to acids in the pH range at which the titration usually is carried out, even at such high temperatures as 50°C.

The titration curve of wool (keratin) as a function of the temperature of the system has been determined by Steinhardt *et al.* (25) at 0 and 50°C. Their data show that the combination of acid with wool is practically independent of the temperature, whereas the uptake of alkali is greatly increased by temperature increase. If the heats of reaction for the hydrogen and hydroxyl ions interacting with wool are calculated from these data, it is found that the heat of reaction for the combination of the protons with keratin is very small, whereas the loss of protons in the alkaline range involves energies of the order of $+10$ kcal. per mole. It is interesting to know that the heat of ionization of organic acids generally is small, between $+1$ and -1 kcal., whereas substituted ammonium ions show values of about $+12$ kcal. A straight confirmation of the ampho-ionic concept of protein reactivity is thus presented by these findings. They prove that the acid titration of proteins consists in the back-titration of carboxyl groups, whereas the alkaline curve represents the hydrolysis and discharge of the ionized basic groups.

In recent work (26a) on the titration curves of collagen at 10, 20, and 30°C. in the pH range of 2 to 12, with the time of interaction 8 hours, it was found that the reaction of hydrochloric acid with collagen was independent of the temperature, as shown by Fig. 21. However, systems of acids containing anions of marked affinity for the basic protein groups showed marked temperature dependence, the fixation being decreased with augmented temperature. Such systems are represented by polymetaphosphoric and lignosulfonic acids, and by sulfonic acids of acid dyestuffs. The curves for the lignosulfonic acid fixation by collagen at 10 and 20°C. are included in Fig. 21. It is to be noted that the fixation at 20°C. is markedly lower than that at 10°C. This temperature dependence is an additional proof of the participation and fixation of the anions of the acid in the reaction with collagen, and, in fact, it is a measure of the degree of affinity of the acid for collagen and also a measure of the degree of irreversibility of the fixation of the anion by the protein. It should be made clear that these findings pertain to systems at attained equlibrium. For reaching that state in a heterogenous system, the rate of diffusion is one of the main factors, which shows the reverse temperature dependence, however.

9. CALCULATION OF THE HEAT OF REACTION FROM TITRATION CURVES

An approximate calculation of the heat of reaction resulting from the interaction of proteins with acids (proton) is feasible from the titration curves obtained at two different temperatures (27). These should be selected in an interval in which the ionization constants of the carboxyl groups of collagen are not markedly affected by temperature changes, or only slightly so. For wool, this range is from 25 to 50°C. Since wool is resistant to acids in the pH range 1 to 5 even at the highest temperature given, the titration curves at 25 and 50°C. can be used. This is not the case with collagen and the suitable range narrows down to 0 to 25°C., in which range, however, the ionization constants of the carboxylic groups show a marked temperature dependence.

The calculation is based on the fact that the pH values of the titration curve corresponding to half-saturation of collagen with an acid, e.g., hydrochloric acid, is equal to the mean value of the pK of the carboxyl group. The difference between the pK values, given as $\Delta \log K$, is related to the difference in heat of reaction, ΔH, at the two temperatures, T_1 and T_2, according to the equation:

$$\Delta H = 4.5787 \cdot \frac{T_1 \times T_2}{T_2 - T_1} \cdot \Delta \log K.$$

This equation is evidently an integrated form of the van't Hoff equation.

The values obtained for the heat of ionization of the carboxyl groups of wool keratin are of the order of 2 kcal. per mole of reactant. The corresponding value for the basic groups is about 12 kcal. per mole of reactant. No figures are available for collagen. Because of its relatively low stability toward acids and alkalis at higher temperatures, such determinations would probably be of a low order of accuracy. However, it is probable that they are not very far from the figures of wool keratin, since the number of ionic groups of the two proteins are of about the same order of magnitude and are of similar type.

As mentioned earlier, the great difference in heat of reaction and temperature dependence of reactions involving the anionic groups, on the one hand, and the cationic protein groups, on the other, can be used to ascertain the protein groups involved in reactions of the proteins with other agents, such as tanning agents. A condition *sine qua non* is that the agent itself is not altered by the temperature increase of the system. Such complications are shown in the reaction of collagen with solutions of basic chromium salts. The composition, structure, hydrolysis, electrical charge, and complex formation of the chromium salts are greatly altered by raising the temperature of the solution, the diminished stability of the solutions of basic salts of higher temperature being especially important for their irreversible fixation by collagen. Thus, although this reaction is specifically directed toward the charged carboxylic groups of collagen and hence should be expected to be only slightly dependent on the temperature, the reverse holds true. On the other hand, in the interaction of formaldehyde with collagen, the basic protein groups are mainly involved. In this instance, the tanning agent is not affected by the temperature of the medium of the reaction. The irreversible fixation of formaldehyde by collagen is greatly *increased* and the tanning effect improved considerably by raising the temperature of the system. This is in perfect agreement with the type of reaction it represents—inactivation of the basic protein groups, which possess high heat of reaction and marked temperature dependence, as already mentioned. In the reaction between collagen and acidic systems in which the

TABLE 9

HEATS OF REACTION OF ACIDS AND BASES WITH WOOL (27)

Reactant	Temperature Range, °C.	ΔH, kcal./mole
0.1 N hydrochloric acid alone	0–25	2.4
	25–50	−0.2
Hydrochloric acid at constant ionic strength, 0.2 N	0–25	3.9
	25–50	0
Hydrochloric acid at constant ionic strength, 0.5 N	0–50	1.3
Sulfuric acid	0–50	0.5
Naphthalene-β-sulfonic acid	0–25	3.6
	25–50	2.2
Dodecyl sulfonic acid	25–50	3.2
Picric acid	0–25	6.6
Orange II acid	25–50	>11.3
Sodium hydroxide at constant ionic strength, 0.2 N	0–25	13.7
	25–50	12.2

anion of the acid is irreversibly fixed, the temperature function is evident. This is also known from quantitative work on sulfonic acids of dyestuffs reacting with wool, e.g., with Orange II. Table 9 contains some instructive data on the heats of reaction of acids and bases with wool in different temperature ranges. Among the acids listed, the acid of Orange II is to a large extent irreversibly fixed. The degree of affinity of the anions of the acids for the cationic protein group, which forms the series chloride, sulfate, naphthalene-β-sulfonate, dodecyl sulfonate, picrate, and Orange II sulfonate, manifests itself in increasing values of the heats of reaction. The high value of this property for the reversible reaction of alkali with the cationic protein groups is also reflected in the NaOH reaction.

As already explained, the differences between the heats of reaction of the various acids must be attributed in the main part to the heat of reaction of the *anions* with the protein, since the heat of ionization of the carboxylic groups of the keratin structure is very small and similar for all acids. Steinhardt et al. (25) consider that the heat of reaction of hydrochloric acid with wool can be largely attributed to the entropy change accompanying the transfer of protons from the dilute external solution to the more concentrated phase formed within the fibrous structure. It is interesting to note that Speakman and Stott (28) have estimated the heat of reaction of wool with hydrochloric acid at 0°C. by direct calorimetry. They obtained a value of 3.56 kcal. per mole, which is in fair agreement with the data of Steinhardt and his associates, considering the complicated experimental conditions and the temperature difference.

Some recent data on collagen, shown in the curves of Fig. 21, on the heat

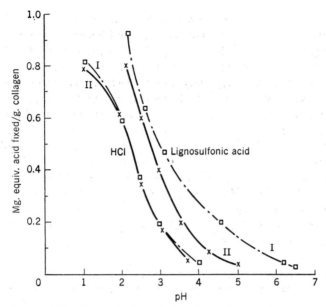

Fig. 21. The combination of hydrochloric acid and lignosulfonic acid with collagen: I, at 10°C.; II, at 20°C.

of reaction of collagen with some polyacids, determined by Larsson and the author on hide powder in the temperature range 10 to 30°C., are the only information available on the collagen system. These data show the same trend as those of wool (26a).

The sorption of polymetaphosphoric acid (mean molecular weight 3600) and a high-molecular fraction of lignosulfonic acid (mean molecular weight 4500) by collagen (lightly formolized hide powder) was determined at temperatures of 10, 20, and 30°C. as a function of the pH value and acid concentration of the solutions at attained equilibrium. The resulting data of the series with hydrochloric acid and lignosulfonic acid are shown by the curves of Fig. 21. The log plots of the data in Fig. 21 give log $[D]_{sol.}$, the log of the hydrogen ion concentration of the residual solution, as a function of log $[D]_{coll.}$, the log of the concentration of hydrogen ions in the solid phase of collagen. The heat of reaction was calculated from the data on the concentration of the acid in the external solution which is in equilibrium with the same amount of acid in the solid phase at two different temperatures, by means of the following equation:

$$\Delta H = \frac{R \times T \times T_1}{T_1 - T} \cdot \ln \frac{[D[_{sol.}}{[D_1]_{sol.}}$$

The straight-line log relation of the free acid of the solution to the sorbed acid of the substrate should be noted. A mean value of $-\Delta H_0$ of 7.3 kcal. was obtained for polymetaphosphoric acid, and 6.8 kcal. per equivalent for lignosulfonic acid. Since release of a proton from the charged cationic protein groups involves heat of reaction of the order of 12 to 14 kcal. per mole and since a direct discharge may be assumed to have the same heat effect, it follows that about half of the cationic protein groups should be directly involved in the fixation of the polyvalent anion. Half the number of the anionic groups are probably compensated electrostatically by long-range forces of the electropositive groups of collagen. The probable reason is unfavorable steric conditions, which limit the accessibility of the cationic protein groups for the numerous anionic sites of the large polyacid molecule. Hence, the degree of the affinity of the polyacid anion for the cationic groups of collagen cannot be estimated by this method. Instead, it may be used for an approximation of the degree of direct interaction of the cationic protein groups (26a).

10. The Reaction of Strong Acids in Moderately Concentrated Solutions with Collagen

In the preceding discussion the systems of strong acids–protein have all been operated in a pH range down to 1 to 1.5, at which acidity the protein has attained its maximum capacity for the binding of acid by electrovalent forces. From the curve of the uptake of hydrochloric acid by collagen, it is evident that with further increase of acid concentration additional amounts of hydrochloric acid are fixed by collagen, in spite of the complete discharge of the carboxylic ions. With the indirect method usually employed, it is very difficult to estimate with the necessary degree of accuracy the amount of additional acid fixed by collagen from acid solutions of very high concentration, even in the concentration range 1 to 2 M since only a small fraction of the acid combines with collagen and the effect of the hydration of collagen is very great. It is probable that this additional fixation is located at the peptide bond. By resonance of the peptide group, its basic character is strengthened and attraction of protons should be possible. It seems more likely that the molecule of hydrochloric acid as such is coordinated to the peptide bond, and, indeed, there are certain indications that this is the case. Thus, for instance, it is found that equilibration of collagen by hydrochloric acid in solutions made 1 to 2 M in sodium chloride, forming a pickle system in which swelling of the protein is eliminated, slightly increases the hydrothermal stability of the collagen (measured by temperature of shrinkage) in hydrochloric acid concentrations less than normal. The increased shrinkage temperature, compared to that of neutral pelt of pH 5 to 7, may be ascribed to the dehydrating effect of the salt-acid combination on collagen which brings the protein chains closer together (probably augmenting the strength of interchain crosslinks of the hydrogen bond type). However, in the corresponding salt-acid system of HCl concentrations greater than $1M$, an abrupt fall in the curve of shrinkage temperature is recorded. If the pelt is treated for a few days in, for instance, a solution made $2 M$ in hydrochloric acid and sodium chloride, then neutralized and brought back to the isoelectric state, it will be found that it has undergone irreversible changes. For instance, it is permanently swollen and possesses greater capacity for fixation of agents which are supposed to be attached to the peptide bonds of collagen by coordination. The nature and behavior of collagen treated *without swelling* in the strong solution of hydrochloric acid is similar to that of pelt pretreated in concentrated solutions of lyotropic salts. It is considered likely that these changes mainly involve irreversible rupture of crosslinks of the hydrogen bond type between adjacent peptide links. This effect of higher concentrations of hydrochloric acid is independent of the neutral salt concentration above a certain minimum value required for elimination of the swelling of collagen. It is apparently a specific molecular effect, probably due to association and coordination of the molecules of hydrochloric acid on the peptide bonds, resulting in a partial irreversible rupture of the stabilizing crosslinks located at these points. The phenomenon is an example of the dual nature of the action of electrolytes in concentrated solutions of proteins: (1) the ionic stoichiometric binding of hydrogen ions and the compensation of the corresponding anions of the acid, which is the primary and regular reaction in all instances; and (2) the molecular attachment of hydrochloric acid, or acids generally, particularly the weak carboxylic acids, to nonionic protein groups by coordination. This reaction, which requires high concentrations of acid, appears to compete with the hydrogen bond bridge existing between adjacent peptide bonds of neighboring collagen chains. It leads to irreversible alterations in the protein structure, most remarkably to the freeing of coordination-active loci on the peptide bonds.

11. THE ACTION OF WEAK ACIDS

The interaction of weak acids with collagen, for instance acetic acid, which has been most thoroughly investigated, in the pH range from the isoelectric point of collagen to an equilibrium pH of about 3 follows the curve given for strong mineral acids which form reversible systems, such as hydrochloric acid. The coinciding curves indicate the reaction of the weak acids in solutions of the pH range given to be the removal of protons by the carboxyl ions of collagen. There is evidently no marked affinity of the anions of the weak acids for the cationic groups of collagen, nor any appreciable effect of the nonionized acid in the range of low hydrogen ion concentration. With decreasing pH of the system, the fixation of the weak acid, acetic acid, increases very sharply, as Fig. 22 shows. The maximum fixation of hydrogen ions by collagen generally is reached by hydrochloric acid and strong mineral acids in the pH range 1.2 to 1.5. There is no indication of such a maximum being approached by acetic acid at pH 2. A fixation of approximately 2.0 mg. equiv. of acid per gram of collagen is shown by Fig. 22. This pH value corresponds to a 3 M solution of acetic acid. There is no use attempting to extend the curve to still lower pH values, in view of the large errors involved in determination of the amount of acid fixed even at pH 2. With increasing concentration of acetic acid, the amounts of acetic molecules increases. At pH 2, for instance, with a solution of 3 M acetic acid about 99 % of the acid exists in the form of molecules of acetic acid. Hence, it is plausible to assume that the additional removal of acetic acid by collagen from concentrated solutions of the acid is in the form of un-ionized acid. It has been shown that the swelling of collagen in acetic acid at a final pH of 2 is very much larger than that produced by hydrochloric acid at this pH, about 50 % larger. Moreover, the acetic acid-treated speci-men (pelt), subsequently freed from acid and brought back to the isoelec-tric state, shows a large permanent swelling, more than twice that of the

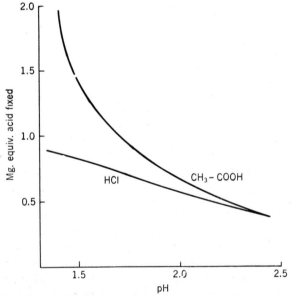

Fig. 22. The combination of hydrochloric and acetic acids with collagens from solutions of low pH values.

isoelectric untreated pelt (blank), whereas the corresponding pelt pretreated in hydrochloric acid shows only a slight permanent swelling, not more than 15 % greater than that of the untreated pelt. The shrinkage temperature of the acetic acid-pretreated pelt, in the neutralized state, was 12 degrees lower than that of the original skin. Evidently, the pretreatment of collagen in concentrated solutions of the weak acid impairs the forces stabilizing the collagen structure. In view of the finding that such pretreatment will result in increased reactivity of collagen toward agents reacting with nonionic protein groups, (probably the peptide bonds by means of coordination, typified by vegetable tannins), apparently the groups predominantly involved in the fixation of molecular acetic acid are the —CO—NH— groups. Since the main part of these groups of the original collagen probably is present in intramolecular or interchain compensation, forming hydrogen bonds, the carboxyl hydrogen of acetic acid may compete with the —NH— group of the chain for the coordination of the CO— groups of the peptide bond on the adjacent chain. Thereby a fairly extensive rupture of the cross-links between adjacent peptide chains will be produced by coordination of the acetic acid molecules on the peptide bonds. This opening up of the structure will be facilitated and made partly permanent by the marked swelling that takes place simultaneously. If the acetic acid is removed, water molecules will take its place (hydration). No restoration of hydrogen bonds in the collagen structure should be expected to occur because of the unfavorable steric conditions of the adjacent peptide links created by the swelling and the partial permanent disorganization of the collagen lattice. The effect of acetic acid on collagen will be further discussed in the chapters on swelling and tanning, particularly the effect of pretreatment of collagen on its fixation of tanning agents.

The view that acetic acid is fixed in the molecular form by collagen, probably on its peptide bonds, from concentrated solutions of the acid receives some support from a comprehensive study of the combination of wool protein with weak acids, carried out by Steinhardt, Fugitt, and Harris (25). They find an increased uptake of weak organic acids at high concentrations of acid. It is shown that the degree of this additional sorption of acid is a rough measure of the amount of *nonionized* acid that has combined with keratin, possibly by solvating it in competition with water. The experimental support for this is as follows: (*1*) The increased uptake of any one of the weak acids of the eight investigated is approximately proportional to the concentration of nonionized acid; (*2*) the increased uptake of any one acid at a given pH value is not fixed, but varies with the concentration of the weak acid. Hence, these investigators emphasize that it is the concentration of the weak acid rather than the hydrogen ion concentration, which is significant for the extent of combination, since the acid is largely taken up

TABLE 10

RELATIVE AFFINITIES OF NONIONIZED ACIDS FOR WOOL PROTEIN (0°C.)

Acid	pK	Partition Quotient	Acid	pK	Partition Quotient
Propionic	4.9	0.3	Benzoic	4.2	11
Acetic	4.7	0.4	p-Nitrophenol	7.1	20
Glycolic	3.8	0.6	2,4-Dinitrophenol	4.0	50
Formic	3.7	0.7	2,6-Dinitrophenol	3.6	60
Monochloroacetic	2.8	1.8	2,6-Dichloro-4-nitrophenol	~5	100
Dichloroacetic	1.3	2	2,4,6-Trichlorophenol	6.0	100

in the molecular form. The tendency of weak acids to combine with wool protein in the form of molecules is given in Table 10. The values are expressed as the partition ratio between the molecular and ionic fixation of the acids by wool at a point where 0.2 to 0.3 mg. equiv. of acid is fixed as undissociated acid by 1 g. of keratin. The range of the affinities of the molecular form of the various acids for wool is approximately 300 to 1.

As mentioned earlier, the figure of the heat of combination of strong acids, such as hydrochloric acid, with wool is of the order of 1 to 2 kcal. For acids with anions of high affinity for the cationic protein groups (irreversibly fixed), the values are found to be about 12 kcal., probably indicating in the latter instance the energy of the reaction of the basic protein groups. Steinhardt and his co-workers (25) made an estimate at two different temperatures, 0 and 25°C. They found about 0.3 kcal. per mole of acid. This result supports the view that the combination of wool with molecules of a weak acid involves the replacement of water in the protein by molecules of the acid, i.e., a process of selective hydration. The heat of hydration of proteins is large, but, as the authors point out, the replacement of one hydrated molecule by another which is held to the protein only slightly more firmly would probably involve very small heat changes, such as those found. The value arrived at also proves the absence of anion affinity of the weak acids for the protein.

B. SYSTEMS INVOLVING PARTLY OR MAINLY IRREVERSIBLY FIXED ACIDS

1. INTRODUCTION

It has repeatedly been stressed that in the systems of typical strong acids interacting with proteins, such as the hydrochloric acid–collagen system, the anions do not possess marked affinity for the cationic protein groups, the anions of the acid being electrostatically compensated by and associated with the electropositive groups of collagen. Investigations of the uptake of hydrochloric acid by globular proteins have shown, however, that a small part of the chloride ions may be bound to the protein (29). It is also worthy of notice that in the two principal concepts of the adsorption of acids and bases by proteins the views on the state of the anions of the acid are diametrically opposite. Thus, according to the proponents of the Donnan theory, no combination of chloride ions with the protein should occur, all the ions being dissolved in the internal aqueous solution without restrain. The opposite view is taken by Gilbert and Rideal (24), in their attempt at a quantitative treatment of the reaction along thermodynamic lines. They consider that the internal solutions cannot be conceived as a normal aqueous solution, and they base their concept on the prerequisite that all the anions in the solid protein phase are associated with the positively charged basic groups of the protein. The curious fact is that both these concepts apparently explain a number of experimental facts equally well in reactions of the hydrochloric acid–protein type. This is not surprising, since this system is reversible. Of course, any choice between the two opposing views is superfluous for problems connected with systems in which partly or mainly *irreversible* fixation of the anions of the acid by the protein takes place. However, in that event the concept based on the Donnan equilibrium is not applicable, and neither is the straight thermodynamic approach to the problem.

It has also been mentioned that the large heat of reaction of acids of complicated structure, such as aromatic sulfonic acids, the dyestuff Orange II especially, compared to the practically zero heat of combination of hydrochloric acid (protons) with proteins, is a measure of the degree of interaction of the anions of the acid with the protein. From a practical point of view such an irreversible combination of tanning agents and acid dyestuffs of the sulfonic acid type with collagen and textile proteins has long been realized by those familiar with tanning and textile dyeing processing.

2. The Effect of the Anions

To limit our discussion to the tanning field, the formation of stable compounds between anions of large molecules and collagen was first recognized in the fundamental researches of Wilson and Thomas and their co-workers (30), who introduced the physicochemical approach to practical protein chemistry as applied to tanning processes. The outstanding work of Otto on the irreversible fixation of dyestuff anions by collagen and tanned collagen has done much to clarify the problem (31). It was noted by Meyer and Fikentscher (31a) that wool combines stoichiometrically with acid dyes, and later by Felzman (32) that the maximum fixation of acid dyestuffs containing free sulfonic acid groups by collagen was stoichiometric, governed by the content of basic protein groups. In further studies of these systems, including chrome- and vegetable-tanned skin collagen, Otto found that the maximum dyestuff fixation was reached at different final pH values, depending on the dyestuff. It was indicated that the constitution and size of the dyestuff molecule was responsible for the behavior. The highest pH value at which the maximum dyestuff fixation is reached is called the pH limit of the dyestuff. Thus, Otto found for Cotton Scarlet extra, a simple acid dye, a maximum fixation of 0.84 mg. equiv. of dye per gram of collagen, with a pH limit of 1.5, whereas the more complicated anion of Acid Anthracene Brown RH gave the figure of 0.95 mg. equiv. at a pH of 2.0.

As a general rule it holds that, the greater the affinity of the dyestuff anion for collagen, the higher the pH limit. By comparative experiments with vegetable-tanned collagen the maximum fixation of the dyestuff was maintained, although the pH limit was considerably decreased. Thus, for Cotton Scarlet a final pH of 1.3 was required for inactivation of all basic protein groups by the dye, and the corresponding value for the anthracene dye was 1.4. The different behavior of vegetable-tanned collagen is considered to be connected with the inactivation of nonionic protein groups (peptide bonds) by the tannins. The latter protein groups are assumed to stabilize the dyestuff anion attached to the electropositive groups of untreated collagen by means of coordination of some substituent in the dye molecule on these groups (through π electrons). The vegetable tannins interact with the peptide bonds (hydrogen bonding), and hence no additional valency forces are available for the secondary fixation of the dyestuff anchored on the basic protein groups of the vegetable-tanned collagen. Otto has elaborated on his theoretical treatise of the dyeing problems, to be further considered in another connection.

Since the initial reaction is ionic, but the resulting compound between dyestuff and protein totally lacks ionic character, it appears that the first-formed electrovalent bond is changed into a covalent-coordinate one, which means neutralization of the oppositely charged components. This will in its turn disturb the equilibrium between free and compensated basic groups; the latter are considered to exist mainly in the form of salt links, and, accordingly, an additional amount of reactive electropositive protein groups will be freed. Hence, the reaction with the dyestuff will proceed until complete interaction and discharge of the basic protein groups is accomplished.

The high pH limit of the acids of the dyestuffs, which contain anions of great affinity for the nonionic protein groups through coordination-active sites on the aromatic compounds, is probably in a great measure due to the participation of secondary stabilizing forces that also account for the fastness of the dyestuff. The modern theory of the resonance of extensively conjugated aromatic compounds and the concomitant formation of weak dipoles in their molecules (function of the π electrons), introduced into leather chemistry so convincingly by Otto, appears to give a satisfactory explanation of these complicated systems. Hence, it is possible that the multipoint attachment of the dyestuff anions on the oppositely charged ions and the participation of auxiliary forces by the dipoles may give a joint effect, resulting in the formation of bonds of a degree of stability resembling that of the covalent bond.

Moreover, at pH values in the acid range near the isoelectric zone, a considerable fixation should be expected to occur. Even the possibility that the attachment of anions possessing extremely great affinity for the cationic protein groups will take place in the pH range on the alkaline side of this point must be considered. Such reactions are realized by the high-molecular lignosulfonic acids and some synthetic tannins of the sulfo acid type (33). The participation of coordinate reactions involving coordination-active, nonionic groups in these structures, for instance the hydroxy groups, may in part be responsible for the fixation, and the presence of the coordination-active groups may also assist in the stabilization of the anion reacting with the cationic protein groups. Figure 23 presents a graphical illustration of the influence of the degree of affinity of the anion of the acid on its combination with collagen as a function of the final pH, the uptake of hydrochloric acid being compared with the *irreversible* fixation of high-molecular lignosulfonic acid and a sulfo acid synthetic tannin (33).

3. RELATIVE AFFINITY OF THE ANIONS

The most elaborate work on the participation of anions in the combination of protein with acids has been carried out by Steinhardt and his associates (25) in comprehensive investigations of the reactivity of wool. Since some of the fundamental aspects of their researches have an immediate bearing on the corresponding problems met in tanning and in the behavior of collagen, a brief discussion of their findings and theoretical conclusions seems appropriate.

The combination of a great number of organic acids of different strength, including all those given in Table 10, with wool as a function of the final pH (at 0°C.) was determined. A striking feature of these curves is the wide range of the positions, with regard to the pH coordinate, in which the titration curves fall. In comparing the affinity of different acids for proteins, it is advisable and convenient to select the state at which the protein substrate is half-saturated with acid. Then the equation of the change in the chemical potential, $\Delta u°$, is simplified to

$$-\Delta u° = 4.6\, RT \cdot \text{pH}_{\text{mid}}.$$

TABLE 11

AFFINITY OF ACIDS FOR WOOL AT 0°C. (34)

Acid	$pH_{mid.}$	Total Affinity, kcal.	Anion Affinity, kcal.
Hydrochloric	2.1	− 5.3	—
Sulfuric	3.0	−11.4	−0.8
Sulfuric (at 22°C.)	2.9	−12.1	−0.8
Trichloroacetic	2.6	− 6.5	−1.2
Benzensulfonic	2.5	− 6.2	−0.9
p-Toluenesulfonic	2.5	− 6.3	−1.0
Naphthalene-β-sulfonic	3.2	− 7.9	−2.6
Anthraquinone-β-sulfonic	3.6	− 9.1	−3.8
o-Nitrobenzenesulfonic	2.7	− 6.8	−1.5
2,4-Dinitrobenzenesulfonic	3.0	− 7.6	−2.3
Chromic acid (as monobasic)	3.3	− 8.2	−2.9
Picric	3.7	− 9.3	−4.0
1-Naphthol-2,4-dinitro-7-sulfonic	4.1	−10.1	−4.8

where $pH_{mid.}$ is the pH value at which the amount of acid bound is half the saturation value. Thus, for wool 0.45 mg. equiv. per gram of protein is found, and this value also applies to collagen.

Hence, a simple method of estimating the relative affinity of any acid for proteins is afforded by annotating the pH value of the midpoint of the titration curve. Table 11 gives the pH at 50% saturation with acid as a measure of the affinity of a number of acids for wool and the total affinity of the acids and of their anions.

In ascertaining the $pH_{mid.}$ values of the titration curves of hydrochloric acid, lignosulfonic acid, and sulfo acid syntan at their interaction with collagen (Fig. 23), the values obtained are, respectively, 2.4, 4.5, and 5.5, demonstrating the exceedingly high affinity of the tanning agents for collagen. Values of $pH_{mid.}$ of the same order have been found in titration of wool with free acids of dyestuffs, as reported in Vickerstaff's monograph (34). Since the estimation of the affinity of high-molecular acids for collagen is of interest and value, the method of obtaining and calculating the last two columns of Table 11 is instructive. The total affinity of any protein for any particular acid is the sum of the affinities of the proton and the anion. Since the affinity of the proton is constant, in view of its independent interaction with the carboxyl ions, the different acid affinities must be due to differences in anion affinity. From a strictly scientific point of view, it is impossible to assess the contribution of each ion to the affinity. Nevertheless an approximation of the affinity of the anion of various acids should be of value. It is

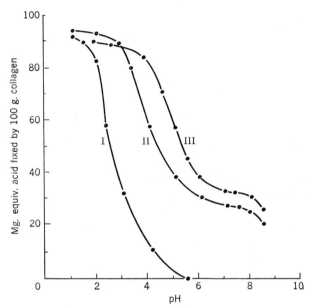

Fig. 23. The combination of hydrochloric acid (I), lignosulfonic acid (II), and sulfonic acid syntan (III) with collagen as a function of the pH values at equilibrium.

necessary to select as a standard an ion with a low but definite affinity. The most suitable standard is apparently the chloride ion, since its affinity for proteins is less than that of any other acid anion so far investigated and, further, since hydrochloric acid is the standard for constructing titration curves of proteins. Then all other anions will show positive values of their affinity. The pH of half-saturation of wool with hydrochloric acid varies but little with the temperature, the figure being 2.2 at 0°C., and 2.1 at 25 and 50°C. If the value of $pH_{mid.}$ is inserted in the equation for the chemical potential (p. 127), the total affinity of hydrochloric acid for keratin is about -5.3 kcal., if the anion affinity is set at zero. The values of the anion affinity are then obtained by subtracting the figure of the proton affinity (hydrochloric acid) from the total affinity of the particular acid figured from the value of the $pH_{mid.}$ of the titration curve, according to the standard equation referred to earlier.

The data of Table 11 show clearly that the affinity of acids for this particular protein will increase with increasing molecular weight of the acid or by introduction of weak dipolar groups possessing coordinative potency. This is particularly well illustrated in Otto's studies of the combination of dyestuffs with collagen (35). With increasing number of sulfonic acid groups of monoazo dyestuffs, such as Fast Reds, with one, two, three, or four sulfonic acid groups at the numbers given in the nuclei, the pH limit of maximum binding of the dyestuffs is reached at final pH values of 2.0 for the monoacid, at pH 1.6 for the disulfonic acid, and at pH 1.3 for the tri- and tetrasulfonic acid compounds. Apparently by the charging of the dyestuff molecule with strongly acidic groups, the effect of the weak polar forces of the type of coordination valencies inherent in the aromatic nucleus is gradually weakened, and the influence of the ionic valency forces will come to the fore. The stability and irreversibility toward water of the dyestuff–collagen compounds formed reaches the optimal values in the combination of the monoacid dyestuff with the protein, indicating the importance of the secondary effect of weaker valency forces (π electrons) for the anchorage and fixation of the sulfo acids on collagen. This problem will be further discussed in the chapters on synthetic tannins and dyeing in "The Chemistry of Tanning Processes."

The fixation of polyacids by collagen offers very interesting but exceedingly complicated problems, as yet little understood. Instructive examples are the small molecule of an acid dyestuff of the Fast Red type containing four sulfonic acid groups, on the one hand, and such large molecules as those present in the high-molecular fraction of lignosulfonic acids, with ten to twenty sulfonic acid groups in the molecule, with molecular weights of the order of a few thousand, on the other. The interaction of four sulfonic acid groups held within a restricted area of the dyestuff molecule with four cationic protein groups hardly seems possible. The analytical data are in complete accord with and satisfy the maximum acid-binding capacity of collagen. This implies the complete discharge of the protons of the acid by the carboxyl ions of collagen. However, no information is obtained regarding the direct discharge of the sulfonic acid groups of the irreversibly attached anion of the dyestuff molecule, or whether these groups are only partially discharged, leaving an excess of negatively charged sulfonic acid groups in the collagen-dye compound formed.

It would appear still more difficult to accommodate a molecule of the size of the lignosulfonic acid mentioned within the fibrils and obtain inactivation of the numerous negatively charged sulfo acid groups on accessible cationic sites on the collagen protofibrils. Although the maximum irreversible fixation of this type of high-molecular sulfo acid by collagen closely corresponds to the acid-binding capacity of the basic groups of collagen, these data say nothing about the extent to which the sulfo acid groups have interacted with their oppositely charged partners. Neither does the lack of binding of decinormal hydrochloric acid by collagen with maximum content of bound lignosulfonic acid constitute a proof of the complete inactivation of the cationic protein groups, in view of the afore-mentioned fact that the carboxyl ions of collagen determine the reaction. On the contrary, it is likely that only a few of the sulfo groups are discharged by direct attachment to the cationic groups of collagen, the main part being compensated by some long-range effect, and some possibly remaining charged. These intricate questions will be further discussed in the chapter dealing with the mechanism of fixation of lignosulfonic acids by collagen.

In this connection, the accessibility of the ϵ-amino groups of the lysine residues of collagen to the fluorodinitrobenzene reagent is of interest. Sykes (36) found that only about 75% of the total number of these groups were accessible to and reacted with the Sanger reagent. Porter (37) had earlier found incomplete reaction of the ϵ-amino group in several globular proteins to DNFB reagent, which was considered to be due to steric hindrance. Prior to Sykes' work, Bowes and Kenton (38) found that only about half of the lysine amino groups were reacting with the DNFB reagent, although they were completely diazotized by nitrous acid. It was first thought that this sluggishness in reactivity was due to nonreactivity of a proportion of the ϵ-amino groups. In a recent investigation by Bowes and Moss (39) the possibility is suggested that the incomplete reactivity is due to decomposition of the ϵ-DNP lysine during the hydrolysis of the DNP collagen.

REFERENCES

1. Ames, W. M., *J. Sci. Food Agr.* **3**, 579 (1952).
2. Grassmann, W., Endres, H., and Steber, A., *Z. Naturforsch.* **9b**, 513 (1954).
2a. Grabar, P., and Morel, J., *Bull. soc. chim. biol.* **32**, 630, 643 (1950).
3. Atkin, W. R., and Campos, J. M., *J. Intern. Soc. Leather Trades Chem.* **8**, 406 (1924).
4. .Speakman, J. B., and Hirst, M. C., *Trans. Faraday Soc.* **29**, 148 (1933).
5. Retterova, E., "Progress in Leather Science," Vol. 1, p. 87. BLMRA, London, 1946.
6. Steinhardt, J., and Harris, M., *J. Research Natl. Bur. Standards* **24**, 335 (1940).
7. McLaughlin, G. D., and Adams, R. S., *J. Am. Leather Chem. Assoc.* **35**, 44 (1940); **37**, 76 (1942).
8. See Küntzel, A., in "Handbuch der Gerbereichemie" (W. Grassmann, ed.), Vol. I, Part 1, p. 555. Springer, Vienna, 1944.
9. Mörner, K. A. H., *Z. physiol. Chem.* **18**, 225, 471 (1894).
10. Gustavson, K. H., *J. Am. Leather Chem. Assoc.* **42**, 569 (1947); *J. Phys. & Colloid Chem.* **51**, 1181 (1947).
11. McLaughlin, G. D., and Cameron, D. H., *J. Phys. Chem.* **41**, 961 (1937).
12. See McLaughlin, G. D., and Theis, E. R., "Chemistry of Leather Manufacture," pp. 466–469, 506–510, 514–523, 528–535. Reinhold, New York, 1945.

13. Theis, E. R., and Blum, W. A., *J. Am. Leather Chem. Assoc.* **37**, 553 (1942); Theis, E. R., *ibid.* **39**, 319 (1944); see Lollar, R. M., *ibid.* **43**, 542 (1948); **45**, 401 (1950).
14. Theis, E. R., *J. Biol. Chem.* **154**, 87 (1944); **157**, 7 (1945); Theis, E. R., and Jacoby, T. F., *ibid.* **146**, 163 (1942); **148**, 105 (1943).
15. Atkin, W. R., "Stiasny Festschrift," p. 13. Roether, Darmstadt, 1937.
16. Thomas, A. W., and Foster, S. B., *J. Am. Chem. Soc.* **48**, 489 (1926).
17. Gustavson, K. H., *J. Am. Leather Chem. Assoc.* **42**, 313 (1947).
17a. Lipsitz, P., Kremen, S. S., and Lollar, R. M., *J. Am. Chem. Assoc.* **44**, 371 (1949).
17b. Armstrong, D. M. G., *in* "Nature and Structure of Collagen" (J. T. Randall, ed.), p. 91. Butterworths, London, 1953.
18. Bowes, J. H., and Kenten, R. H., *Biochem. J.* **43**, 358 (1948); Bowes, J. H., *Research* **4**, 155 (1951).
19. Lichtenstein, I., *Biochem. Z.* **303**, 13 (1939).
20. Vickerstaff, T., "The Physical Chemistry of Dyeing," p. 228. Oliver and Boyd, London, 1950.
21. Kekwick, R. A., and Cannan, R. K., *Biochem. J.* **30**, 227 (1936); Cannan, R. K., *Chem. Revs.* **30**, 395 (1942); *Ann. N. Y. Acad. Sci.* **41**, 243 (1941); *J. Biol. Chem.* **142**, 803 (1942).
22. Speakman, J. B., and Hirst, M. C., *Trans. Faraday Soc.* **29**, 148 (1933); Speakman, J. B., and Stott, E., *ibid.* **30**, 539 (1934).
23. Peters, L., and Speakman, J. B., *J. Soc. Dyers Colourists* **65**, 63 (1949).
24. Gilbert, G. A., and Rideal, E., *Proc. Roy. Soc.* **A182**, 335 (1944).
25. Steinhardt, J., Fugitt, C. H., and Harris, M., *J. Research Natl. Bur. Standards* **30**, 123 (1943); Steinhardt, J., *Ann. N. Y. Acad. Sci.* **41**, 287 (1941).
26. Olofsson, B., *J. Soc. Dyers Colourists* **68**, 506 (1952).
26a. Larsson, A., and Gustavson, K. H., *J. Soc. Leather Trades Chem.* **39**, 112 (1955).
27. Vickerstaff, T., see ref. 20, pp. 83–118, and particularly pp. 284–308.
28. Speakman, J. B., and Stott, E., *Trans. Faraday Soc.* **31**, 1425 (1935); **34**, 1203 (1938).
29. Scatchard, G., Scheinberg, I. H., and Armstrong, S. H., *J. Am. Chem. Soc.* **72**, 535, 540 (1950).
30. See Wilson, J. A., "The Chemistry of Leather Manufacture," Vols. 1 and 2. Chemical Catalog Co., New York, 1928, 1929.
31. Otto, G., *Collegium* **1933**, 586; **1935**, 371; **1938**, 164.
31a. Meyer, K. H., and Fikentscher, H., *Melliand Textilber.* **7**, 605 (1926).
32. Felzmann, C., *Collegium* **1933**, 373.
33. Gustavson, K. H., *Svensk Kem. Tidskr.* **56**, 14 (1944); *Ing. Vetenskaps Akad. Handl.* **No. 177** (1944); *Discussions Faraday Soc.* **No. 16**, p. 109 (1954).
34. Vickerstaff, T., ref. 20, p. 303.
35. Otto, G., *Das Leder* **4**, 1 (1953).
36. Sykes, R. L., *J. Soc. Leather Trades Chem.* **36**, 267 (1952).
37. Porter, R. R., *Biochim. et Biophys. Acta* **2**, 105 (1948).
38. Bowes, J. H., and Kenten, R. H., *Biochem. J.* **55**, 735 (1953).
39. Bowes, J. H., and Moss, J. A., *in* "Nature and Structure of Collagen" (J. T. Randall, ed.), pp. 199–207, Butterworth, London, 1953.

CHAPTER 6

The Internal Linking of the Collagen Molecule

1. INTRODUCTION

The interchain and intermolecular forces of the collagen structure which give raise to the cohesion of the molecule, inter- and intrafibrillar, are generally considered to be of two main types, directed valency and undirected valency. Directed valency consists in (*1*) electrovalency, located at polar side chains with opposite charge, forming a saltlike crosslink, and (*2*) coordinate valency between various weakly polar groups, such as the peptide bond and hydroxy and amide groups, forming crosslinks by hydrogen bonding. The undirected valency forces are of the nature of coulombic or van der Waals forces. In view of the almost complete lack of knowledge of the steric conditions of the collagen chains, such as the distances between the reactive groups, the discussion of this subject must necessarily consider possibilities and suggestions rather than state actual facts. The recent introduction of the helical structural concept makes the task still more difficult. Many of the present ideas will probably have to be radically modified in the near future. This presentation will therefore follow the more traditional lines of approach.

The stabilization of the collagen molecule is probably due to a number of different types of lateral links, of which *the electrovalent salt link* will be discussed first. This is exemplified by the lysine–glutamic acid saltlike crosslink (1):

$$\diagdown\!\!\!\!\!\!\!\!\!\!_{\diagup}\, CH \cdot CH_2 \cdot CH_2 \cdot CH_2 \cdot CH_2 \cdot NH_3^+ \cdot O^- CO \cdot CH_2 \cdot CH_2 \cdot CH \!\!\!\!\!\!\!\!\!\!^{\diagup}\!\!\!\!\!_{\diagdown}$$

In the dry fiber, its length is about 10 Å., in hydrated collagen about 16 Å (2). Since there is no sharing of electrons in this link, the distance between the oppositely charged groups may be altered within certain limits without breaking the crosslinking. The strength of this link will largely depend on the distance between the charged groups and the dielectric environment. Thus, in the fully hydrated state of collagen, the water dipoles associated with the charged groups will diminish the strength of the crosslink. It is obvious that this rather weak crosslink is easily opened by acids and bases or by any agent interacting with any of the side chains involved in its formation. Thus, acids discharge the carboxyl ions and destroy the cohesive forces, and alkalis exert the same effect by the discharge of the ammonium ions.

The suggestion of the existence of saltlike crosslinks in keratin was first advanced by Speakman and Hirst (1). It was later applied to collagen by Lloyd (3). The main evidence for the existence of this type of link was the finding by Speakman and Hirst (1) that the amount of work required to stretch wool fibers is reduced in acid solution, as compared with water, in direct proportion to the acid concentration. The effect is attributed to the rupture of the salt link by discharge of the carboxyl ion of keratin. It has also been suggested that the salt link of collagen may be converted into the —CO—NH— group, resulting in a covalent crosslink between adjacent chains, on excessive drying of skin at extreme heat by a process of anhydride formation (3). The difficulty of wetting back strongly dried skins has been assumed to be connected with such an alteration (3).

By the action of solvents of low dielectric constant, such as alcohols, the dipolar forces are impaired, which change should be expected to facilitate the discharge of the groups by the passage of the proton from the cationic to the anionic groups. The final result would be a coordinate link (hydrogen bond):

$$\overset{\diagdown}{\underset{\diagup}{}} CH(CH_2)_3 \cdot CH_2 : \overset{H}{\underset{H}{\overset{..}{N}}} : \; \rightarrow \; H : \overset{..}{\underset{:\overset{..}{O}:}{O}} : C : CH_2 \cdot CH_2 \cdot C\overset{\diagup}{\underset{\diagdown}{H}}$$

The increased thermal stability of collagen pretreated in ethanol, as evidenced by a marked increase in the shrinkage temperature of the collagen fiber, should thus be explainable, since this coordinate link would be much stronger than the original ionic crosslink, being fixed in direction and length to hold the structure firmly. From evaluation of the relative importance of the two types of directed valency forces as contributors to the hydrothermal stabilization of collagen, it is indicated that the participation of the saltlike links is relatively unimportant compared to that of the coordinate type of links.

2. COORDINATE LINKS OF VARIOUS TYPES (HYDROGEN BOND)

The direct carbimino backbone link, $\overset{\diagdown}{\underset{\diagup}{}} C :: O : \; \rightarrow \; H : \overset{..}{\underset{\diagdown}{N}} :$, and its reso-

nance forms have already been discussed. Pauling and Niemann (4), who were the first to apply the concept of hydrogen bonding to proteins methodically, point out that interactions of this type, although individually weak with a bond energy of a few kilocalories, can by combining their forces of several hundred bonds in long polypeptide chains stabilize such large structures as protein molecules. In collagen every fourth backbone link is a

CO—N= group, which means a gap in the regularity of hydrogen bonds. Since part of these non-hydrogen-bonded links are formed by hydroxyproline residues, other interesting possibilities of hydrogen bonding are suggested, as will be shown later. Since the water molecule is a typical dipole, it might be expected that water molecules would sever hydrogen bonds by association with the CO and NH groups. This is apparently not the case. In such high polymers as drawn nylon fibers, in which hydrogen bonds are the only type of crosslink, water has no effect on its strength. The link is not opened by ordinary organic solvent. The only rupturing agents are those possessing strong coordinate reactivity, i.e., the tendency to form hydrogen bonds, such as the acetic acid molecule and phenols. Also lyotropic agents, such as urea and certain salts, compete with the internal hydrogen bond to be hydrogen-bonded to the carbonyl group; in fact, their "peptizing" effect is founded on this property.

Hydrogen bonds are formed not only between peptide linkages but also between other groups of the collagen molecule. One of these groups furnishes the hydrogen ion, and the other group, containing nitrogen or oxygen, furnishes the lone electron pair, the negative charges of which attract the positively charged hydrogen ion. Since there are far more peptide linkages than other groups capable of forming hydrogen bonds, and since they are sterically favored, it is likely that the majority of the hydrogen bonds of collagen are located at the peptide links. Chemical evidence (4a) has been presented

to substantiate the presence of interchain links of the type —OH— —OC$\diagup^{HN}_{\diagdown}$

In Huggins' helical model of collagen, this type of bond is assumed also (4b).

A typical hydrogen bond, verified experimentally by ultraviolet spectrography, is formed in proteins containing tyrosine, probably between its hydroxyl group and a free carboxyl group of an adjacent side chain (5). Since collagen contains only a slight amount of tyrosine, this type of bond cannot be important, possibly linking the hydroxy and carboxyl groups (6), or the hydroxy–carbonyl link mentioned. In collagen, the hydroxyamino acids account for about one-sixth of the side chains. The linking of the hydroxy groups of hydroxyamino acids with carboxyl ions, previously mentioned, is indicated in some globular proteins (Klotz, 6). Other suggested links are those between the amide group and the carboxylic group, and between the amide group and the serine residue. Collagen of fishskin shows a considerably lower degree of stability than mammalian skin collagen, as mentioned earlier. For instance, the hydrothermal stability of skin of deepwater fishes measured by the shrinkage temperature is about 25 degrees lower than that of collagen of bovine skin (8). This was originally interpreted to imply that the hydrogen bond crosslinking of the chains of fish-skin collagen is less developed than that of the mammalian type, at a time when no definite information as to the amino acid composition on fish skin collagen was available. Since then, figures of the analysis of fish collagen show considerably less hydroxyproline than the generally accepted figure for mammalian collagen (7, 8, 8a). It is possible that the low content of this imino acid has a direct bearing on the low degree of internal organization of fishskin collagen, as the crosslinking by means of hydrogen bonds from the hydroxyproline residue to the carbonyl oxygen of an adjacent keto-imide link should be impaired in the teleostean collagen. Dr. P. Alexander has pointed out to this author that the fact that collagen is insoluble in concentrated solutions of lithium bromide, which dissolves straight hydrogen–bonded fibrous proteins (silk), suggests the presence of a very strong interchain crosslink in collagen, probably an ester bond, —O—CO—. Certain anomalies in the reactivity of collagen are in accord with this suggestion.

There is some chemical evidence pointing to participation of the guanidyl residue of gelatin and collagen in the internal linking of the protein structure. It has been shown by Roche and Blanc-Jean (9) that the Sakaguchi reaction, which is specific for the guanidyl group, is not quantitative for some globular proteins which appear to contain a part of their arginine residues in the "masked" state. Gelatin shows the same tendency, as demonstrated by Grabar and his associates (10), who also suggest that the hydroxyl groups of hydroxyproline, serine, and hydroxylysine probably are involved in the blocking of the guanidyl group of gelatin. As to collagen itself, the extremely high degree of alkalinity required for discharge of the electropositive arginine residues is difficult to understand unless some type of interaction of the guanidyl group has taken place with some other protein groups such as the carboxyls or the hydroxy groups of hydroxyamino acids. It is somewhat parallel to the high alkalinity required to split the tyrosine–carboxyl–hydrogen bond of certain globular proteins. In addition to the ineffectiveness of the Sakaguchi reaction, the great difficulty experienced in the deamination of the arginine residue of collagen by nitrous acid–extremely low pH values and prolonged time of reaction being necessary, as first established by Speakman and Stott (11)—may be cited in support of the theory of some type of stabilization of the guanidyl group by its interaction with some other side chain of collagen.

Some important arguments in support of this view have been advanced by Grabar and Morel (10). For instance, if the guanidyl group of gelatin is destroyed by oxidation with hypobromite or partially degraded by means of ultrasonic vibration, it loses its gel-forming power. It is interesting to note that, by addition of arginine to gelatin solution, the setting of gel will be inhibited when amounts of at least 2 moles of arginine per 100 g. of gelatin are present. Evidently the arginine molecules compete with the arginine residues of the gelatin for the other group, forming the site of the original crosslink in gelatin. Addition of hydroxyamino acids such as hydroxyproline has no effect. The inhibition is reversible; neither the removal of the ε-amino group of the lysine residue by diazotization nor the inactivation of these groups by the dinitrofluorobenzene reagent of Sanger has any effect on the gel-forming power of gelatin. In the ultrasonic treatment of gelatin in slightly acid solution, losses of arginine and hydroxyproline were incurred.

From comprehensive investigations of the conversion of collagen to gelatin, Ames (12) concludes that in the making of gelatin from collagen by means of the acid process a special type of crosslink is broken. The strong ester link suggested by Alexander may be involved. Ames suggests that this stable link may be supplied by the ammonium ion of a side chain and a carboxyl group, forming a —CO—NH— link by condensation. Ames has also assumed the existence of crosslinks in which an amide group is shared between two carboxyl groups (—CO—NH—CO—). The formation of the last-named bond appears unlikely, since the end carboxyls of glutamic and aspartic acids are probably not involved in peptide bond formation, because this type of bond is not cleaved by proteinases (Grassmann and Schneider, 13), which is the case with an ester bond (13a).

In any event, the chemical evidence and the general behavior of collagen point to some immobilization of the chemical reactivity of the arginine residue of collagen. It is likely that the crosslinks formed on the guanidyl groups govern the stability of collagen to an appreciable extent.

At the present state of our knowledge, it appears that numerous crosslinks of weakly polar forces, probably of the hydrogen bond type, and a rather limited number of electrovalent crosslinks formed by the attraction of oppositely charged strong ionic side chains are the main valency forces stabilizing the collagen structure. The presence of an exceedingly strong interchain bond is likely (Alexander).

An evaluation of the relative importance of the two types of directed valency forces may be obtained by measuring the hydrothermal stability of collagen, most conveniently the temperature of instantaneous shrinkage, after treatments with agents which are specific for the groups involved. Thus, β-naphthalene sulfonic acid will inactivate the ionic protein groups almost completely, thereby eliminating the saltlike crosslinks, *without swelling* the collagen and not interfering appreciably with the coordination activity of the peptide groups (14). The change in shrinkage temperature effected by such inactivation may be applied for the evaluation of the degree of intermolecular cohesion of the collagen lattice due to electrovalent interaction of polar R groups. It will be found that the shrinkage temperature of mammalian collagen (65 to 68°C.) is decreased by 12 to 16 degrees by this treatment (14). For comparison, it is of interest to note that by pretreatment of bovine collagen in solutions of agents with a specific action on coordinate links, such as the crosslinks of the hydrogen bond type—for example, 6 to 8 M solutions of urea or 2 M solutions of sodium perchlorate—shrinkage will occur at room temperature. This means a lowering of the shrinkage temperature by about 50°C. (14). Accordingly, it is evident that the main stabilizing forces of mammalian collagen depend on the type of coordinate crosslinks, probably bridges of hydrogen bonds. The data indicate that they are responsible for at least three-fourths of the internal cohesion, the rest being probably supplied by the saltlike crosslinks. This figure refers to collagen of mammalian corium.

For the collagen of the skin of bone fishes (*Teleostei*), particularly those of deep-water habitat, the nature of interchain compensation and intermolecular linking appears to differ considerably from the type described for the bovine corium, not only in the fact that the shrinkage temperature of the fish collagen is located in the temperature range 35 to 45°C., compared to 60 to 70°C. for mammalian collagen (8). Particularly instructive and typical in this respect is the different effect of anionic agents which are attracted to the basic groups of collagen on the two types of skin proteins and also the contrasting effect of high-molecular anions on the mammalian and the teleostean collagens, which bind these anions irreversibly and apparently without disturbance of the normal valency partition on the nonionic protein groups, such as the peptide linkages (15, 16).

As an illustration of the first type of reaction, the effect of the anionic detergent sodium dodecyl sulfate in 5 % aqueous solution and of pH about 7 is of interest (15). The structural characteristics of the bovine skin were not detrimentally affected by this treatment, which lasted for 48 hours. The only change detectable was a slight lowering of the shrinkage temperature by 1 to 2 degrees, practically within the range of the experimental variations. The collagen of codfish skin was almost completely solubilized (about 80 %). These experiments may be interpreted to prove that by breaking of the salt links of fish collagen through the discharge of the cationic protein groups by the large anion of the detergent, resulting in elimination of the electropositive site of attraction, the strength of the fiber structure is destroyed, because only weak crosslinks or other cohesive forces are left after the destruction of the ionic crosslinks. Practically all the collagen goes into solution. In mammalian collagen, on the other hand, the severing of these electrovalent crosslinks does not lead to any great impairment of the stability of the structure. The elimination of the salt link is shown by a lowered T_s and a minor loss of collagen by solubilization, if a high degree of swelling is simultaneously produced. The fiber structure is left intact, however, and by removal of the agent the original properties of collagen are largely restored. The related behavior indicates the secondary importance of the hydrogen bridge formation in fishskin collagen and its dominating importance for the mammalian type of collagen. Complete inactivation of the basic groups of fish collagen by nonswelling naphthalene sulfonic acid results in complete loss of fiber strength. Bovine collagen showed a decrease of 12 to 16 degrees in the shrinkage temperature, but hardly any loss in fiber strength.

The second type of interaction, i.e., the irreversible fixation of an anion by the cationic protein groups, specific for these groups and not interacting with the coordination active groups of collagen, is exemplified by the binding of polymetaphosphoric acid (molecular weight about 3000) by the two types of collagen (16). By complete inactivation of the basic groups of mammalian collagen, its tensile strength is slightly increased and also its shrinkage temperature, whereas cod collagen after the identical treatment lost 90 to 95 % of its original fiber strength, and the shrinkage temperature was elevated by 1 to 2 degrees. In this instance, greatly impaired tensile strength of the structure was obtained by simple inactivation of the acidic and basic protein groups under conditions leading to dehydration, the opposite of swelling. It is remarkable that hydrothermal stability does show the opposite trend. It was shown by Highberger (17), in his important investigations of formaldehyde tannage, that the mechanical strength of bovine skin fibers in the dry state is lowered by formaldehyde tannage, although the shrinkage temperature is considerably increased. This finding led him to question the validity of the concept of crosslinking as applied to aldehyde tannage. In commenting on Highberger's paper, this author pointed out (18) that the two properties—tensile strength of the fibers and hydrothermal stability—may be functions of entirely different factors. The bridging of polypeptide chains and protofibrils may be conceived as effecting hydrothermal stabilization of the collagen lattice, whereas the tensile strength of the fibers may not be governed by the crosslinking of these units, but instead depend on the cohesion of fibrils and fibers. Speakman (19), Sykes (20), and Mitton (21) have also presented evidence difficult to reconcile with the hypothesis of the degree of crosslinking governing the tensile strength of collagen fibers.

The lack of knowledge of the fine structure of collagen, particularly the distance between the reactive groups on the chains in the protofibril, and on the surface of the protofibril as well as in the interior and the surface of the larger units, such as fibrils and fibers, makes any explanation of these findings highly speculative. Very likely the large polymetaphosphate anion is interacting by multiple attachment to the basic protein groups. There are reasons to believe that, because of the presence of the regularly inter-spaced numerous —O— bridges of the polymetaphosphate molecule, a certain flexibility of the long-chain molecule is achieved, which would facilitate reactions with a number of the active protein groups on adjacent chains. The main argument for the occurrence of crosslinking is supplied by the documentation of the increased shrinkage temperature. Complete inactivation of the ionic linkages *without* swelling would mean a lowering of the shrinkage temperature by 12 to 16 degrees. Evidently the crosslinking more than makes up for the loss in salt links caused by the discharge of the ionic protein groups. The distance between polypeptide chains of hydrated collagen, which is of the order of 16 Å., should then be bridged by the fixed phosphate chains. This discussion pertains to the intermolecular linking of polypeptide chains and protofibrils. Quite different spatial conditions are probably encountered in reactions with the surface layer of the fibrils and fibers. The gap between these units is believed to be too wide to be bridged. It may then be that the surface protein chain of these larger units is covered by a single phosphate chain. This would lead to the discharge of only a fraction of the negative sites of the large phosphate chain by the cationic groups of the surface layer of the fibril and fiber. Since any cohesive forces on these electrovalent groups would be eliminated by the combination taking place, the residual negative charge of the surface layer, imparted by the phosphate fixed, would be expected to increase the gap between the larger units by repulsion. This would be especially disastrous to the mechanical strength of the fishskin, which apparently is stabilized mainly by salt links. These ideas are expressed by the schematic picture of Fig. 24.

3. SOME PHYSICAL PROPERTIES OF COLLAGEN FIBERS AND LEATHER

The question of the cohesive forces operating between the various units of the collagen structure draws our attention to the connection between structure and mechanical strength of the individual fiber or fiber bundles and skin as a whole. The principles of these important problems will now be briefly discussed.

The significance of the intermolecular and interchain linkings of collagen can be stated in a general way: The sum total of physical properties of the structure, such as insolubility, flexibility, and tensile strength, is determined by the degree of mutual interaction between constitutional structural units. The behavior of the protein is directly related to the number, kind, and distribution of the different bonds which hold the collagen molecule together.

The energy required to break the crosslinking bonds that result in rear-

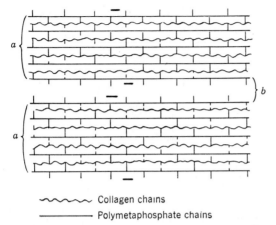

~~~~~ Collagen chains

————— Polymetaphosphate chains

FIG. 24. Schematic idea of the molecular organization of collagen (fishskin) in combination with polymetaphosphate, a representing micelles with phosphate chains riveting together the individual protein chains. The intermicellar gap, b, is assumed to be too wide for bridging by the —POO— ions of the phosphate chain. The surface layers of a will take on negative charge, resulting in widening of the gap, b, by repulsion. The decrease in strength due to the loss of the polar attraction of original collagen will thus be further accentuated.

rangement of chains by denaturation or to separate them mechanically will, apart from the influence of the bond strength, depend also on the environment of the protein. This has been strikingly demonstrated in Lundgren's researches on feather keratin (22). Thus the mechanical behavior of collagen fibers is highly sensitive to variations in the solvent environment. Water has a pronounced influence on the forces operating between the fibers of collagen. For instance, the tensile strength of dry fibers of skin is considerably lowered by swelling of the fiber bundles.

Figure 25 summarizes the various forces acting on a fiber network surrounded by solvent, according to Lundgren (22). The osmotic swelling force, in addition to the mechanical deforming force and the thermal kinetic force, tends to disperse the chains. Opposing these destructive forces are the constructive ones holding the network together, the cohesion of the structure. Further, there is a small contribution by the hydrostatic force of the solvent acting on the fiber. The corresponding changes in energy of the fiber–solvent system may be represented by the equation:

$$\Delta F_s + f\,\Delta L + T\,\Delta S = \Delta E + P\,\Delta V = \Delta H$$

where ΔF_s is the free energy of solvation, i.e., the free-energy decrease involved in the interaction of collagen with the solvent; $f\,\Delta L$ is the mechanical work of deformation, f being the applied force and ΔL the resulting

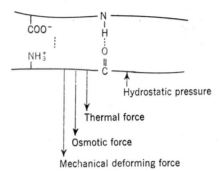

FIG. 25. Schematic representation of dispersive and cohesive forces in the fiber network of proteins in the aqueous system (Lundgren, 22).

elongation; $T \Delta S$ is the change in kinetic energy of the system, T being the absolute temperature and ΔS the change in entropy; ΔE is the change in the fiber network energy; and $P \Delta V$ is the hydrostatic work done, P being the hydrostatic pressure and ΔV the change in volume of collagen.

In view of the different spatial conditions offered by the collagen weave in the form of macro, micro, and molecular units to an interacting agent, particularly tanning agents, the effect of the introduction of these agents on the different properties of the particular units might be expected to manifest itself quite differently in the intermolecular range and among fibers, to name the extremes. The positive effect of crosslinking by the agent would be increased hydrothermal stability, since this is governed by the behavior of the smallest units which offer conditions for crosslinking. The agent introduced, not being able to reinforce the larger units of the order of fibers, would then, in consequence of the reduced number of active sites on the surface chains of the larger units (due to the combination with the agent), decrease the mechanical strength of the fiber. Hence, the term stabilization of the protein structure should not be used indiscriminately; the particular stabilization concerned should be specified.

It can be stated that the tensile strength of the fiber bundles of corium is not a function of the number and strength of the crosslinking bonds of the molecular units, the cohesion of the fiber being an additional factor. Hence, a direct comparison of the shrinkage temperature and the mechanical strength of fibers is not permissible (18). In fibers in equilibrium with water, its dipole nature will probably influence the internal cohesion, especially the strength of the attraction between oppositely charged R groups, affecting the relative strengths of the wet and dry fibers. The distance between the ionic groups is also widened by hydration of collagen. Fiber strength generally decreases with increased moisture content. Drastic drying may lead to markedly increased strength, possibly caused by conversion of ionic crosslinks to covalent links, as mentioned earlier (3). Some water of constitution (bound water), which amounts to about 20 % of the weight of collagen, must be lost in the drying of collagen in the form of chrome leather, for instance, to a moisture content of about 12 %. It is not known if this water is withdrawn from the ionic groups or from the weakly polar groups, such as the peptide groups. It has been assumed, originally by Huggins (23), that the water molecule forms the link between internally

compensated peptide groups, as $\diagdown N \cdot H \cdots O \cdot H \cdots O : C \diagup$, the additional
$$ \diagup H \diagdown$$

water taken up by collagen being coordinated on the molecule of water, functioning as a vehicle for crosslinking.

In a discussion of the mechanical properties of skins and fiber bundles, the issues are frequently confused in that the tensile strength and the degree of elongation of a strip of the whole skin or leather are applied as a measure of the effect of the tannage on the corresponding properties of the fibers. However, data on the strength of skin pieces cannot be used to evaluate the influence of various types of processing, such as tanning, on the strength of the fibers, since the tensile strength measured on a strip of skin really gives the strength of the fiber weave. This aspect of the problem, with due consideration to the effect of various tanning agents on simple fiber bundles, has been particularly stressed by Jovanovitz (24), Chernov, (25) Grassmann (26), and Mitton (27).

Skin has a netlike weave of microscopically fine, endless fibers with a random arrangement. The stretch-force curve (Fig. 26) is S-shaped (28). At first the curve is flat, with a large increase in force producing considerable stretch. This first portion corresponds to the straightening out of the netlike weave of fiber bundles. The next part of the curve is steep, where a large augmentation of force produces relatively little stretch, followed by a flat portion, in which a large force imparts a large stretch. These portions of the curve correspond to the elongation of the tissue itself. The influence of tanning agents on the strength of the fibers should be tested on fiber bundles. It is advisable to tan pieces of the neck of a steer hide with flesh and grain removed or tendons, and after complete tannage to tease out fiber bundles by means of a pincette. The tanning of simple fiber bundles often results in case-hardening of the fibers (24).

As already mentioned, the resilient properties of leather are due to the interweaving of its fiber bundles and may be expected to vary with the principal direction of weave. The elasticity of the leather, denoted as the resilience of the structure, varies with the topographic structure of the skin. The butt part, with the fiber weave vertical to the grain surface, shows the lowest degree of deformation on repeated stretchings; the belly portion,

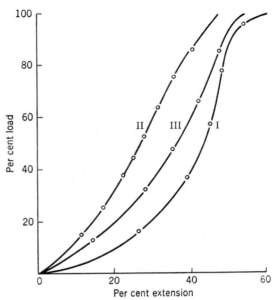

FIG. 26. The degree of extension of fibers of: I, untanned skin (pelt); II, vegetable-tanned leather; III, chrome-tanned leather; on application of a load.

with a horizontal weave pattern, shows the properties of a plastic body. By exposing leather for one hundred repeated stretchings at a load 0.3 of the breaking stress, the increment of elongation, Δl, was determined on samples from the butt, shoulder, and belly portions of a vegetable-tanned steer hide. The following formula was then applied:

$$\Delta l = \frac{(l_{100} - l_1)100}{l_1 - l_o}$$

where Δl = the increment of elongation; l_o = the original length of the strip; l_1 = its length after the first stretching; and l_{100} = its length after the hundredth stretching. The values obtained were: for the butt, 0; for the shoulder, 40; for the belly, 57 (25). Some data on the mechanical properties of the most important fiber materials are given in Table 12.

Although the present discussion is not intended as a general treatise on tanning processes, it seems desirable to outline briefly the main findings as to the effect of tanning processes on the fiber strength of collagen. These findings were based on investigations of single fiber bundles, taken from steer hide, Achilles tendon, kangaroo tail tendon, and rat tail tendon.

Since measurements of tensile strength are referred to the cross section of the fiber, which is very difficult to estimate accurately, the strength of the fiber bundles is better expressed as the mean breaking length (MBL)

TABLE 12

MECHANICAL PROPERTIES OF FIBERS (28)

Material	Tensile strength, kg./mm.²	Mean Breaking Length, km.	Elongation at Break-age, %
Silk	65	—	31
Nylon (drawn)	55	—	25
Collagen (steer hide)	51	39	35
Cotton	44	29	11
Wool	18	14	35

in kilometer. This implies an expression on a weight basis. The results are calculated from the formula:

$$\text{MBL} = \frac{B \times L}{1000W}$$

where B = the breaking load in grams; L = the length of the fiber in millimeters; and W = its weight in grams.

In the earlier investigations of Jovanovitz (24) and Chernov (25), it was found in testing dry fibers that vegetable tannage decreased the tensile strength of the fiber bundles, whereas chrome tannage improved this property. In these experiments, the dry strength of the fibers was determined, since measurement of the wet strength is difficult. It is worthy of notice that the vegetable-tanned *leather* shows greater tensile strength than chrome-tanned *leather*. This is probably due to different weave patterns of the leathers, and different hide substance content.

In view of the risk of case-hardening in tanning of single fiber bundles, a complication noticed long ago by Jovanovitz (24) and more recently by Mao and Roddy (29), the conflicting results obtained by different investigators are not surprising. Thus, Highberger (17), who tanned teased single fiber bundles and examined the dry fibers for strength, found drastic impairment of the tensile strength after tanning with formaldehyde, the decrease being about 65 % of the original value. The fixation of vegetable tannins by the fiber bundles also lowered their strength. Similar results on kangaroo tail tendon, tanned as fiber bundles, has been reported by Compton (30), who found that formaldehyde tanning decreased the MBL from 31 km. to 9 km. (0.4 millimole of formaldehyde fixed by 1 g. of collagen). On the other hand, according to Mao and Roddy (29), who stress the importance of the method of tanning and who tanned "gross pieces" of tendon and teased out the tanned fiber bundles for MBL determinations, the incorporation of tanning agents into the fiber structure does not affect the tensile strength of the fiber bundles, tested after air-drying and the usual conditioning. For untreated bundles and for specimens teased out from "gross pieces" tanned by means of basic chromium salts, vegetable tannins, and formaldehyde, the MBL values were in the range 25 to 26 km. According to these data, the dry strength of the original collagen fibers is not altered by the incorporation of tanning agents. Their finding is in harmony with the view already mentioned, which assumes that interchain cross-linking by tanning agents governs the hydrothermal stability, as evidenced by the shrinkage temperature. According to this concept, the cohesive forces between the larger units should not be affected materially by cross-linking which cannot take place between fibers because of the unfavorable steric conditions, i.e., too wide a gap to be bridged.

In view of the fact that the results of the "gross-piece" technique do not agree with the data obtained from single fiber bundles tanned as such, Mao and Roddy suggest that the data from the latter method of tanning do not include the effect of the fiber relationship as it occurs in skin. In the skin structure, the collagenous fiber bundles are present as an interlocking network with little interspace. This network serves as a filter and delays an otherwise too rapid uptake of the tanning agent, whereas the single fiber bundles come into immediate contact with the tanning agent and are more rapidly tanned, particularly on the surface. Mao and Roddy believe that the "gross-piece technique" more closely simulates the behavior of whole skin in tanning and hence better serves the purpose of studying the effect of tanning processes on fiber structure.

The investigations referred to have all measured the tensile strength of the fiber bundles in the *dry* state. However, the influence of various tanning agents on the strength of the *wet* fibers should be more informative for comparison with the corresponding effect on the hydrothermal stability (shrinkage temperature). Measurements of the mechanical strength of wet and dry synthetic fibers prepared from globular proteins such as casein, ovalbumin, gliadin, and zein, have been reported. The investigations of Nutting and his co-workers (31) are especially informative. They found the tensile strength of highly oriented dry artificial fibers of ovalbumin to be decreased by formaldehyde treatment from 19 to 16 kg. per square millimeter, whereas the strength of wet fibers was improved from 10 to 15 kg. The corresponding figures for the same type of fibers treated with quinone were 19 and 18 kg. in the dry state, and 10 and 15 kg. for the wet fibers. Thus, these types of tannage slightly decrease the tensile strength of the dry fibers but increase their wet strength approximately 50%. In this instance, under comparable conditions, the mechanical strength and the hydrothermal stability of synthetic fibers in a fully hydrated state were both increased by tanning.

In a paper by Jacobson and Lollar (32), the effect of various treatments, including tanning, on the wet strength of kangaroo tail tendon tanned and employed as bundle aggregates has been investigated. The wet strength of the fibers increased after treatments with basic chromium sulfate, mercuric acetate and tetrahydroxytriphenylmethane, whereas it decreased after formaldehyde tannage.

It should be noted, however, that the unknown factor in investigations of the breaking strength of macrofibers is the longitudinal slip involved in the distribution of the strain on various elements of the fibrils, fibers, and fiber bundles. Under the ordinary conditions of measurement of the tensile strength, the elastic elongation is very small (7 to 10 %), and rupture occurs at a load which corresponds to a tensile strength of 10 to 12 kg. per square millimeter. Of course, the mechanism of this rupture does not involve the breaking of the main polypeptide chain (covalent bonds) which would require a load of the order of 300 kg. if the rupture involved the weakest covalent linkage, the —C—N— bond of 1.4-Å. length, with an energy of 49 kcal. per mole (33). This is nearly thirty times as high as the observed tensile strength. It is probable that the fiber bundles and fibers under stress rupture by breaking the lateral cohesive forces between the fibers. Then the fibrils can glide over each other, with consequent rupture of the fiber.

The problem of the effect of various treatments of collagenous fibers on their tensile strength has not yet been solved. From the experimental material presented, in spite of its heterogenity, it may tentatively be concluded that the action of tanning agents of the type presumed to be crosslinking agents of polypeptide chains and protofibrils does not materially affect the mechanical strength of the larger skin units such as fibers and fiber bundles.

The hydrothermal stabilization of collagen in tanning will be discussed in connection with the shrinkage and denaturation of collagen (p. 227).

4. The Hydration of Collagen

Proteins contain two types of hydrophilic groups which are capable of binding water through electrostatic forces and by hydrogen bond formation: (1) the polar side chains and (2) the oxygen and nitrogen atoms of the peptide bond. The number of the latter is generally greater than that of the side chains. In collagen about every fourth residue of the backbone contains a CO=N— group, and hence an uncompensated carbonyl group of the opposite peptide bond, which makes for easy hydration of these groups. The most strongly intermolecularly compensated —CO—NH— groups may not readily function as coordinators of water molecules. A number of the ordinary peptide bonds of collagen which has received alkaline pretreatment and has thus been exposed to swelling forces should be capable of functioning as centers of hydration. This point will be further discussed.

Bull ((34) has claimed that nylon illustrates the fact that peptide carbonyl and imido groups have little affinity for water. Although hexamethylene-diamine and adipic acid supply about 900 moles of CO— and NH— groups per 10^5 g. of nylon, they bind only about 100 moles of water in the weight given. However, by no means does the low degree of hydration of this polyamide constitute evidence for the behavior of the peptide bonds of ordinary proteins toward water in general, in view of the strongly developed hydrogen bonding of the opposite —CO·NH— groups in the nylon chains, with the close approach made possible through the close packing of paral-lelly aligned chains under the most favorable steric conditions, i.e., with the small hydrogen atom as the only side group. The behavior of silk fibroin toward water is similar to that of nylon for the very same reason, although the less strongly developed internal compensation of the peptide bonds of silk, and the presence of ionic groups and some bulkier side chains, makes the affinity of this protein for water greater than that of nylon.

The S-shaped curve which is obtained by plotting the amount of moisture sorbed by collagen from air of different degrees of relative humidity after established equilibrium shows some interesting characteristics (35) (Fig. 27). In the first part of the curve, the water adsorption increases rapidly with the increase in vapor pressure. The next section of the curve shows a much slower slope and a more linear dependence up to 65% humidity. Finally, in the part of the curve corresponding to high relative humidity, the uptake of moisture by collagen increases very rapidly with the aug-mented vapor tension.

A certain minimum amount of water in intimate association with the protein appears to be required for the maintenance of the physical proper-ties of collagen and leather (tanned collagen) at an optimal level. This water may be considered to be bound water which in many respects is similar to the water of constitution of crystalline substances and hence may be considered as the water of constitution of the protein lattice in its natural state. The amount of bound water in the form of water of hydration of collagen appears to be about 20% of the weight of the protein.

In collagen in the fully hydrated state, the peptide chains or protofibrils are freed from the restriction in motion prevailing in the dry state, which probably explains the fundamental function of water for the physical properties of collagen. Bull (34) suggests that first a layer of water mole-cules is taken up between two planes of the protein molecule. This fraction represents the first part of the curve of sorption. Since this layer of water is shared by neighboring protein chains, it should be tightly bound. The straight intermediate part of the adsorption curve then represents a meas-ure of the completion of a second layer of water molecules between the protein planes. It is interesting to note that Bull finds the water of hydra-

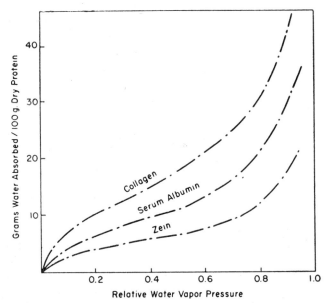

FIG. 27. Adsorption of water vapor by dry proteins. From F. Haurowitz, "Chemistry and Biology of Proteins," p. 91, Fig. 24. Academic Press, New York, 1950.

tion to be about 21 % of the weight of the protein. Further, his data indicate that most of the heat, up to the 20 % hydration level, is involved in the combination of the polar groups with water which leads to forcing these residues apart. It has been mentioned earlier that the distance between adjacent polypeptide chains of dry collagen, on the side of the electrovalent links, is about 10Å. By hydration this distance increases to 15 to 16Å., and hence Bull's theory is in harmony with the X-ray findings on this particular point. Since the water of hydration of proteins is independent of the pH value of the medium in which collagen is equilibrated, the conclusion seems justified that all bound water is not held by electrostatic forces by the ionic groups, which vary considerably in number with the pH value.

Pauling (36) believes that for some proteins the initial water adsorption takes place to the extent of one water molecule per polar side chain capable of forming hydrogen bonds. There is good agreement between the number of molecules of water initially sorbed by the proteins and the number of their polar groups. For collagen with a mean residue weight of 93, the presence of one molecule of water attached to each residue would mean approximately 20 % water of hydration on the basis of dry protein, which was the amount experimentally obtained. It is interesting to note, as Pauling points out, that the amount of water adsorbed initially by collagen, or 530 moles per 10^5 g. of protein, is much larger than the number of polar side chains, which is about 330, and somewhat smaller than the total number of polar groups including the peptide bonds available on links opposite to the peptide bond-forming proline and hydroxyproline residues. This fact supports the suggestion that these particular carbonyl groups of the peptide bond are capable of binding water to a degree of stability comparable with that of the polar side chains. Pauling seems inclined to the view that peptide carbonyl and imide groups usually do not bind water because of their mutual interaction by hydrogen bond formation. Further, he believes that water is bound by carbonyl groups which are not coupled by hydrogen bonds with imide groups such as are present in collagen (adjacent to CO—N= links).

It appears to the author of this book that the function of the peptide bond in water binding by hydrogen bonding has been too lightly dismissed. It must be emphasized that there is no doubt that part of the hydration of collagen and proteins generally occurs at the ionic groups by hydrogen bonding, in view of the X-ray evidence showing extension of the gap between the protein backbone of the partners in the salt link on wetting of collagen. However, the salt links are few in number, and only a small part of the bound water can be accommodated by these strongly ionic side chains. The main argument against the participation of the carbonyl and imide groups of the peptide bond in hydration is the fact that polyamides, such as nylon, evidently bind only small amounts of water. However, nylon should by no means be considered as a prototype of fiber proteins of the collagen class, since the hydrogen bonds of nylon are much stronger than those of collagen. However, by introducing a copolymer into the polyamide chain of nylon, some degree of structural irregularity is forced on the chains, which makes for solubility of the modified nylon in hydroxyl-containing solvents such as methanol (37). The polyamide obtained by spinning the methanol solution of the modified nylon into water, in appearance very much like ordinary hide powder, contains in equilibrium with air of 60% relative humidity about 5% water on the basis of the dry weight of stock (37). With a mean residue weight of about 115, an amount of water of 16%, based on the weight of the polyamide, should represent the state of each —CO·NH— group coordinating with one molecule of water. Allowing for the small amount of water taken up by terminal groups, about every third —CO—NH— group of the modified polyamide should be hydrated. Hence, in the case of collagen, apart from the water binding of the strongly polar side chains and the free carbonyls in proximity to CO—N= groups, the hydration of some of the ordinary —CO—NH— groups appears reasonable, particularly in limed collagen.

The free energy, ΔF, required to transfer 1 g. of water molecules from the vapor state to the protein surface is given by the equation:

$$\Delta F = \frac{RT}{M} \int \frac{a\,dx}{x}$$

where R is the gas constant, a is the weight of water sorbed by 100 g. of protein, x is the relative vapor pressure of water, and M is the molecular weight of water.

From the sorption curves at two temperatures, the differential heat of adsorption, ΔH, can be calculated by means of the Clapeyron-Clasius equation:

$$\Delta H = 2.3R \frac{T \times T_1}{T_1 - T} \log \frac{P_1}{P}$$

where P and P_1 are the vapor pressures of water in equilibrium with the collagen at the absolute temperatures of T and T_1. In these calculations, the log of the vapor pressure is plotted against the amount of water adsorbed. The value of the heat adsorption varies somewhat with the temperature and the extent of water adsorption, i.e., according to the relative humidity. Below a water content of 20% of the weight of collagen, the figure averages 13.5 kcal. per mole.

As already mentioned, the hydration of dry collagen probably occurs in steps of various energy content, involving protein groups of different degrees of strength and reactivity. This was indicated in the experimental studies of Kanagy (35) and Wollenberg (38), who investigated the heat of wetting of unlimed hide substance between 0 and 60°C. The heat of wetting showed a strong temperature dependence, with values from about 50 cal. per gram of protein at 0°C. to about 16 cal. at 60°C. The value for limed hide is about 40 cal. at 15°C. The heat of adsorption of collagen found was of the order of 13 kcal. per mole. Since the heat of adsorption of moisture decreases rapidly with temperature increase, the sorption of water will decrease with increasing temperature of the system. This has some practical consequences for the use of leather.

As to the sorption isotherm of collagen, and some related fiber proteins shown in Fig. 27, the equilibrium between collagen and air of 60% relative humidity corresponds to 20% moisture on the basis of collagen, or a quantity about equal to one molecule of water on each amino acid residue. Formation of water bridges between adjacent peptide bonds intermolecularly compensated, as suggested by Huggins (23), the originator of the concept of hydrogen bridges, is a possibility, as is also the binding of the water molecules jointly by two adjacent groups of the same amino acid residue, e.g., the guanidyl groups (Pauling, 36).

The water present as water of hydration is considered to be incapable of functioning as a solvent for electrolytes and nonelectrolytes. Using the latter class of substances, such as various sugars, Eilers and Labout (39) found values of about 20 % for the water actually bound to collagen. The degree of hydration was independent of the pH value of the system, in the pH range 1 to 10. Neutral salts of anions placed ahead of the chloride ion in the lyotropic series, for example, sulfate, decreased the hydration, whereas neutral salts beyond the chloride ion in this series tended to increase the bound water. The Dutch investigators' figures indicate that chrome tannage will increase the degree of hydration, and vegetable tannage will tend to decrease this property. However, the nonsolvent technique is not reliable for the estimation of the hydration of leather, since secondary reactions between tanning agents and the indicating substances cannot be wholly eliminated, according to this author's personal experience (37).

It appears that the best method available of establishing the degree of hydration, combining simplicity with a fair degree of accuracy, is the determination of the equilibrium moisture content of collagen and leather after prolonged conditioning of the stock in an atmosphere of 55 to 65 % relative humidity at 25°C. Holland (40) has used this method, evidently with great satisfaction. The importance of the degree of hydration of collagen for the properties of leather is now fully realized. Conditioning of leathers at 60 to 65 % humidity has a beneficial influence on their working qualities, independent of the type of tannage. Wilson (41) has proved that the moisture content of leather has a marked effect on its various physical properties, such as tensile strength, grain flexibility, stretch, area, and resilience. The moisture content of sole leather is an important factor in wear; soles of low moisture content show loss of wearing quality. Chrome-tanned upper leather with moisture content insufficient to secure complete hydration of its collagen generally develops brittleness of the grain membrane and loss in fiber strength. Holland found 20 % water of hydration, on the basis of collagen, in ordinary hide powder. From his study of the moisture content of gelatin as a function of the vapor pressure, Katz (42) obtained values of 20 to 21 %. Bull's figures (34) are of the same order of magnitude. The amount of water in chrome leather was 21 % also. The degree of hydration of collagen was lowered by vegetable tannage, values of 13 to 17 % being recorded.

During the hydration of proteins, the total volume of the system decreases, and hence the process can be followed dilatometrically. Theis and his co-workers (43) have applied this method in studies of the hydration of gelatin and collagen as a function of the hydrogen ion concentration. Unfortunately, they interpreted their results to imply that the hydration decreases with decreasing pH, and that the degree of hydration of proteins is a function of hydrogen ion concentration of the system, reaching its maximum at the isoelectric point. However, the dilatation observed at decreasing pH values of the system hide substance—hydrochloric acid solutions, from the isoelectric point to the pH of maximum swelling, or to a pH of about 1.5, is *not* a measure of the hydration of the protein, as Theis *et al.* state. Recalculation of Theis dilatometric figures has shown (44) that the removal of protons from the acid solution by the protein, which results in complete discharge of the carboxylic ions, is accompanied by a dilatation of 10 ml. per mole proton (44), which closely agrees with the theoretical value of 12 ml. (45). Actually, the hydration of proteins is independent of the pH value.

REFERENCES

1. Speakman, J. B., and Hirst, M. C., *Nature* **128,** 1073 (1931); *Proc. Roy. Soc.* **A132,** 167 (1931); *Trans. Faraday Soc.* **29,** 148 (1933); **30,** 539 (1934); **31,** 1425 (1935); **32,** 897 (1936); Astbury, W. T., "Fundamentals of Fibre Structure," Oxford University Press, London, 1933.
2. Astbury, W. T., and Marwick, A., *Nature* **128,** 309 (1932); Astbury, W. T., *Trans. Faraday Soc.* **29,** 139 (1932).
3. Lloyd, D. J., Marriott, R. H., and Pleass, W. B., *Trans. Faraday Soc.* **29,** 554 (1933).
4. Pauling, L., and Niemann, C., *J. Am. Chem. Soc.* **61,** 1866 (1939).
4a. Gustavson, K. H., *Acta Chem. Scand.* **8,** 1299 (1954).
4b. Huggins, M. L., *J. Am. Chem. Soc.* **76,** 4045 (1954).
5. Crammer, J. L., and Neuberger, A., *Biochem. J.* **37,** 302 (1943).
6. Klotz, I. M., and Urquhart, J. M., *J. Am. Chem. Soc.* **71,** 1597 (1949); Klotz, I. M., *Cold Spring Harbor Symposia Quant. Biol.* **14,** 97 (1950); Klotz, I. M., and Ayers, J., *Discussions Faraday Soc.* **No. 13,** 189 (1953); for an excellent review see Klotz, I. M., *in* "The Proteins" (H. Neurath and K. Bailey, eds.), Vol. 1, Part B, pp. 788, 789, 792. Academic Press, New York, 1953.
7. Neuman, R. E., and Logan, M. A., *J. Biol. Chem.* **184,** 299 (1950).
8. Gustavson, K. H., *Svensk Kem. Tidskr.* **65,** 70 (1953).
8a. Borasky, R., and Takahashi, T., private communications.
9. Roche, J., and Blanc-Jean, G., *Compt. rend.* **210,** 681 (1940).
10. Grabar, P., and Morel, J., *Bull. soc. chim. biol.* **32,** 643 (1950); Morel, J., and Grabar, P., *ibid.* **32,** 630 (1950).
11. Speakman, J. B., and Stott, E., *J. Soc. Dyers Colourists* **50,** 341 (1934); cf. Plimmer, R. H. A., *J. Chem. Soc.* **127,** 2651 (1925).
12. Ames, W. M., *J. Soc. Chem. Ind.* **63,** 200, 234, 277, 303 (1944).
13. Grassmann, W., and Schneider, F., *Biochem. Z.* **273,** 452 (1934).
13a. Schwert, G. W., Neurath, H., Kaufman, S., and Snoke, J. E., *J. Biol. Chem.* **172,** 221 (1948).
14. Gustavson, K. H., *Biochem. Z.* **311,** 347 (1942); *Advances in Protein Chem.* **5,** 353 (1949); *Acta Chem. Scand.* **4,** 1171 (1950).
15. Gustavson, K. H., *Acta Chem. Scand.* **4,** 1171 (1950); see also Pankhurst, K. G. A., *J. Soc. Leather Trades Chem.* **37,** 312 (1953).
16. Gustavson, K. H., *J. Am. Leather Chem. Assoc.* **45,** 789 (1950); *J. Soc. Leather Trades Chem.* **33,** 332 (1949); Gustavson, K. H., and Larsson, A., *Acta Chem. Scand.* **5,** 1221 (1951).
17. Highberger, J. H., *J. Am. Leather Chem. Assoc.* **42,** 493 (1947).

18. Gustavson, K. H., *J. Am. Leather Chem. Assoc.* **43**, 741, 744 (1948).
19. Speakman, J. B., *J. Soc. Leather Trades Chem.* **37**, 37 (1953).
20. Sykes, R. L., *J. Soc. Leather Trades Chem.* **37**, 294 (1953).
21. Mitton, R. G., and Nattrass, E. F., *J. Soc. Leather Trades Chem.* **34**, 299 (1950).
22. Lundgren, H. P., *Advances in Protein Chem.* **5**, 305 (1949).
23. Huggins, M. L., *Chem. Revs.* **32**, 195 (1943); *Ann. Rev. Biochem.* **11**, 28 (1943).
24. Jovanovitz, J. A., *Collegium* **1932**, 215; Jovanovitz, J. A., and Alge, A., *ibid.* **1932**, 222.
25. Chernov, N. W., *J. Intern. Soc. Leather Trades Chem.* **20**, 121 (1936).
26. Grassmann, W., *Kolloid-Z.* **77**, 205 (1936).
27. Mitton, R. G., *J. Intern. Soc. Leather Trades Chem.* **29**, 169 (1945); see also ref. 21, and Nice, G. R., *ibid.* **35**, 17 (1951).
28. Grassmann, W., *Das Leder* **1**, 57 (1950).
29. Mao, T. J., and Roddy, W. T., *J. Am. Leather Chem. Assoc.* **45**, 131 (1950); Roddy, W. T., *ibid.* **47**, 98 (1952).
30. Compton, E. D., *J. Am. Leather Chem. Assoc.* **44**, 140 (1949).
31. Senti, F. R., Copley, M. J., and Nutting, G. C., *J. Phys. Chem.* **49**, 192 (1945); Nutting, G. C., Halwer, M., Copley, M. J., and Senti, F. R., *Textile Research J.* **16**, 599 (1946); Senti, F. R., *Am. Dyestuff Reptr.* **36**, 230 (1947).
32. Jacobson, J. H., and Lollar, R. M., *J. Am. Leather Chem. Assoc.* **46**, 7 (1951).
33. See Highberger, J. H., *J. Am. Leather Chem. Assoc.* **42**, 493 (1947); Pauling, L., "The Nature of the Chemical Bond." Cornell University Press, Ithaca, N. Y., 1940; Meyer, K. H., and Mark, H., "Der Aufbau der hochpolymeren organischen Naturstoffe." Akademische Verlagsges., Leipzig, 1930.
34. Bull, H. B., *J. Am. Chem. Soc.* **66**, 1499 (1944).
35. Kanagy, J. R., *J. Am. Leather Chem. Assoc.* **45**, 12 (1950).
36. Pauling, L., *J. Am. Chem. Soc.* **67**, 555 (1945).
37. Gustavson, K. H., unpublished data; see also Gustavson, K. H., and Holm, B., *J. Am. Leather Chem. Assoc.* **47**, 700 (1952).
38. Wollenberg, H. G., *J. Soc. Leather Trades Chem.* **36**, 172 (1952).
39. Eilers, H., and Labout, J., *in* "Fibrous Proteins," p. 30. Society of Dyers and Colourists, Leeds, 1946.
40. Holland, H. C., *J. Intern. Soc. Leather Trades Chem.* **27**, 207 (1943).
41. Wilson, J. A., "The Chemistry of Leather Manufacture," Vol. 2. Chemical Catalog Co., New York, 1929.
42. Katz, J. R., *Ergeb. exakt. Naturw.* **3**, 316 (1924).
43. Theis, E. R., and Neville, H. A., *Ind. Eng. Chem.* **21**, 377 (1929); **22**, 64, 66 (1930).
44. Gustavson, K. H., *Ind. Eng. Chem.* **23**, 1298 (1931); *J. Am. Leather Chem. Assoc.* **27**, 40 (1932).
45. Weber, H. H., *Biochem. Z.* **218**, 1 (1930); Weber, H. H., and Nachmansohn, D., *ibid.* **204**, 215 (1929).

CHAPTER 7

Swelling of Collagen, Donnan Effects

1. SWELLING

The swelling of insoluble proteins and gels has been studied mainly in collagen of skin and gelatin gels in solutions of acids and bases. In the early investigations, and even in the majority of more recent contributions, the degree of swelling has been measured in terms of the amount of water taken up, which has been estimated by the increase in weight of the substrate. This method is quite satisfactory for gels. For the collagen of skin, which possesses a highly orderly structure, the mechanism of swelling should be considered (i.e., apart from the amount of solution imbibed by the substrate) in relation to the volume changes, by determining the changes in fiber length and width. These changes are typical results of the swelling, which is due to alteration of the electrostatic conditions of the ionic protein groups. This important point has been emphasized by Lloyd particularly (1). Such dimensional data will give a measure of the degree of structural organization of the fiber which shows anisotropic properties.

The effect of structural restraint on the degree of swelling is evident when the collagen fiber of native hide, containing about 33 % protein and 67 % water, is compared with a gelatin gel of corresponding protein content (2). The latter shows much greater swelling because the intermolecular forces are not able to act against the inflow of water, as is the case in the fibrous structure with its strong cohesive forces (see Fig. 28). The free water in the fiber weave of corium is considerably less than the free water in the gelatin jelly of equal protein concentration. The constrictive effect of the fiber weave of the hide on the swelling of collagen is very strong. Thus, isolated fiber bundles of oxhide will take up about twenty times their weight of water at the point of maximum swelling, whereas the whole hide takes up only three to four times its own weight of water (3).

The degree of swelling may be determined by noting the increase in weight of the swelled substrate; in this way fibers and gels may be compared. The effect of the degree of the molecular organization of various protein fibers may then be established. This is graphically illustrated in Fig. 28, which shows the degree of swelling of the substrate in terms of the amount of water associated with the dry fibers, on equilibration in solutions of hydrochloric acid and sodium hydroxide, as a function of the pH value (4). For comparison, the curve of the swelling of a gelatin gel (12 %) is

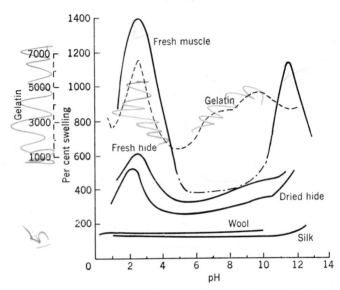

FIG. 28. The degree of swelling of various fibrous proteins as a function of the pH values of the equilibrated solutions.

included, on an ordinate reduced to one-tenth of the scale shown for the fibers. These data have been selected with regard to the different degrees of orientation and stability of the structures, decreasing in the order: silk, keratin, collagen, muscle fiber, and gelatin gel. The curves are of interest from the following points of view: The closely packed strongly hydrogen-bonded silk fibroin, practically devoid of acid- and base-binding groups, and the extremely stable keratin structure, stabilized by means of the covalent —S—S— bridge and strong hydrogen bonds, are practically inert to the swelling action of hydrogen and hydroxyl ions in the pH range 1 to 12. In view of the low content of ionic groups in the silk fibroin, this inertness to acids and bases would be expected. On the other hand, in the case of keratin, with its fair degree of acid- and base-binding power, conditions for swelling are present. Its nonappearance is caused by the efficient cross-linking of the chains. Collagen, which lacks the covalent interchain bridge and is not so effectively internally stabilized as keratin, and which also contains a fair amount of strong ionic groups, comparable to that of keratin, is more susceptible to the swelling action of acid and bases than keratin. In the muscle proteins, the less-developed internal cohesion makes for large swelling. And, finally, the gelatin gel, without definite structural characteristics or any definite scheme of orientation, swells enormously. Since gelatin and collagen possess practically identical capacities for binding of acids and bases, the difference in resistance of the two proteins to swelling agents is an outstanding example of the governing importance of the internal cohesion of proteins in controlling their behavior and properties (4).

Some other interesting points are: (1) the gradual change in the general form of the curves, with the maximum becoming less and less conspicuous and finally disappearing; (2) the formation of a zone of stability in a more or less wide pH range around the pH value of the isoelectric point, in which variations of pH have hardly any influence on the extent of swelling. A certain minimum concentration of H and OH ions appears to be necessary for breaking the internal compensation of ionic side chains, the salt links, in the isoelectric zone. Hence, the number and the strength of these links will in part determine the extent of the isoelectric zone. The water associated with the proteins in this range is not water of swelling. The latter is therefore not correctly measured by the curves. In fact, the free water associated with and due to the swelling of proteins should be measured by taking the curve at the isoelectric zone as the base level, i.e., by letting this part of the curve coincide with the abscissa. The water of collagen in the isoelectric state is composed of water of hydration and water mechanically held in the interstices of the skin.

At this point, it is advisable to point out that, apart from the osmotic swelling in solutions of acid and bases, associated with the strongly ionic protein groups and their charges, another type of swelling, the lyotropic, has to be recognized, which is due mainly to interactions of ions and molecules with the protein with nonionic bonds, probably crosslinks of the hydrogen bond type. In *osmotic swelling*, the fibers decrease in length but increase in diameter. In *lyotropic swelling*, on the other hand, only the width of the fibers increases, as a result of the lessened cohesion and the separation of the component fibrils. The swelling of collagen in neutral solutions, for instance in lyotropic neutral salts, is of the latter type, whereas both types of swelling are to be found in the effect produced on collagen by solutions of weak acids, such as acetic acid at pH values in the vicinity of 2. In strongly alkaline solution, particularly of bivalent metal hydroxides such as calcium hydroxide, of pH values greater than 10, the lyotropic swelling of collagen plays an important part, in addition to the osmotic effects and the alterations in the ionic and coordinate crosslinks which occur on prolonged interaction and which are partly irreversible.

The absorption of water by the protein in the swelling of skin treated in acid and alkaline solutions has long been recognized in leather manufacture as occurring in two different ways: (1) swelling of the type of the plumping effect, which imparts a turgent and translucent appearance to the skin on treatment in acid or alkaline solutions in the absence of dissolved neutral salts; (2) swelling under absorption of water by the skin, resulting from its treatment in neutral solutions of certain salts, in which case the skin remains flaccid and opaque. The fibers of plumped skin are glassy and pressed together, whereas in salt-swelled skin the fibers are split into fibrils and the fiber weave is loose. The plumping effect is further characterized by a shortening of the fibers, which can be completely reversed by loading the fiber; about 1 kg. per square millimeter suffices. The swelling which takes place in solutions of lyotropic neutral salts at pH values corresponding to the isoelectric zone of collagen, which also may accompany the pure osmotic effect of plumping by acids and bases, leads only to an increase in the width of the fiber. Moreover, lyotropic swelling of the fiber is not reversed by loading of the fiber. It can only be partially reversed by removal of the lyotropic agent; a more or less marked *permanent* swelling effect is produced. Another difference between swelling by plumping and lyotropic swelling by salts is that the former is depressed by the addition of neutral salts to the solution, and usually it is completely reversible. If the swelling is unduly prolonged, however, concomitant irreversible changes in the structure take place.

The swelling of skin in solutions of weak acids of moderate concentration, for instance in a 3 M solution of acetic acid of pH about 2, involves both the electrostatic or osmotic effect, and the lyotropic or Hofmeister effect (5). In this instance the lyotropic effect dominates. In fact, it is then not a specific ion effect but a specific molecular effect, since the un-ionized acid is the effective swelling agent, probably by competing with the peptide groups involved in the intermolecular linking of the protein chains, which results in a partial rupture of the hydrogen bond crosslinks and association of acetic acid molecules with the freed CO— groups of the —CO—NH— bond (6).

In solutions of strong bases, such as sodium hydroxide, the osmotic effect is more marked and the lyotropic effect less prominent, provided that the treatment is not unduly prolonged. In that event, the marked swelling and contraction of the fibers will lead to severance of crosslinks and furthermore will create unfavorable steric conditions for the re-forming of the crosslinking on reduction of the swelling. These effects are secondary, and hence they are not directly related to the swelling associated with the reactivity of the ionic protein groups. By treating skin in alkaline solutions of moderately strong bivalent bases, such as calcium hydroxide, the Hofmeister effect predominates. The splitting of the fiber into its constituent fibrils is one of the most important changes brought about by the alkali, and in fact this change in fiber structure is one of the great advantages derived from liming of skin in the manufacture of leather.

Table 13 summarizes the various factors of the osmotic effect and the lyotropic effect which take part in and affect the swelling and cohesion

TABLE 13

OSMOTIC (DONNAN) AND LYOTROPIC SWELLING OF COLLAGEN (7)

Action of	Effect of Osmotic Swelling	Effect of Lyotropic Swelling
Hydrogen ions	Maximum swelling at pH 2, reduced at lower or higher pH	At high concentrations cohesion is impaired
Neutral salts	Reduced swelling	No effect
Nonionized acid (molecular effect)	—	Weakened cohesion
Temperature increase	Increased swelling	Weakened cohesion
Specific ion effects { Valency of anion	Increasing valency, less swelling	—
Affinity of anion for collagen	Increasing affinity, reduced swelling	—
Lyotropic effect	—	As a rule, the cohesion is reduced, depending on the position of the anion in the lyotropic series

of collagen in solutions with pH values below the isoelectric point of limed collagen (7).

In the evaluation of swelling by the customary method of observing changes in the weight of the substrate, there is no means of distinguishing between water uptake caused by increased osmotic pressure and that due to diminished cohesion within the collagen structure. However, from indirect evidence it is often possible to ascertain which type of swelling is dominant. In the technology of leather, the dimensional changes are of greater importance than changes in weight, since the former can be correlated with a number of physical properties of the final leather, particularly the smoothness of the grain, its tightness, and the stretch and extensibility of the skin structure. Furthermore, from the theoretical point of view, it is important to ascertain the shape and the size of the fiber structure. Lloyd early realized the significance of this problem. The graphs of Fig. 29, taken from a paper by Lloyd, Marriott, and Pleass (8), show the influence of the pH values of the solutions (hydrochloric acid and sodium hydroxide) on the volume, length, and width of single collagen fiber bundles, in both the fresh and the dry state. The much lower swelling of the dry fibers is noteworthy, as is also the fact that the maximum swelling property of the dry fibers is attained at a decidedly lower pH value than for the fresh wet fibers. This is probably due to the greater internal cohesion of the dry fibers. The width of the fiber bundles increases over the greater part of the pH range covered,

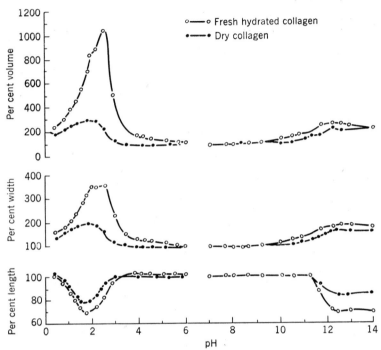

FIG. 29. Changes in length, width, and volume of collagen fiber bundles on equilibration with solutions of various pH values, adjusted with HCl or NaOH.

whereas the length decreases. Since collagen contains a fair amount of rather strong positively and negatively charged side chains, which at the maximum state of charge partially compensate and attract each other, a certain potential of H and OH ions is required for severance of this internal compensation by the discharge of the corresponding oppositely charged groups. The freeing of these ionic groups will lead to the establishing of a Donnan membrane potential inside the fibers. This will in turn lead to an inflow of water for equalization of the concentration of ions inside the substrate and in the external solution. These changes may be expected to distort the structure, by twisting the fibrils, shortening their length, and expanding them across their diameter. The fibrils are restrained by the structural environment and hence will be pressed together. This is shown by the turgidity and translucense of the swelled skin, which is described by the leather technologist as the plumping of the skin.

2. The Donnan Effects (9)

The osmotic swelling that is due to the presence of charged protein groups may be considered a result either of the Donnan membrane equilibrium set up or of the alterations of the electrical charge on the protein. The freeing of charged groups by discharge of their oppositely charged partners by means of H or OH ions is accompanied by electrostatic repulsion of the charged groups carrying the same sign of charge. Water is thus allowed to flow into the gaps formed in the partly disorganized structure. This concept has been developed mathematically by Tolman and Stearn (10), and the application of the Donnan membrane equilibrium by Procter and Wilson (11) represents a classical contribution to the chemistry of leather.

It seems to the author that the idea of the electrostatic mechanism advanced by Kuhn and Katchalsky (12) for polymethacrylates may have a counterpart in the swelling of collagen. It may be of greater value than the Donnan concept, which is not applicable to some of the most important reactions of collagen.

Since the equations for the Donnan equilibrium are treated in most textbooks on the physical chemistry of proteins (13) and the Procter-Wilson extension of the Donnan effect has received its due attention in the literature on the chemistry of leather, particularly in Wilson's monumental monograph (14), only the essentials of the theory will be outlined here.

In the reactions of insoluble proteins such as collagen with acids or bases in aqueous solution, conditions exist for the establishment of the Donnan equilibrium between collagen and the external solution, because there are present nondiffusible ions in the protein network (e.g., charged NH_3^+-groups in the case of an acid system) and diffusible anions in the acid. The presence of the nondiffusible ions leads to an unequal distribution of the diffusible ions between the solid phase and the external solution. This is illustrated by the following tabulation, showing the distribution of the concentrations of the various ions within the collagen structure and in the solutions of hydrochloric acid after equilibration of the system. The concentrations are given in millimoles per liter.

DISTRIBUTION OF H AND CL IONS BETWEEN COLLAGEN AND SOLUTIONS AT EQUILIBRIUM

Collagen		Solution	
Ion	Concentration	Ion	Concentration
Collagen$^+$	z	H^+	x
H^+	y	Cl^-	x
Cl^-	$y + z$		

Even in his early work (15), Procter recognized that gelatin combines with hydrochloric acid to form an almost completely ionized chloride. He also conceived the resulting equilibrium to be a special case of the Donnan membrane equilibria. In the subsequent development of the swelling theory by Procter in collaboration with Wilson (15), independently by Burton (16); and by the Wilsons (17), it was proved that the system could be treated quantitatively according to the laws of physical chemistry on the simple assumption that hydrochloric acid combines with the protein to yield a highly ionizable chloride.

The ionic distributions given above are derived from the following reasoning. The ions of hydrochloric acid interdiffuse into the collagen structure, some of the hydrogen ions combining with the carboxyl ions of collagen, the corresponding chloride ions being electrostatically compensated by the cationic protein groups but present in the form of ions. Consequently the solution inside the collagen network will contain more chloride ions than hydrogen ions. Therefore the Donnan equation is applicable. The law of mass action gives the equation $x^2 = y(y + z)$, since the product of the concentrations of hydrogen and chloride ions must be equal in the external solution and in the collagen phase. In the equation given, the product of equals is equated with the product of unequals, from which it follows that the sum of the unequals is greater than the sum of the equals: $2y + z > 2x$. If the excess of diffusible ions of the solid phase is e, then it follows that $2y + z = 2x + e$. The difference in the distribution of the ions between the two phases gives rise to a difference in osmotic pressure and also to an electrical potential difference between the two phases. This potential difference is governed by the equation:

$$E = \frac{RT}{F} \log_e \frac{y}{x}$$

This equation, expressed in volts, is of fundamental importance in the theory of membranes and protein behavior.

According to the Wilsons (17), the chloride ion inside the collagen network tends to diffuse out into the external solution, since its concentration in the solid phase is greater than in the external solution. However, the chloride-ions cannot diffuse without dragging their protein cations with them, and this is hindered by the cohesive forces of the collagen structure which resist the outward pull. This force is equal to the excess of anions, e. According to Hooke's law, $e = CV$, where C is a constant corresponding to the bulk modulus of the protein and V is the increase in volume, in milliliters per millimole of collagen. The importance of the cohesion of the structure was first recognized by Procter and Burton (16). With the value of the bulk modulus and the equilibrium constant of the system known, the distribution of any strong acid in reversible equilibrium with collagen can be calculated. The real difficulty is the approximation of C, which varies with the properties of collagen, its previous history, and the temperature.

Another difficulty is the postulate of the nonreactivity of the anion with collagen.

The equalization of the distribution of ions in the system can as easily be conceived as being a result of the water induced to flow into the collagen structure in order to reduce the concentration of the anions in the solid phase. The water flowing into the capillary spaces of collagen will produce swelling.

When the original equation given above is presented in the form $e = 2y + z - 2x$, it is evident that the value of z, the positive charge of collagen (the degree of discharged carboxyl ions), is a function of the hydrogen ion concentration of the system. On the addition of acid, the value of z will at first increase rapidly, until all the carboxyl ions have been discharged, i.e., until all cationic protein groups have been freed. By an additional increase in the hydrogen ion concentration, z will remain constant but the value of x will increase. Accordingly, the value of e will first increase until a maximum is reached, and then decline. The maximum value of e coincides with the pH value of the maximum swelling of collagen, a condition that is considered by many to be one of the strongest experimental supports of the Procter-Wilson concept. The depressing effect of neutral salts on the swelling, for instance that of sodium chloride, is also satisfactorily explained by this theory, since as x increases, the value of e decreases. In other words, the difference in anion concentration between the two phases will be reduced. Of course, the osmotic effect of the added salt is a contributing factor.

The Procter-Wilson concept also accounts for the fact that the swelling power of a dibasic strong acid such as sulfuric acid is only about half that of hydrochloric acid of identical pH value. In this case, the concentration of sulfate ions of the equilibrated solution is equal to $x/2$, and that of the collagen structure is equal to $(y + z)/2$. By inserting these values in the equation for e, the value of e is obtained and hence a measure of the degree of swelling. The system collagen–strong base solutions can be treated in the corresponding manner. The difference in swelling of collagen by sodium hydroxide and by calcium hydroxide at a common pH may be explained by the same reasoning as was given for the acid system, as will be shown. It should be noted, however, that the agreement between theory and experiment is less satisfactory in alkaline solutions and, above all, that the neutral salts, such as sodium chloride added to a solution of sodium hydroxide, do not reduce the swelling of collagen. It should also be realized that there are other means of explaining the swelling action of strong acids and bases on collagens, for example by the electrostatic theory, particularly on the basis of the Kuhn-Katchalsky model (12).

TABLE 14

OSMOTIC SWELLING OF PELT (SKIN) BY NaOH AND Ca(OH)$_2$

Time of Treatment, Days	Osmotic Swelling, %		Ratio of Swelling, NaOH:Ca(OH)$_2$
	NaOH	Ca(OH)$_2$	
1	159	83	1.91:1
2	154	85	1.81:1
7	149	102	1.46:1

The swelling of skin in saturated solutions of calcium hydroxide, usually in the form of a suspension of lime, is important both theoretically and practically, in view of its technical application in unhairing and conditioning of skins and hides in the manufacture of leather. The investigations of Marriott (18) have contributed materially to our knowledge of this complicated system. By treating pieces of pelt in lime water ($N/20$ calcium hydroxide) and in solutions of $N/20$ sodium hydroxide for various length of time, the degrees of swelling due to osmotic effects produced by the two alkalis were determined from the water adsorption, expressed as percentages of the original air-dried weight of the pieces of collagen, with due correction for the water which was absorbed by the pelt in plain water (pH about 6). Some typical data of the final results are shown in Table 14 (18).

It was found that the swelling of the specimens in the solution of sodium hydroxide remained constant after the fourth day, whereas the pieces in lime water continued to swell for the duration of the treatment. It is also worthy of note that the initial swelling accomplished in a 1-day treatment by sodium hydroxide is almost twice as large as that found for calcium hydroxide, as required by the Procter-Wilson theory. The initial reaction thus follows the valency rule of Loeb (18). After prolonged treatment in lime solution, the additional swelling of the pelt leads to a reduced ratio of swelling of about 1.5:1. The secondary swelling of skin produced by calcium hydroxide and divalent bases generally is due to at least two independent reactions. First, liberation of carboxyl groups by deamidation takes place more freely and easily in the treatment of collagen in solutions of bivalent bases than in the systems with univalent bases. This results in a breaking up of the interchain crosslinks in which the amide groups are involved and also to a greater uptake of cations. Second, calcium hydroxide has a specific effect on the protein and a tendency to form complexes with hydroxy groups, which probably is connected with its lower degree of ionization, its complexing power, and the bivalency of the cation. Marriott found that the solution of sodium hydroxide set free 0.14 mg. equiv. of ammonia per gram of collagen, compared to 0.33 mg. equiv. set free by calcium hydroxide.

The amounts of cations removed by collagen were 0.57 and 0.76 mg. equiv., respectively.

Marriott (18) was also the first to investigate the differences in swelling produced by bases of sodium and calcium, noting the increase in thickness and the shortening of the length of the fibers treated in solutions of sodium hydroxide at pH values > 12. On the other hand, in a corresponding solution of calcium hydroxide the fiber bundles do not contract in length, nor do they contort to the same extent or so rapidly as when monovalent bases are used. The limed fiber gradually begins to show fine striations due to separation of the constituent fibrils, changes which probably are partly the cause of the continuous increase in the water absorption by skin during the liming treatment. Marriott suggested that the reason for the comparatively slow reaction of skin with calcium hydroxide is possibly connected with the difficulty a bivalent cation would have in finding suitably placed pairs of anionic protein groups, compared with the ease with which a univalent cation can combine with the acidic groups of the rigid collagen lattice.

A tentative hypothesis was advanced by Marriott (18) to account for the lack of contortion and the splitting of fibers by lime solutions. The osmotic pressure exerted by the sodium salt of collagen will produce a localized pressure, bringing about a local bulging of the backbone, which will result in a shortening of the fiber. On the other hand, according to Marriott the bivalent calcium ions will distribute themselves so that each one shares two acidic groups of collagen. Hence, the osmotic pressure due to the calcium ions will be active over a larger area and will only slightly contract the fiber.

In these various explanations of the different degrees of swelling of collagen produced by uni- and bivalent bases of pH values > 10, it seems to the author that the mechanism of the interaction of alkali with the protein has not received the attention it deserves. The main reaction is discharge of the cationic protein groups, and the electrostatic balance of the cations by the anionic groups of collagen. For a cation such as sodium, no problem exists. As for the calcium ions, there appears to be no possibility of bringing two carboxylic ions of collagen into its valency sphere. The result may be imagined to be electrostatic compensation by means of the nearest carboxyl ions and other weakly negatively charged groups such as the enolized form of the peptide bond. This competition with the partners of the opposite peptide bonds forming a hydrogen bridge may be expected to weaken the link or even to rupture of some of these links, which will be favored by the osmotic swelling. This reaction would proceed slowly, and the lyotropic effect of the lime solution would first be noticeable after prolonged treatment of the skin in lime solution. These alterations are probably due to this electrostatic effect which is not a molecular effect of the

Hofmeister type but actually a specific ion effect of an electrostatic nature and intimately bound up with the valency of the cation and the steric conditions of the collagen lattice, particularly with regard to the distance between adjacent carboxyl groups, and the unipointal attachment (compensation) of Ca^{++} on the carboxyl ions of collagen.

The complexing power of the calcium ion with hydroxy amino acids is probably involved in the action of lime on collagen, as suggested by Phillips (19). Physiologists have long attributed to dissolved proteins the power to form un-ionized complexes with calcium ions. This combination has been characterized in numerous instances by the mass-action law constant (20). Even in dilute solutions, divalent cations, such as calcium, form only partially ionizable complexes with anions of carboxylic acids (21). The results of the researches of the Schmidt-Greenberg school on complex formation between the calcium ion and the hydroxyamino acids and proteins rich in such residues also support the view of this secondary type of fixation of calcium by collagen.

The brilliant application of the Donnan effect to the explanation of the protein swelling by Procter and Wilson denotes the first successful attempt to establish the physicochemical behavior of proteins on a thermodynamic basis. Its greatest importance lies in the introduction and development of the physicochemical method of reasoning and techniques in protein chemistry, especially with regard to tanning processes. Because of the originality and fundamental features of this innovation, it can safely be stated that the Procter-Wilson concept forms the cornerstone for our understanding of these processes, although it must be realized that subsequent findings have proved the phenomena involved to be not quite so simple as originally thought and not amenable to strictly mathematical analysis. Among the pioneers, the name of Jacques Loeb (22) is outstanding. His brilliant experimental investigations and strict scientific reasoning have probably been the greatest single contribution in this field. Moreover his lucid form of presentation and his critical attitude toward the occultism prevailing in the "colloidal" approach to protein behavior at the time of his investigations focused attention on the importance of the physicochemical approach.

A great deal of the criticism of the Procter-Wilson theory appears to be based not so much on the inherent faults and shortcomings of this concept as on misunderstandings and insufficient familiarity with the original postulate. Certain aspects of Küntzel's (23) objections to the osmotic swelling theory apparently are of that sort. The originators of the theory were fully aware of the limitation of their equations when applied to complicated systems. Thus, complete ionization of the protein compound formed is a prerequisite, and it is to be noted that only the strong acid hydrochloric acid and the strong base sodium hydroxide were used in the original investigations. Hence, the concept itself cannot be blamed for occasional failures connected with this deficiency—for instance, the failure to account for the swelling of proteins in systems containing electrolytes which are not completely ionized or in systems of strong acids with anions of marked affinity for the cationic protein groups by which they are irreversibly fixed. At the time of the promulgation of the swelling theory based on the Donnan effect, some forty years ago, the important role played by molecular and specific ion effects in the internal structure and cohesion of fibrous proteins of the collagen type, and hence in the degree of swelling, was only superficially recognized. However, Burton and Wilson's emphasis on the importance of the value of the bulk modulus takes into consideration the changes in internal cohesion of the substrate. Even an approximation of the degree of cohesion is not possible in general, and consequently a mathematical approach to the problem is useless. It is evident that swelling phenomena involving both osmotic and lyotropic effects, resulting in alterations of the cohesion of the protein, do not obey the simple equations of Procter and Wilson, and attempts to introduce correction factors and additional terms to the equations would make them too unwieldy for practical use. It is interesting and quite illuminating to note that the uptake of acid by solid proteins is claimed to be equally well described and accounted for by the Procter-Wilson theory as by the recently developed Gilbert-Rideal concept (24), and also by the concept of Steinhardt (25), although the fundamental conditions for these theories are diametrically opposed. The Donnan theory assumes all anions of the solid phase to be free, existing as ions electrostatically balanced by cationic protein groups only, whereas the Gilbert-Rideal concept is based on the presumption that all anions of the protein phase are combined with the protein. Steinhardt postulates separate affinity constants for the proton and anion of an acid. This is an excellent illustration of the point that there are many ways in which a phenomenon can be satisfactorily explained. It has aptly been pointed out by Lloyd (26) that the Procter-Wilson equations are not invalidated by the statement that they cannot be applied without modifications to systems in which the factor of structure is an integrating part. This is self-evident, since both the Donnan and the Procter-Wilson equations were worked out for diffusion of ions into a volume sufficiently large for surface forces to be neglected, and not for diffusion into a set of capillary tubes, which skin nearly represents. It is therefore obvious that, as soon as structure factors become prominent in the system, the simple calculations based on the Donnan effect can no longer be applied in their original form. The higher the restraint imposed on the structure of the solid phase, the less free water will be present, which accordingly implies introduction of new and unknown factors into the simple equations.

However, they are several instances of definite failure of the Procter-Wilson concept, as first pointed out by Küntzel (23). Only a few major ones will be mentioned. One of the most serious is the inability of neutral salts, such as sodium chloride, to depress the swelling of hide in solutions of sodium hydroxide; this has been mentioned previously. It is interesting to note that salts of dibasic acids, for instance sodium sulfate, markedly depress this swelling. The failure of sodium chloride is probably not due to any countereffect of the lyotropic type, because common salt in the rather low concentrations in which the swelling-depressing action should be forthcoming, and which are used, does not show any marked lyotropic effect during the short time necessary for demonstrating the effect of the salts on the swelling of collagen. In the case of calcium chloride, which, when added to the system collagen–saturated solution of calcium hydroxide, greatly increases the swelling produced by the hydroxide itself, the lyotropic effect apparently is active (splitting of fibers and fibrils, impairment of interchain crosslinks).

On the whole, the influence of neutral salts of various valency combinations or alkaline solutions containing a common cation on the swelling of collagen cannot be explained by any concept heretofore advanced. It should be noticed that the issue concerns systems containing a common cation of hydroxide and neutral salt. In systems with unlike cations, the cation interchange and displacement will further complicate the problem. Thus, the criticism of Küntzel as to the alleged failure of the Procter-Wilson theory to explain the increase in swelling of collagen induced by the addition of sodium chloride to hide in equilibrium with calcium hydroxide solution is not valid. In this instance, the exchange of bivalent calcium ions of the collagen for univalent sodium ions of the solution should increase the swelling in consequence of the partial formation of a system with univalent cations, which should theoretically at the corresponding pH value be capable of about twice the degree of swelling of the system with bivalent cations. In reality, the swelling of bivalent systems is more than predicted, because of the specific effect of the calcium ion on collagen, which leads to diminished internal cohesion of the structure and to separation of the fibril within the fiber. The difficulties encountered at such high pH values as those exceeding 13, represented by solutions of calcium hydroxide sharpened with depilating agents, such as sodium sulfide, are mainly due to the changes of the intermolecular linkage by the hydroxyl ions, and first of all to a partial rupture of crosslinks of the hydrogen bond type. These alterations are in part permanent. They are evidenced by increased reactivity of the limed hide to ionic and coordinate agents (27), the deamidation which occurs giving rise to a greater number of carboxylic groups, as was first shown by Marriott (28), and the swelling resulting in an increased number of available loci of coordination on the ruptured coordinate crosslinks on the —CO—NH— bonds (27).

Another example of the inadequacy of the Procter-Wilson swelling concept occurs in the pickling process. When skin is treated in a solution composed of hydrochloric acid of pH ~1 and sodium chloride in a concentration greater than 1 M per liter, the water content of the skin is reduced to a value considerably less than that originally present. The neutral salt eliminates the swelling by equalization of the chloride distribution between skin and solution. But an additional factor is involved, the dehydration of the skin, which is similar to the effect produced by acetone or alcohol. The electrostatic concept provides a reasonable explanation of this effect, although purely qualitative. It is worthy of note that such a high degree of dehydration of the skin cannot be produced by immersing the neutral pelt in a concentrated solution of sodium chloride. Apparently, not only complete inactivation of the carboxyl ions and the freeing of the charged cationic groups of collagen but also the presence of a certain concentration of chloride ions (>0.5 M per liter) is required in this peculiar dehydration, which forms the basis for the preservation of skins by pickling.

The system collagen–acid–salt offers many interesting aspects, some of which are of practical interest and hence will be briefly mentioned. From the point of view of the electrostatic concept of swelling, the effect of neutral salts is due to their discharge of the protein. Thus, the water content of isoelectric collagen which contains an equal number of positively and negatively charged groups associated with water is decreased by treatment with a saturated solution of sodium chloride, which yields a leatherlike product on dehydration. This drying-out is believed by some people to be due to the removal of free water within the interstices of the skin, and further to removal of the water held by the charged protein groups through their discharge. The water is still more effectively removed by the salt from collagen that has its acid-binding capacity satisfied. The electrostatic theory explains the effective water removal from collagen on the discharge of the protein by the combination of chloride ions with the cationic protein groups (Gegen-ion effect). The chloride ion of hydrochloric acid should have a similar effect. However, the addition of hydrochloric acid to make the system >0.5 M in chloride ion does not by any means bring about the same effect as a solution of 0.5 M sodium chloride on collagen of maximum content of hydrochloric acid. The probable reason is that hydrochloric acid commences to show lyotropic effects in the concentration mentioned.

REFERENCES

1. Lloyd, D. J., *J. Intern. Soc. Leather Trades Chem.* **17**, 208, 245 (1933).
2. Lloyd, D. J., and Phillips, H., *Trans. Faraday Soc.* **29**, 132 (1933).

3. Kaye, M., and Lloyd, D. J., *Proc. Roy. Soc.* **B96,** 294 (1924); Bowes, J. H., *J. Soc. Leather Trades Chem.* **33,** 176 (1949).
4. Lloyd, D. J., and Marriott, R. H., *Trans. Faraday Soc.* **32,** 932 (1936); Marriott, R. H., *Biochem. J.* **26,** 46 (1932); Lloyd, D. J., Marriott, R. H., and Pleass, W. B., *Trans. Faraday Soc.* **29,** 554 (1933).
5. Gustavson, K. H., *Biochem. Z.* **311,** 347 (1942).
6. Gustavson, K. H., *Svensk Kem. Tidskr.* **55,** 191 (1943).
7. Balfe, M. P., *in* "Progress in Leather Science," Vol. 1, pp. 86–94. BLMRA, London, 1946.
8. Lloyd, D. J., Marriott, R. H., and Pleass, W. B., *Trans. Faraday Soc.* **29,** 554 (1933).
9. Bolam, T. R., "The Donnan Equilibria," Bell, London, 1932.
10. Tolman, R. C., and Stearn, A. E., *J. Am. Chem. Soc.* **40,** 264 (1918).
11. Procter, H. R., and Wilson, J. A., *J. Chem. Soc.* **109,** 307 (1916).
12. Katchalsky, A., Künzle, O., and Kuhn, W., *J. Polymer Sci.* **5,** 283 (1950); Katchalsky, A., *J. Polymer Sci.* **7,** 393 (1951).
13. Schmidt, C. L. A., "The Chemistry of Amino Acids and Proteins." Thomas, Springfield, Ill., 1938; Cohn, E. J., and Edsall, J. T., eds., "Proteins, Amino Acids and Peptides." Reinhold, New York, 1943.
14. Wilson, J. A., "The Chemistry of Leather Manufacture," Vol. 1, pp. 129–180. Chemical Catalog Co., New York, 1928.
15. Procter, H. R., *Kolloid Beihefte* **2,** 243 (1911); *J. Am. Leather Chem. Assoc.* **6,** 270 (1911); *J. Chem. Soc.* **105,** 313 (1914); Wilson, J. A., *J. Am. Chem. Soc.* **38,** 1982 (1916).
16. Procter, H. R., and Burton, D., *J. Soc. Chem. Ind.* **14,** 404 (1916); *J. Intern. Soc. Leather Trades Chem.* **2,** 114 (1916).
17. Wilson, J. A., and Wilson, W. H., *J. Am. Chem. Soc.* **40,** 886 (1918).
18. Marriott, R. H., *J. Intern. Soc. Leather Trades Chem.* **17,** 178 (1933).
19. Phillips, H., *J. Intern. Soc. Leather Trades Chem.* (*Symposium, London*) p. 17 (1933).
20. Drinker, N., Green, A. A., and Hastings, A. B., *J. Biol. Chem.* **131,** 641 (1939).
21. Cannan, R. K., and Kibrick, A., *J. Am. Chem. Soc.* **60,** 2314 (1938); Greenwald, J., *J. Biol. Chem.* **124,** 437 (1938); **135,** 65 (1940); see also Greenberg, D. M., *Advances in Protein Chem.* **1,** 121 (1944).
22. Loeb, J., "Proteins and Theory of Colloidal Behavior," McGraw-Hill, New York, 1922.
23. Küntzel, A., *in* "Handbuch der Gerbereichemie" (W. Grassmann, ed.), Vol. I, Part 1, pp. 602–605. Springer, Vienna, 1944; see also Stiasny, E., "Gerbereichemie," pp. 173–199. Steinkopff, Dresden, 1931.
24. Gilbert, G. A., and Rideal, E., *Proc. Roy. Soc.* **A182,** 335 (1944).
25. Steinhardt, J., *Ann. N. Y. Acad. Sci.* **61,** 287 (1941).
26. Lloyd, D. J., and Shore, A., "Chemistry of Proteins," pp. 380–381. Churchill, London, 1938.
27. Gustavson, K. H., and Widen, P. J., *Collegium* **1926,** 562.
28. Marriott, R. H., *J. Intern. Soc. Leather Trades Chem.* **12,** 216, 281, 342 (1928); **15,** 25 (1931).

CHAPTER 8

Lyotropic Effects

1. Introduction

The lyotropic phenomena in protein behavior have been mentioned frequently. The specific ion and molecular effects on collagen are of utmost importance, although they have been and still are a neglected factor in the technology of leather manufacture, the probable reason being the difficulty of assessing these effects and distinguishing them from other influences.

In tanning, various types of lyotropic effects must be recognized. A few practical examples will be given. The presence of small amounts of calcium chloride or magnesium chloride in the common salt used for preserving and curing of skin will, on prolonged storing of such salted skins, lead to losses in protein by degradation, probably mainly through the association of calcium chloride in the molecular form with the peptide bonds, an effect due to the concentrated solutions of chlorides present in the cured skin. In the soaking of skins, compounds of lyotropic power may be added to assist the hydration and wetting of skins. Such compounds are polysulfides, thiocyanates, and salts of hydroxycarboxylic acids. In the liming of skins, the calcium ion opens up crosslinks of the hydrogen bond type, as a result of electrostatic intervention with the weakly polar peptide groups. In the washing and deliming of the limed skin, the choice of deliming agent is very important, since the accumulation of the deliming agents in the interstices of the skin results in rather high concentrations of these compounds in the hide structure, in spite of only small percentages being employed. Thus, the use of ammonium chloride as a deliming agent *per se* or as an adjunct to and constituent of the bating agent in the bating of skin will result in a softer and looser type of leather than is the case when ammonium sulfate is employed. The specific action of acids, such as sulfuric acid gradually added and acetic acid, will also be evident in the leather produced. The same considerations apply to the pickling process. In chrome tannage, specific ion effects on the protein are not apparent, but the influence of the type of anion of the chromium salt enters instead. It is also well known that the type of swelling which the skin has undergone prior to chrome tannage, and which usually involves lyotropic effects in the preparatory processes, will have an effect on the final leather and may even cause the fixation of chromium complexes to take a diverse course. These specific effects are even more important in vegetable tanning, since the fixation of the vegetable tannins and the nature of the fiber weave are profoundly affected by such effects, those imparted to collagen previous to tannage as well as those induced during the tanning process. The nature of the nontannins, the neutral salts and the acid present or added for adjustment of the pH value, will to a marked extent determine the character of the final leather, as the important researches of the British Leather Manufacturers' Research Association have proved (1).

The "hot pitting" process in the manufacture of sole leather, in which the tanned leather is submitted to a concentrated solution of vegetable tanning extract, acidified by weak organic acids, at an elevated temperature probably also involves lyotropic effects (2). The combination of the weak acids and the high temperature apparently causes a slight denaturation of collagen (the incipient shrinkage of Pankhurst), which results in the formation of additional sites of binding for the vegetable tannins. If the treatment is prolonged excessively or if the temperatures and pH values approach the critical zone of fiber stability, the fiber strength of the leather is endangered.

The lyotropic effect is generally most pronounced in neutral solutions in which the specific effects of the ions or molecules do not have to compete with the powerful hydrogen and hydroxyl ions. This applies to lyotropic agents of the neutral salt type, such as calcium chloride and thiocyanates. In the case of weak acids, such as acetic acid, their action is bound to the molecules and not to the anion, and hence they require the presence of hydrogen ions and anions in equilibrium with large amounts of un-ionized acid, i.e., low pH values. The same reasoning also applies to agents present as hydroxides, their lyotropic action being exerted at high alkalinity.

2. NEUTRAL SALT EFFECTS

The effect of neutral salts on collagen in its isoelectric range is of fundamental importance. As a rule, salts with weakly hydrated ions, e.g., thiocyanates, are strongly adsorbed by collagen from aqueous solution, whereas those with strongly hydrated ions, such as the sulfates, show a negative adsorption owing to their dehydrating effect on collagen. Thus, sodium thiocyanate is strongly adsorbed by collagen and in concentrations exceeding 1 M has a strong swelling effect on this protein, large amounts of which are brought into solution. A 2 M solution will give a threefold swelling, compared to the initial water content of native collagen. The shrinkage temperature of the collagenous fibers is so drastically lowered that shrinkage takes place in treatments with solutions of a 2 M NaCNS solution even at room temperature, which means a decrease of the shrinkage temperature of approximately 50 degrees. A solution of 1 M sodium sulfate, which salt is only slightly taken up by collagen, will dissolve less of the collagen than water does if used in toluene-saturated state (employed as a blank) and dehydrates the protein. The shrinkage temperature of the original fiber is not lowered; on the contrary it is slightly elevated. These salt effects are not discernible at low concentrations, for instance at 0.1 M. Our present knowledge favors the view that the effect is due chiefly to the molecules of the salt, and hence not to the ions. It is evident that the most effective lyotropic salts are those which in concentrated solution are only partly ionized, such as the bivalent metal chlorides of calcium and barium. This must unquestionably be true for the action of nonpolar substances and nonelectrolytes, such as sucrose and glucose. Sucrose in a 1 M solution will increase the swelling of collagen by more than 100 %. In all instances, the change of the dielectric constant of the solution probably is a contributing factor.

It was first noticed by Wilson, through practical tannery experience, that solutions of certain neutral salt, for instance calcium chloride, added in high concentration, badly damaged skins. The first scientific investigation of this peculiar destructive action of certain neutral salts on hide substance was carried out by Thomas and Kelly (3) in the hope of throwing more light on the science of curing skins. The experiments were carried out with 50-g. portions of hide powder, covered with 1-l. portions of c.p. salt solutions in stoppered bottles, covered with toluene at room temperature. At the intervals of time noted on the abscissas of their figures, showing the loss of hide substance as a function of the length of treatment, aliquots of solutions were withdrawn and the filtrates subjected to the Kjeldahl process for determination of nitrogeneous substances gone into solution. From these figures the percentage of the destruction of hide substance was calculated.

The most remarkable finding is that all the halides are able to bring collagen into solution, and that sulfates, and also thiosulfates (3), inhibit the "peptization" of collagen, making it less than in pure sterile water. The concentration of the salt also enters into the picture in different ways. With chlorides of Li, K, and Mg, the destructive effect on collagen is augmented with increasing concentrations of salt, whereas with calcium chloride the maximum effect is obtained in 2 to 3 M solutions. In the case of sodium iodide, the 2 M solution is most destructive.

Figure 30 shows the effect of time on the solubilization of hide powder by various salts in 4 M solution, except as otherwise noted, in comparison with the loss of hide substance incurred in water. The most interesting fact is the effective conservation of hide by means of saturated solutions of sodium sulfate. Hardly any collagen is broken down during treatment for as long as 170 days at 37°C., whereas more than 30 % of the original collagen

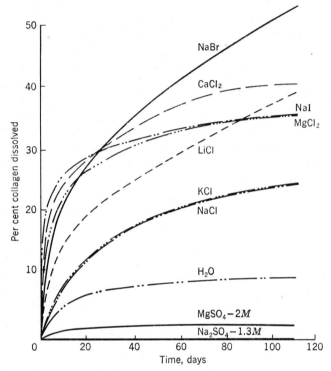

FIG. 30. The lyotropic effect of various neutral salts in solutions of 4 M strength on hide powder, measured by the degree of solubilization of the collagen.

is lost from the blank kept in water covered with toluene, and as much as 80 % of the hide powder kept in a solution of magnesium chloride.

Wilson (4) even proposed the use of sodium sulfate as a hide preservative to take the place of common salt which, in the concentrated solutions that are formed in the brine of hides, may have a destructive action on hide substance. However, many other properties of the curing agent must be considered. A very important one is the degree of the bactericidal power of the curing salt. Common salt possesses this property to a fair degree, whereas sodium sulfate is lacking in this respect. Another drawback of the sulfate is its strong hygroscopic property, which will have bad practical consequences, particularly in curing and storing hides in moist and warm climates. For these reasons, among others, sodium sulfate has not found extensive application as a curing agent. Quite recently, magnesium sulfate has been advocated.

The results obtained for a great number of neutral salts in concentrated solutions under sterile conditions at fairly constant pH values in the isoelectric range of collagen are typical of the Hofmeister ion series. However, under the conditions of these experiments (and this applies also to the lyotropic action of neutral salts on collagen in general, which effect is intimately bound up with *concentrated* solutions of the salts), the swelling and solubilizing effects of these agents are not caused by any specific ion or pair of ions. On the contrary, they are mainly due to the influence of the molecule of the salt on the protein, *a molecular effect*. Hence, the Hofmeister ion series loses its significance.

Thomas and his co-workers (3), as well as Wilson (4), use the term hydrolysis to describe the destructive effect of lyotropic salts on collagen, but they offered no explanation of their findings. It should be noted, however, that the phenomena are not hydrolytic in the original meaning of the word, since that would imply that scission of primary valency occurs in the solubilization. This is not the case, or, if so, only to a slight extent, the main solubilization being caused by rupture of a weaker type of bond, probably hydrogen bonds, electrostatic crosslinks, and van der Waals forces. The word peptization, which in itself is not very satisfactory as a general term, was coined by the older colloid chemists for processes of the type involved in the destruction of collagen by neutral salt solutions, and it is etymologically acceptable for present usage.

In the second edition of his monograph, Wilson (4) discusses the probable reasons for the hydrolysis of hide substance by various neutral salts, basing his explanation on some suggestions advanced by the author of this book in 1926 (5), as a prelude to an investigation of the effect of pretreatment of collagen (hide powder) with solutions of neutral salts of a lyotropic nature on its reactivity. At the time of these investigations, in the middle 1920's, some new ideas of the architecture of the proteins were being evolved. On the whole, our knowledge of proteins had at that time not advanced very far beyond the fundamental concept that proteins are built up from long chains of polypeptides, advanced by Emil Fisher in the early years of this century. The history of lyotropic salt effects depicts the development of protein chemistry during the past three decades, and a brief account therefore seems justified.

With regard to collagen, Stiasny (6) had suggested that the original concept of Herzog (7) was generally applicable to all proteins. It was stated that the huge protein molecule was not formed from long polypeptide chains. The building units were conceived to be smaller chains of polypeptides, simple cyclic compounds of the type of dioxopiperazines or small peptones which were held together by forces of secondary valency type to form the huge protein molecule. Previous to that time, the nature of high-molecular substances had been neglected from the point of view of structural chemistry, because of their lack of crystallizability and of other fundamental physical constants easily measured. Now the general trend of thought centered on the possibility that small primary valency compounds, such as diketopiperazines, may be the building stones of proteins, with secondary valency forces considered as responsible for the association of these smaller units into the large protein molecule. Bergmann (8) particularly had produced evidence pointing in that direction, since simply by adjusting a solution of certain isomeric forms of diketopiperazine to a certain pH value he had been able to bring about the formation of high-molecular compounds showing certain of the characteristics of proteins. Waldschmidt-Leitz and Schaeffner (9) had proved, however, that the diketopiperazines were resistant to proteolytic enzymes, in contrast to the behavior of proteins. Hence, their findings were in support of the classical concept of proteins as polypeptide chains. On the other hand, Bergmann *et al.* (10) had been able to show that the proteinlike substance obtained by polymerization of simple diketopiperazines was easily split by proteinases, and hence that by polymerization the original diketopiperazine structure was converted into an entirely different product. Bergmann was one of the strongest advocates of this view at the time. Also, it should be added he was one of the first major investigators to recognize its shortcomings and to admit that the concept was inadequate in the light of the new experimental evidence resulting from the work of a number of scientists, including Astbury, Meyer, Mark, Weber, Staudinger, and Sponsler. Meyer and Mark (11) were the first to show that silk contains extended primary protein chains of high-molecular weight and were able to interpret the X-ray diagram of the silk fibroin lattice. Furthermore, they could show that protein fibers generally are built up from stretched primary valency chains. Fundamental contributions were supplied by the lucid researches of Astbury (12). These researches represent the early development of the chemistry of high-molecular compounds based on the concept of long molecular chains of primary valency linking, a concept which is still the generally accepted one.

In the first explanation of the dispergating effect of lyotropic neutral salts on hide substance, the problem was considered from the point of view that collagen may be a secondary valency aggregate of smaller units of the peptone type, owing to the breaking of a part of the links holding the units together. This in turn would result in swelling, hydration, and dissolution of the freed smaller units. The formation of coordination compounds, so-called molecular compounds, between the simple peptones and the lyotropic neutral salt, exemplified by calcium chloride, was considered to be the initial reaction of the competition for the coordination bonds and valencies of the protein.

In the discussion of the work of Thomas and his school (3), it was pointed out that Loeb (13) had already found this specific ion effect on gelatin gel, noting increased solubility of the gel in the presence of calcium chloride, and decreased solubility by neutral sulfates in concentrations greater than $M/32$. Loeb's data showed ion series similar to those observed by Thomas and Foster (3), corresponding to the Hofmeister series. In fact, Loeb concluded that the solubility of gelatin in water is not controlled by the Donnan equilibrium and does not show "the characteristics of colloidal behavior." A case of peptization seemed to him most likely. The salts would probably influence the secondary valency forces between gelatin and water, and a possible explanation based on the Langmuir-Harkins concept of the orientation of molecules was suggested.

It was stressed by the present author (5) that this particular neutral salt effect is not a question of hydrolysis, i.e., a severing of primary valency forces. On the contrary, it is a problem of secondary valency partition between the protein units themselves and between these units and the molecules of the neutral salt. It was pointed out that a number of definite chemical compounds between neutral salts and amino acids had been isolated by Pfeiffer (14) in crystalline form, as, for instance, those of glycine (Gl) and calcium chloride: $CaCl_2$–1 Gl; $CaCl_2$–2 Gl; $CaCl_2$–3 Gl. The formation of these addition compounds was restricted to halogen salts and related compounds. They have been definitely proved to be molecular compounds, that is, coordination compounds with coordination on the central atom of the metal of the salt, on the one hand, and the oxygen atom of the carboxyl group of the amino acid, on the other. A most important fact is that the neutral salts which form such compounds in the solid state all cause a considerable increase in the solubility of the amino acids, such as diketopiperazine in the salts mentioned, which in fact is strong evidence for their nature as molecular compounds.

Based on the ideas given in this outline, the explanation of the neutral salt effect on collagen, resulting in destructive action, was as follows. The neutral salts of coordinate potency compete with the protein subunits for the sites of the secondary valency forces, which in modern terminology are hydrogen bonds, schematically represented by the following formula:

RCH	RCH		RCH		RCH
CO-----HN	+ $CaCl_2$	—CO--$CaCl_2$	+	HN	
NH-----OC		NH		OC	
HCR	RCH		HCR		RCH
Collagen		Solubilized fragment		Collagen	

The extent of the interaction of salts and proteins will depend on the strength of the forces operating between the subunits of collagen and the strength and stability of the secondary valency compound formed between the salt and any individual protein unit. A weakening and partial breaking up of these intermolecular forces will result from the combination, and a part of the smaller units will be segregated and go into solution. The parallelism for calcium chloride, with regard to its pronounced tendency to form stable addition compounds with amino acids and its highly destructive action on collagen, was pointed out.

From these theoretical deductions, it was predicted that, as a result of the lyotropic action of salts on collagen, its reactivity toward agents which involve secondary valency forces (coordination) for their fixation should be greater than that of the original collagen, since additional sites of coordination on the collagen would be formed by the treatment. To express this concept in modern terms, a part of the crosslinks of the hydrogen bond type in collagen should be ruptured and additional —CO—NH— groups freed from their interchain compensation and made available for binding of the coordinating agents

$$—CO \cdot NH— \qquad —CO \cdot NH—$$
$$\vdots \qquad \vdots \qquad \rightarrow$$
$$—NH \cdot CO— \qquad —NH \cdot CO—$$

and also

$$—CO \cdot NH \rightarrow \qquad —CO \cdot NH \rightarrow$$
$$\vdots \qquad \rightarrow$$
$$HO \qquad HO$$
$$\vert \qquad \qquad \vert$$
$$\underline{\qquad} \rightarrow \qquad \underline{\qquad} \rightarrow$$

Since the neutral salt treatment does not alter the ionic valency capacity of collagen, agents reacting strictly electrovalently with the protein should not be affected by the pretreatments (15). Chromium salts of the cationic type with only a few chromium atoms in the complex (such as the 67% acid chromium sulfate and chloride), chromium compounds containing aggregated complexes (later found to be largely nonionic), vegetable tannins, and simple acids and bases were investigated (15) as to their affinity for specimens of hide powder which had been pretreated in solutions of various neutral salts. Some typical examples are given in the following tables.

Table 15 shows the loss of hide substance incurred on 14 days' treatment of 100-g. portions of standard hide powder in 1-l. portions of 1 M solutions of various neutral salts, covered with toluene, with final pH values adjusted to the range 5.7 to 6.0, at room temperature. The treated speci-

TABLE 15

TREATMENT OF HIDE POWDER IN 1 M SOLUTIONS OF NEUTRAL SALTS (15)

Treated in M Solution of	Loss of Collagen, % of Original Amount	pH at Equilibrium in Treatment with 0.01 N Sulfuric Acid
Na_2SO_4	1.6	2.62
$Na_2S_2O_3$	1.2	2.62
$MgSO_4$	1.6	2.62
H_2O (blank)	4.9	2.62
NaCl	7.8	2.61
KCl	7.0	2.62
$MgCl_2$	9.3	2.62
KBr	14.4	2.62
KJ	16.8	2.63
$BaCl_2$	14.9	2.63
$SrCl_2$	21.1	2.62
$CaCl_2$	31.9	2.63
KSCN	24	2.63

Increasing peptization for cations in the order: Ca > Sr > Ba > Mg > Na, K.
Increasing peptization for anions in the order: CNS > J > Br > Cl > SO_4 , S_2O_3 .

mens were washed free from the salt and acetone-dehydrated. Portions of the dehydrated hide powder equal to 1.8 g. of collagen were treated with intermittent shaking in 200 ml. of 0.01 N sulfuric acid of pH 2.06 for 12 hours. The pH values of the equilibrated solutions served as a measure of the acid-combining capacity of the treated hide powder specimens and are included in the table.

The pH values show that the neutral salt treatment has not altered the reactivity of collagen for hydrogen ions. Neither was the maximum binding capacity of collagen, applying 0.1 N hydrochloric acid containing 5% w/v sodium chloride, altered by these pretreatments. These findings were interpreted as indication that the peptization of hide powder by these agents does not affect the potency of the electrovalent groups of collagen.

The degree of fixation of chromium compounds of different types is illustrated by the data in Table 16. The solutions contained 0.5 equiv. of chromium, per liter and the time of tanning was 48 hours.

These data pertain to an investigation published in 1926. At that time only qualitative indications of the electrochemical composition of the various solutions were available. By ion-exchange methods, applying the sodium salt of a cationic exchanger, such as Dowex 50, and the hydrochloric acid salt of a quaternary base, the anion exchanger Amberlite IRA-400, the following average percentages of cationic, nonionic, and anionic chromium complexes were found to be characteristic of these types of chromium

TABLE 16

FIXATION OF CHROMIUM COMPOUNDS BY HIDE POWDER PRETREATED WITH NEUTRAL
SALTS (15)

Pretreated in M Solution of	I 67% Acid Cr-sulfate	II 67% Acid Cr-chloride	III 40% Acid Cr-sulfate	IV Sulfito-Cr-sulfate, Containing $3Na_2SO_3:1Cr_2O_3$
Na_2SO_4	11.4	5.1	18.2	16.8
H_2O	11.6	5.2	23.7	20.7
NaCl	11.6	5.1	24.2	21.3
KCl	11.6	5.3	24.1	21.6
KBr	11.8	5.4	26.5	23.7
KJ	11.9	5.5	30.8	26.0
KSCN	12.0	5.6	32.2	31.3
$SrCl_2$	11.8	5.4	27.1	26.2
$BaCl_2$	11.7	5.3	28.4	28.4
$CaCl_2$	11.8	5.4	29.8	30.5

compounds (Nos. I, II, III, and IV, respectively): 96, 4, 0; 100, 0, 0; 80, 15, 5; and 0, 85, 15 (16).

Recent work has shown that sodium perchlorate (17) in solutions of 2 to 4 M is an exceedingly powerful lyotropic agent. Thus, for instance, a 48-hour pretreatment of calfskin pelt in solutions of 1, 2, and 4 M sodium perchlorate had a drastic effect on the chrome fixation of the treated stock from a solution of sulfito-chromium sulfate, 0.8 equiv. of chromium per liter, containing 2.5 Na_2SO_3:1 Cr_2O_3 (86% nonionic and 12% anionic chromium), as the following figures of the amounts of Cr_2O_3 fixed by collagen show. The untreated pelt fixed 11.4% Cr_2O_3 ; the pelt pretreated in the 1 M $NaClO_4$ solution combined with 14.9% Cr_2O_3 ; and the corresponding specimens pretreated in 2 M and 4 M solutions of perchlorate gave 17.8 and 55.7% Cr_2O_3, respectively. The advantages and disadvantages of using pieces of skin (pelt) instead of hide powder for such experiments will be discussed later.

Referring to the data from the tanning experiments of Table 16, it should be noted that solutions I and II represent chromium salts of moderate basicity which contain cationic chromium entirely or nearly so. Solution III contains a good deal of nonionic and anionic complexes in addition to the main constituent of cationic complexes. Finally, the highly aggregated sulfito-sulfato-chromium compound present in solution IV is devoid of cationic chromium, nonionic complexes being the dominant constituent.

According to our present knowledge, the cationic chromium complexes of the type present in solutions I and II are initially reacting with the carboxyl ions of collagen. This initial reaction is hence electrovalent, followed by penetration of the carboxyl group into the chromium complex. The extent of fixation is governed by the number of carboxyl ions available under otherwise identical experimental conditions. The nonionic and anionic chromium complexes probably are fixed mainly by other groups than the carboxyl. The data show that the neutral salt treatment of hide powder has no effect on its fixation of cationic chromium. Thus, they prove that the neutral salt action does not alter the function of the carboxylic protein groups. On the other hand, the fixation of the noncationic aggregated chromium complexes from solution IV is very much affected by treatment with the most effective lyotropic agents, such as the calcium chloride and the thiocyanate, the chrome uptake being increased about 50 %. These findings indicate that nonionic protein groups of collagen are more reactive after lyotropic treatment and may be considered as evidence for an increase in the number of coordination sites in collagen resulting from the action of the hide-dispersing neutral salts. It is probable that the protein groups involved are the peptide linkages originally present in interchain compensation by means of hydrogen bonds. This suggestion is supported by data on the behavior of the vegetable tannins, which are specific for the —CO—NH— groups, toward the peptized hide powder, as will presently be shown. Recent work points to the freed hydroxy groups as sites for the binding of nonionic chromium complexes (sulfito).

Before proceeding any further, it should be pointed out that neutral pelt, i.e., whole pieces of skin, is in many respects superior to hide powder for experiments of this sort. The tissue of skin is more resistant to the action of the neutral salts and more uniform in composition, whereas hide powder contains fractions of various degrees of fineness. The finely divided portions show markedly greater reactivity toward coordination agents and are also more susceptible to solubilization by lyotropic agents than the coarser fractions. Thus, it is quite possible, as the experiments prove, to decrease the reactivity of standard hide powder by lyotropic treatment if the particular conditions favor the solubilization of the highly subdivided fractions which possess a much higher binding capacity for coordination agents, such as solution IV, than the remaining hide powder. This complicating effect of the heterogeneity of hide powder is particularly strikingly illustrated by the influence of tryptic digestion of standard hide powder on the reactivity of hide powder and also by the different reactivities of various fractions of hide powder, sifted to different degrees of fineness, to reagents which coordinate with collagen. In Table 17, data on the fixation of chromium by hide powder of different degrees of subdivision from a solution of cationic chromium complexes and a solution containing preponderantly nonionic complexes are given in terms of the per cent of Cr_2O_3 fixed by collagen on 48 hours' tanning (18).

TABLE 17

INFLUENCE OF THE DEGREE OF SUBDIVISION OF HIDE POWDER ON ITS REACTIVITY
(18)

Hide Powder Fraction	Cationic Chromium in the Form of 63% Acid Cr-sulfate; 0.8 Equiv./l. Cr	Nonionic Chromium in the Form of Sulfito-Cr-sulfate, 3 Na_2SO_3:1 Cr_2O_3 ; 0.6 equiv./l. Cr
Coarse particles retained by sieve of 5 mesh per cm.^{2}	12.0	17.8
Medium particles retained by sieve of 5 to 20 mesh per cm.^{2}	12.2	22.6
Fine particles passing the 20-mesh sieve	12.9	27.0
Ordinary hide powder, not sieved	12.3	23.2

By tryptic digestion of ordinary hide powder (19, 20), the finer fractions apparently are digested first, which leads to a gradual decrease in the amounts of chromium fixed from the sulfito-chromium sulfate by the coarser hide powder remaining after the trypsin treatment. In concluding this discussion of pelt versus hide powder as the substrate for investigations of this type, one main disadvantage of the use of pelt should not be left unnoticed. That is the difficulty of obtaining complete interaction of large complexes of the type of the sulfito-chromium sulfate, particularly as regards even penetration throughout the interior of the skin, which will result in too low values of chrome fixation by the "peptized" skin tissue. In a number of unpublished experiments, the main findings on lyotropic effects on hide powder have been confirmed on skin tissue in the form of whole pieces (pelt).

Only a few representative data from experiments with pelt will be presented here. Isoelectric calfskin pelt in portions of 10 g. of collagen was treated for 7 days at room temperature in 100-ml. portions of 2 M solutions of the neutral salts listed in Table 18. The washed specimens were tanned for 48 hours by means of (1) purely cationic chromium complexes (67 % acid chrome sulfate liquor, 0.4 equiv. of chromium) per liter and (2) nonionic chromium complexes (sulfito-chromium sulfate, 2.5 Na_2SO_3:1 Cr_2O_3 , 0.8 equiv. per liter of chromium). Identical series were run with hide powder, the resulting data being shown in parentheses in the table.

The tremendous increase in chrome fixation by the perchlorate-pretreated pelt from the solution of nonionic sulfito-chromium sulfate must be emphasized. Sodium perchlorate in the concentration range 2 to 4 M is the most effective lyotropic agent in the neutral salt class found in the wide range of salts investigated over many years by the author of this book.

TABLE 18

EFFECT OF PRETREATMENT OF PELT ON ITS BINDING OF CHROMIUM COMPLEXES (17)
(Numbers in parentheses indicate corresponding data on hide powder.)

| | | % Cr_2O_3 Fixed by Collagen from: | |
Pretreated with	Loss of Collagen, % of Original Amount	Cationic chromium	Nonionic chromium
H_2O (Blank)	0.4 (3.1)	10.3 (11.8)	20.7 (29.4)
M Sodium sulfate	0.4 (0.7)	10.4 (12.0)	19.1 (28.3)
Sodium chloride	1.1 (9.6)	10.0 (11.9)	20.7 (33.6)
Sodium perchlorate	83 (26.7)	10.9 (12.9)	76.7 (58.3)
Sodium thiocyanate	80 (—)	11.0 (13.6)	62.0 (59.8)
Potassium iodide	77 (51)	11.8 (13.2)	52.6 (57.7)
M Calcium chloride	5 (25)	10.4 (12.8)	24.8 (37.9)

TABLE 19

THE CONCENTRATION FACTOR IN THE ACTION OF SODIUM PERCHLORATE ON COLLAGEN
(PELT) (17)

Pretreated in Na-perchlorate Solution of Molarity	Loss of Collagen, %	T_s of Treated Washed Pelt	Cr_2O_3, % Fixed by Collagen from:	
			Cationic chromium	Nonionic chromium
0 (blank)	0.2	64	9.7	19.5
0.5	0.8	64	9.7	19.7
1.0	1.5	62	9.7	19.5
2.0	66.8	Shrunk in the pretreatment	10.1	37.8
4.0	59.4	Shrunk in the pretreatment	11.3	50.4

In view of sodium perchlorate being a typical strong electrolyte, considered not to be complex-forming, the series of data shown in Table 19 are of interest, since they give the concentration of the perchlorate at which the lyotropic effect commences. Neutral pelt was pretreated as described above in the solutions given in the table. The chromium salts were those of the previous table.

Evidently, sodium perchlorate in solutions of less than 1 M strength produces no lyotropic effect on collagen, as shown by the figures of the percentage of collagen solubilized in the treatment, the shrinkage temperatures of the treated specimens of pelt, after their conditioning, restoring them to the isoelectric state, and also by the fact that the chrome fixation by collagen is not altered by the pretreatment in this particular instance.

Investigations of Batzer and Weissenberger (21), and of Holm and the present author (22) have definitely proved that the fixation of vegetable tannins of the condensed type takes place mainly on the peptide links. In view of this fact, some data on the effect of the lyotropic changes of hide powder on its irreversible fixation of vegetable tannins are of interest. From a solution of tannin in the form of a 5 % w/v solution of mimosa extract of pH 4.6, the following percentages of irreversibly fixed tannins, based on the weight of collagen, were obtained: blank hide powder fixed, 60; the specimen pretreated in 1 M sodium sulfate, 58; that in calcium chloride, 84; and the hide powder pretreated in potassium thiocyanate, 88. These figures give substantial support to the theory of the nature of the lyotropic effect on collagen advanced in this text. The nonionic sulfito-chromium complexes possess no affinity for the CO·NH— link of the polyamide. Hence, the largely increased fixation of these complexes by collagen on its pretreatment with lyotropic agents and heat denaturation cannot be due to the breaking of the hydrogen bonds crosslinking adjacent keto-imide groups. The rupture of hydrogen bonds in which the hydroxy group partakes is probably responsible for the increased reactivity of the nonionic chromium complexes. This is indicated by the fact that by O-acetylation of bovine collagen the fixation of vegetable tannins, specific for the —CO·NH— link, is increased, whereas the fixation of sulfito-chromium complexes is lowered, probably as a result of the inactivation of the hydroxy groups.

3. THE EFFECT OF CONCENTRATED SOLUTIONS OF UREA

The action of urea on collagen is in many respects similar to that of neutral salts. It appears to be principally a molecular effect. It is worthy of note that the swelling and peptizing action of urea in aqueous solutions of concentrations >4 M, preferably solutions of 4 to 6 M, is not very marked at room temperature (23). Concentrated solutions at temperatures of about 35°C. are recommended for demonstrating the swelling, shrinkage, and peptizing effects drastically. As already mentioned, urea in 6.6 M solution was long ago found to be effective in splitting the molecules of a number of globular proteins into definite subunits (24), probably by dislocation of hydrogen bonds operating between these subunits. Also the fact that urea is a polar compound may contribute to its effective denaturation of proteins, as pointed out in Chapter 1. As an example of the influence of urea in 6 M solution, the following data are of interest (17). After 24 hours of treatment of neutral calfskin pelt in this solution at 35°C., about half of the amount of the original collagen was solubilized. The remaining highly swollen pelt fixed the same amount of cationic chromium as the original pelt, whereas the uptake of the nonionic sulfito-chromium sulfate was 60 % greater and the fixation of mimosa tannins 35 % greater than the corresponding values for the untreated pelt. Although the acid-binding capacity of the original collagen was not changed, the binding of hydrogen ions from solutions of hydrochloric acid in the pH range of 2.5 to 5 at equilibration was increased by the urea treatment, which probably is due to the weakening of the electrostatic attraction between oppositely charged polar groups of some of the salt links by the increased distance between the groups. The carboxyl ions then require a lower hydrogen ion potential for their discharge; i.e., at identical final intermediate pH values the urea-treated collagen with disorganized chains will combine with a greater number of hydrogen ions. Corresponding differences in the titration curves in the pH ranges 2.5 to 5.0 and 6 to 10 are shown by gelatin, fish collagen, and mammalian collagen, with gelatin showing the largest binding of H and OH ions. These data on the effect of urea on collagen are best explained by the lyotropic effect of the compound directed toward nonionic protein groups, probably the peptide bonds, with the oxygen atom of the urea molecule being attracted to the imino group of the —CO—NH— linkage. The detanning action of concentrated solutions of urea on vegetable-tanned leather and the probable role played by the urea of foot perspiration in the damaging of leather will be further considered in connection with vegetable tannage in "The Chemistry of Tanning Processes".

4. The Lyotropic Effect of Weak Acids

This effect has also been definitely established as a molecular one. Acetic acid, as an example of the carboxylic acids, shows a marked tendency for association, not only in the pure liquid and nonassociated solvents but also in the vapor phase and in water. A marked dimerization has also been shown by Katchalsky, Eisenberg, and Lifson (25). The dimer formation of the carboxylic acids is caused by the strong hydrogen bonds formed by the oxygen atom of the carboxyl group. The dimer of acetic acid forms the following structure:

$$
\begin{array}{c}
\text{O—H --- O} \\
CH_3 \cdot C \diagup \qquad \diagdown\!\!\diagdown C \cdot CH_3 \\
\diagdown\!\!\diagdown O \text{-----} HO \diagup
\end{array}
$$

The value of the distance —OH---O of the dimer of formic acid, determined by the electron-diffraction method by Pauling and Brockway (26), is 2.67 Å. The distance from each hydrogen atom to the nearest of the two adjacent oxygen atoms in the dimer of acetic acid is about 1.07 Å., or greater than the corresponding value for ice, as is to be expected in consequence of the increased strength of the hydrogen bond. This can be accounted for by resonance of the molecule to the structure $CH_3 \cdot C \begin{smallmatrix} \ddot{O}-H, \\ \diagup\diagup \\ \diagdown \\ \ddot{O}: \end{smallmatrix}$

which gives a positive charge to the oxygen atom that donates the proton in hydrogen bond formation and thus increases the ionic character of the —OH— bond and the positive charge of the hydrogen atom. Simultaneously the other oxygen atom, the proton acceptor, is given an increased negative charge. The sum total will be a tendency to increase the strength of the —O—H---O— bond.

Evidence for the existence of the dimer of carboxylic acids in dilute aqueous solution has been presented by Katchalsky and co-workers (25) in an investigation of the hydrogen bonding and ionization of carboxylic acids in aqueous solution. Their paper is of the greatest importance in the present problem.

Since the ionic behavior of acetic acid is of general interest, a brief outline will be given. It has long been known that for acetic acid the Debye-Hückel theory is valid only for extremely low concentrations of this acid, which shows pronounced deviation from this equation at dilutions at which the Debye approximation should still hold. It is shown by the authors mentioned that the marked deviation of acetic acid can be satisfactorily accounted for by assuming the presence of the dimeric form of a low degree of ionization. The ionization constant resulting from the modified formula for ionization as a function of the concentration of acid, with due consideration of the dimerization constant, will make K of acetic acid a true constant of the value 1.75×10^{-5}. The dimerization constant of acetic acid, L, is equal to 0.16 in the equation:

$$\log K = \log k - 1.013 \sqrt{\alpha \cdot c} + \log \left[\sqrt{1 + 8L(1 - \alpha)} + 1 \right]$$

where K is the true ionization constant, k is the classical ionization constant, α is the degree of ionization of acetic acid, and c is its concentration. In solutions of acetic acid of 2 to 3 M, as are usually applied in the study of its lyotropic effect, the solution contains more than 99 % of the total acid as molecules, of which a considerable amount exists as the dimer. Hence, in such systems the equilibrium concerns chiefly $(HOCOCH_3)_2 \rightleftarrows 2HOCOCH_3$, with sites for hydrogen bonds available in the monomer.

The lyotropic effect of the carboxylic acids on collagen has long been familiar to the practical tanner, although not as a phenomenon under this name but as a permanent swelling or plumping effect imparted to hides and

TABLE 20

DEGREE OF SWELLING, SOLUBILIZATION, AND HYDROTHERMAL STABILITY OF SKIN AFTER PRETREATMENT BY ACIDS (27)

Treated with:	Final pH	Degree of Swelling in Solution	Solubilized Collagen, % of Original Weight	Degree of Permanent Swelling	Shrinkage Temperature, °C.
0.03 M HCl	2.0	5.8	1.2	4.6	62
3 M HCOOCH$_3$	2.0	8.3	9.7	7.2	55
Water (blank)	5.7	3.0	0.1	3.0	67

skins subjected to the prolonged action of such acids, mainly in connection with vegetable tannage ("hot pitting"). To such an eminent investigator as Loeb, this effect was well known. He drew attention to the fact that acetic acid, among several weak organic acids, does not obey the valency rule in its action on gelatin. The valency rule implies that the same degree of swelling of the protein should be produced by isovalent acids in solutions equilibrated to identical pH values. He found that acetic acid produced a very much larger swelling than hydrochloric acid of corresponding final pH value, and moreover decreased the cohesion of the protein.

From a comprehensive investigation of the effect of acetic acid on collagen, in the form of pelt and hide powder (27), the following findings are of particular interest in this connection. Isoelectric pelt of calfskin was used as the substrate. Table 20 shows the results of comparative series with hydrochloric and acetic acid in regard to the degree of swelling produced by the solutions (in grams of water associated with 1 g. of collagen), the degree of solubilization of collagen, and the permanent irreversible swelling of the treated pelt after the swelling agent was removed and the stock brought back to the isoelectric state. The latter will be a measure of the *permanent* changes of the structure and the cohesion of collagen due to the specific effect of the acid.

The direct swelling produced by acetic acid at pH 2.0 is about 50% greater than that induced by hydrochloric acid, and the degree of peptization of collagen is about eight times as great. Pelt pretreated in acetic acid solution, subsequently freed from acid by neutralization, and made isoelectric shows a large *permanent* swelling. Hydrochloric acid gives only a light permanent change. The degree of organization of the structure is markedly lowered by the acetic acid treatment, as is evident from the decrease in shrinkage temperature of 12 degrees, the corresponding figure for the specimen treated in solution of hydrochloric acid being 5 degrees. The shrinkage temperature is considered to be a measure of the strength of the intermolecular forces of the protein lattice. These data indicate that the swelling produced by acetic acid differs fundamentally from the swelling due to hydrochloric acid, certain irreversible changes in the collagen structure being imparted by the lyotropic agent.

In order to ascertain whether the molecule of the acid or its anion, or both, are responsible for the drastic effect of moderately concentrated solutions of acetic acid on the permanent swelling of collagen, the effect of buffer solutions of sodium acetate–acetic acid of various molarities, adjusted to pH 5.7, were investigated (27). After 120 hours of treatment of pelt in solutions containing 0.25 to 3 M acetate, only 0.1 to 0.6% collagen was solubilized, and the degree of swelling was 3.5 to 3.6, compared to 3.0 for untreated pelt. No permanent swelling was evident. The acetate-treated pelt possessed a binding capacity identical to that of the blank for ionic and coordinate reacting agents. These findings prove the nonparticipation of the acetate ions in the swelling and disorganization of collagen by means of acetic acid. It was deemed of interest to ascertain the nature of the permanent alterations produced by the acetic acid treatment and the binding groups of collagen for the acid. Series of pelt treated in acetic acid of various concentrations for 120 hours were run simultaneously with series in hydrochloric acid in the absence and in the presence of swelling-depressing sodium chloride; corresponding series were run with sulfuric acid. The treated specimens were freed from electrolytes and brought back to the isoelectric state. By including systems with straight solutions of mineral acid and also systems in which the swelling was eliminated by the addition of neutral salt, an evaluation of the changes due to the hydrogen ion itself and to the swelling process was obtained. The isoelectric-conditioned, pretreated specimens were then tanned for 48 hours in chromium salts of two different types: (1) cationic chromium complexes and (2) nonionic sulfito-chromium complexes and also mimosa tannins. The titration curves of the specimens treated in acetic acid were also obtained for the pelt restored to the isoelectric state. Its acid-binding capacity was slightly increased, as measured by fixation of decinormal hydrochloric acid, made $M/2$ in sodium chloride. However, a markedly greater acid binding was present in the pH range 2.5 to 5, probably caused by the swelling and contraction of the protein chains, resulting in increasing the gaps between COO^- and NH_3^+ groups, decreasing the electrostatic interaction, and thus facilitating the discharge of the carboxyl ions of collagen by the hydrogen ions, as described for urea-treated collagen. The alkali binding increased in the pH range 7 to 10, and also the binding capacity for OH ion to some extent. The treatment in 2 to 3 M acetic acid results in some deamidation of collagen, which means an increase in the content of carboxylic groups. This explains the small increase of cationic chrome fixation noted for the acetic acid-pretreated pelt.

TABLE 21

THE EFFECT OF PRETREATMENT OF COLLAGEN IN ACID SOLUTIONS ON ITS REACTIVITY
TO TANNING AGENTS (27)

Pretreated with	Final pH	Dissolved Collagen, %	Cr$_2$O$_3$, % Fixed by Collagen from		Organic Matter, % Taken up by Collagen from Mimosa Extract	
			66% acid Cr-sulfate	Sulfito-Cr-sulfate	Total	Irre-vers-ible
3 M acetic acid	2.0	16	7.3	29.8	164	76
2 M acetic acid	2.2	12	7.1	25.7	164	69
M acetic acid	2.3	7	6.8	24.3	159	74
0.04 M hydrochloric acid	1.9	5	6.8	21.5	135	72
0.04 M hydrochloric acid, containing 5% w/v NaCl	1.9	0.4	6.7	14.7	92	55
0.1 M hydrochloric acid	1.2	4	6.8	19.1	124	67
0.1 M hydrochloric acid, containing 5% w/v NaCl	1.2	0.4	6.4	14.6	93	51
0.05 M sulfuric acid	1.9	3	6.7	17.2	112	63
0.05 M sulfuric acid, containing 5% w/v Na$_2$SO$_4$	1.9	0.4	6.6	14.8	92	51
H$_2$O (blank)	5.7	0.1	6.7	14.6	93	52

The results of these experiments are summarized in Table 21. The comments on these data will be very much the same as those given on the reactivity of collagen pretreated in solutions of lyotropic salts. It is evident that the ionic reaction capacity of collagen is not altered by the action of the acids in swelling or nonswelling systems, as is proved by the fixation of cationic chromium from 66% acid chromium sulfate. However, a slight increase is noted for the specimens pretreated in the most concentrated solutions of acetic acid. This is due to deamidation of collagen, whereby additional carboxyl groups are made available and enter into the reaction. As to the interaction of the nonionic chromium complexes of the solution of sulfito-chromium sulfate, the acetic acid-treated stock shows a very large increase in the fixation of these complexes, particularly the specimen from the 3 M solution, which has doubled its chrome uptake. It is interesting to compare the effect of hydrogen ions in systems allowing free swelling of the substrate and those in which swelling is prevented by the osmotic pressure of the neutral salt added, with respect to the fixation of the coordinating agent of nonionic chromium by the variously pretreated skin tissues. The data show that the changes in the substrate brought about by the swelling govern the degree of the combination of the nonionic chromium with collagen and, further, that the effect of the hydrogen ion, if restricted to the discharge of the carboxyl ions in the pretreatment, exerts no permanent change in the reactivity of collagen. The main alterations concern the nonionic crosslinks, i.e., rupture of the hydrogen bonds. The contraction and disorganization of the collagen chains associated with the swelling are partly irreversible, and fewer interchain crosslinks are present in the swelled stock after it is brought back to the isoelectric state. Accordingly, the swelled substrate contains a greater number of coordination sites on these noncompensated links, probably of the hydrogen bond type, than the original collagen. The increased chrome fixation of the coordinate type is thus explained. It agrees with the view of the nature of the lyotropic effect which has been promulgated in this text.

Concerning the uptake of vegetable tannins (mimosa extract), both the total removal of the constituents of the extract and the amounts of irreversibly fixed tannins are included; the latter are the part of tannins combined with collagen so tenaciously as to resist the prolonged action of water or aqueous solutions of a pH corresponding to that of the tanning bath. Evidently, both types of combination are a function of the permanent degree of swelling, resulting from the lyotropic effect of the acetic acid, and the secondary alterations caused by the osmotic swelling of the mineral acid, which create unfavorable steric conditions for crosslinking of collagen chains and thus make available new sites of reaction in the collagen structure.

In the provocative paper, "Collagen Structure and the Vegetable Tanning Process," Braybrooks, McCandlish, and Atkin (2) stress the governing role of the degree of swelling of the hide in making it accessible to the tannins. The starting point in their discussion is the accessibility of the amino groups to the tannins. The parallelism between the curves showing the effect of the pH value of the systems on the vegetable tannin fixation, on the one hand, and on the degree of swelling of the hide, on the other, is striking. Since any increased reactivity of the ionic groups, such as the amino groups, is not induced by the swelling, with regard to maximal binding capacity, the groups chiefly affected and increased being the nonionic groups of collagen, this view needs to be modified by including the coordinating protein groups, as the groups chiefly affected by the swelling and of vital importance for the fixation of vegetable tannins.

In view of the strong tendency shown by the acetic acid molecule to become hydrogen bonded, the following schematic picture (27) of the reaction of collagen with solutions of acetic acid of concentrations greater than 1 M

seems applicable:

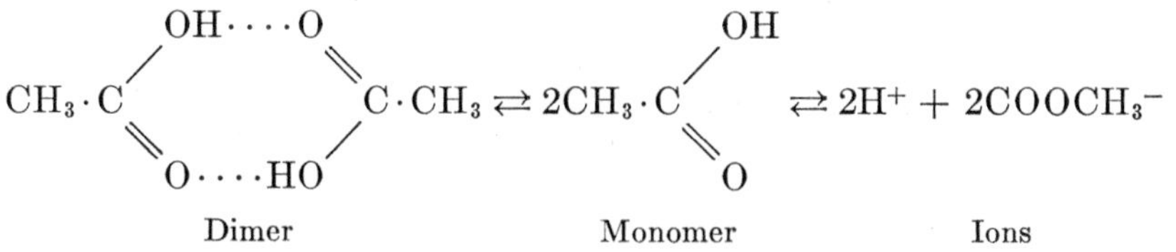

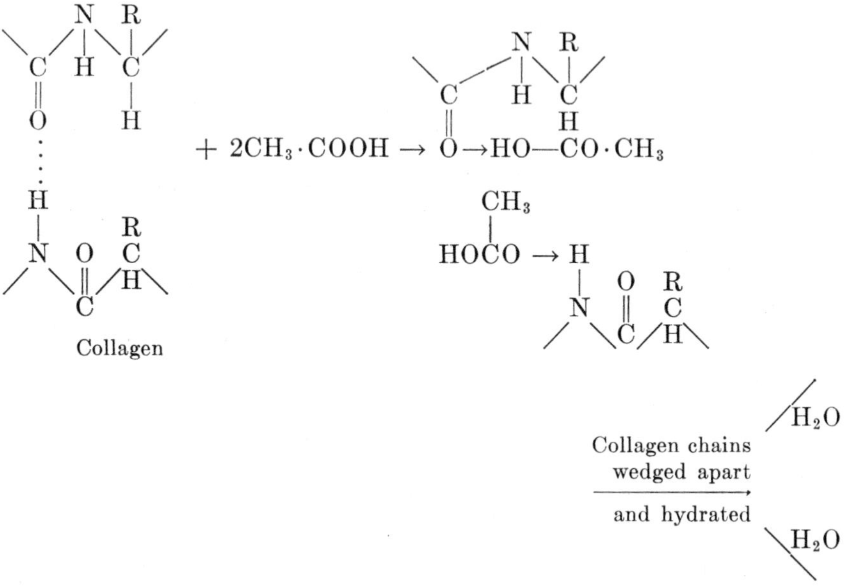

$$CH_3 \cdot C \overset{OH\cdots O}{\underset{O\cdots HO}{\diagup\diagdown}} C \cdot CH_3 \rightleftharpoons 2CH_3 \cdot C \overset{OH}{\underset{O}{\diagup}} \rightleftharpoons 2H^+ + 2COOCH_3^-$$

| Dimer | Monomer | Ions |

$$+ 2CH_3 \cdot COOH \rightarrow \overset{N\ R}{\underset{}{C\ H\ C}} \ O \rightarrow HO - CO \cdot CH_3$$

Collagen

$$HO\overset{CH_3}{C}O \rightarrow H$$

Collagen chains
wedged apart
────────────
and hydrated

This schematic illustration shows how the acetic acid molecules successfully compete with the collagen chains for valency sites on the CO and NH groups of the peptide bonds. The discharge of the carboxylic ions by the hydrogen ions of acetic acid occurs simultaneously, resulting in dislocation of the salt links between chains. However, the main cohesive and inter-chain bridging is due to hydrogen bonds, and the breaking of these links or part of them, followed by the attachment of acetic acid molecules on the CO and NH groups, removes the restraint of the chains. These are prone to take on the most probable and natural configuration of the chains, i.e., the state of disorder. This means giving up of the parallel alignment in parts, and contraction and disorganization of chains is the final result. It may also be conceived as a wedging apart of the collagen chains at the points where acetic acid is combining with collagen. This partial crumpling of the chains, with widening of the distance between sites of interchain crosslinks, is mainly an irreversible process, which only to a slight degree is reversed by applying strain or loads on the fibers. By removal of acetic acid, making the collagen isoelectric, water molecules are taking the sites occupied by acetic acid. An increased hydration of collagen is the final result, and also greater ability for reaction with, and binding of agents specifically directed on, nonionic valency forces in their reactions with proteins.

It then seems safe to conclude that the lyotropic effects of carboxylic acids on collagen are intimately connected with the hydrogen bonding power of the molecules of the acids, and that breaking or weakening of interchain crosslinks of the type of hydrogen bonds is the principal reaction which leads to contraction and labilization of the chains, alterations which are chiefly permanent.

5. THE ACTION OF PHENOLS

Among the lyotropic agents of principally nonionic type, phenol is one of the most interesting and thoroughly investigated. The ionization constant of phenol, 1.7×10^{-10}, is much larger than that of aliphatic alcohols. Pauling (28) attributes this fact to resonance with the structures

which will give the oxygen atom a positive charge. Hence, conditions are favorable for hydrogen bonding to take place with the phenol molecule.

More than forty years ago, Herzog and Adler (29) investigated the sorption of phenols by hide powder and found that the adsorption of phenol did not obey the common adsorption formula. The system collagen–phenol solutions has since been investigated by Küntzel and Schwank (30). They found that an exponential equation of the form $y = a^b$ describes the reaction, in which y = amount of sorbed phenol and a = its concentration in the solution at equilibrium. The value of b was 2.5. In normal adsorptions, the value of b is usually less than 1. If it is assumed that an equilibrium between monomeric and dimeric phenol exists in the stronger solutions and, further, that the main part of the phenol is adsorbed as the dimer, the value of the constant b will be about 2. Then, it is likely that the dimer, which should be a much weaker acid than the monomer, is mainly sorbed by collagen. Very large amounts of phenol are sorbed, or amounts about ten times as great as the stoichiometric maximum value. Thus, from a 5 % solution of phenol, hide powder will take up about 60 % of its own weight.

The sorption does not involve ionic groups of collagen, since the binding of mineral acids and strong bases by collagen is unchanged. It is worthy of note that shrinkage of collagen occurs at room temperature in solutions of phenol containing 8 % phenol or more.

Of particular great interest is the reversal of the sign of the birefringence of the collagen fibers by adsorption of phenol in quantities of at least 20 % of the weight of collagen. This interesting phenomenon was noticed by von Ebner sixty years ago. As mentioned earlier, the collagen fiber shows positive double refraction. By incorporation of various tanning agents into the structure, the degree and sign of the birefringence are in many instances altered. Some tanning agents, particularly some vegetable tannins, may also cause a shift from positive to negative values. Such a reversal is also induced by the adsorbed phenol. The reason is probably the arrangement of the phenol molecules, which possess negative values of double refraction, parallel to the fiber axis of collagen. The magnitude of the negative value of the refraction of the phenol more than outweighs that of the positive value of the fiber. In view of the similar action of certain tannins, a parallel alignment of these in the collagen structure probably takes place on their attachment to the protein.

A comparable case occurs in the textile field (31). Direct dyestuffs of the benzidine class, such as Congo red, attach themselves to cellulose by hydrogen bonding parallel to the main axis of the cellulose molecule, as is evident from the double refraction of the fibers. This can easily be demonstrated by viewing the fibers through a polarizing device, or simply through a piece of Polaroid glass. Most interestingly, azoic dyes arrange themselves on the cellulose fiber with their conjugated chains at right angles to the fiber axis of cellulose. In both instances, the spacing of the sites of the hydrogen bonds in the dyestuff molecule appears to be the deciding factor for the particular mode of orientation to be established by the dyestuff on the fiber. Similar differences in orientation of vegetable tannins, with reference to the main direction of the fibers, are probably the cause of the opposite effects of tannins fixed by collagen on its sign and degree of birefringence. Similar effects are produced by dihydric phenols.

Some foundation for an explanation of the drastic effect of phenol on collagen is supplied by Pfeiffer's investigations of the molecular compounds formed between phenols and anhydrides of amino acids (32). Thus, Pfeiffer has prepared molecular compounds of phenol and sarcosine in the crystalline form, which, according to our present concept of valence, are hydrogen-bonded structures. In sarcosine, the group —CO·N·CH$_3$— takes the place of the —CO·NH— group of proteins; i.e., the imino hydrogen of the sarcosine peptide bond is methylated. Pfeiffer conceived the molecular compound formed between each molecule of phenol and sarcosine to be coordinated on the oxygen atom of the CO groups of the sarcosine ring structure and on the hydrogen atom of the phenol group. Amines give a similar type of compound.

The interaction of phenol with collagen may then be conceived to involve a similar system. The attraction of the phenol molecule to the peptide bond and its hydrogen bonding on the liberated sites of the —CO—NH— linkage, with the resulting rupture of bonds and disorganization of protein chains, should be in line with the cases of lyotropic functioning agents discussed previously. The association of the phenol on collagen is pictured by Küntzel (33) to conform with the schematic formula:

$$
\begin{array}{c}
\text{C} \quad \text{H} \\
\diagup \parallel \diagdown \text{N} \diagup \\
\{ \text{O}_- \}^+ \\
\text{H}_- \quad \{ \quad \}^+ \\
\text{C}\!\!=\!\!\text{CH} \\
\overset{+}{\text{HC}}\diagup \qquad \diagdown \overset{-}{\text{COH}} \\
\diagdown_- \quad \overset{+}{\diagup}\!\!\diagup \\
\text{C}\!\!-\!\!\text{C} \\
\text{H} \quad \text{H}
\end{array}
$$

This represents a mutual attraction of two dipoles. According to Küntzel (33), the lyotropic effect of phenol and the tanning action of polyphenolic vegetable tannins are extremes of the same phenomenon, which meet in the reaction mechanism toward proteins. Both classes of compounds form addition compounds with collagen by coordination on the peptide bonds. The action of the unifunctional phenol leads to disorganization and solubilization of collagen, since it breaks crosslinks of the protein lattice by its combination, whereas the incorporation of polyfunctional polyphenolic tannins into the collagen lattice results in stabilization of the structure, probably through multifunctional interaction of the numerous phenolic groups of one large molecule, with a degree of extension making interaction with adjacent peptide bonds feasible, with neighboring protein chains riveting them together. The unifunctional reaction and the hydrophilic nature of the simple phenol, and the entirely different properties of the polyphenols, contribute to the diametrically opposite effects produced on the protein. Küntzel speculates also about the function of the phenolic groups. He believes that the group itself is not responsible for the affinity of this class of compounds for collagen or for the tanning power of the natural polyphenols. Instead, he believes that the main function of the phenolic group in tanning agents is to induce polarity in the aromatic nucleus. The formation of activated CH groups with alternating positive and negative charge should then be the governing factor in the affinity of the tannins for collagen, and the activated CH groups adjacent to the OH group should be the loci for the binding. The scheme given above would thus apply generally. This rather speculative claim should, according to its originator, give the answer to the question of why other groups than the phenolic one, such as the sulfonic acid group, for instance, are able to induce tanning action in aromatic compounds. The concept seems rather far-fetched in view of the earlier stated possibilities of resonance of the molecule of the simple phenol, which indeed is expected to affect the electron movement and density over the whole benzene ring. The theory of Otto, which is similar to the concept discussed and involves the mobile electrons, the π electrons, advanced for the explanation of the secondary binding of dyestuffs by collagen, will be discussed later.

The reaction between dihydric phenols and collagen is of interest, particularly with reference to the influence of the position of the substituents in the benzene ring (34). It was erroneously claimed by Shuttleworth and Cunningham (35) that intramolecular hydrogen bonding of the adjacent hydroxy groups of the 1,2 derivative, catechol, explains its nonreactivity to collagen. In fact, among the diphenols the ortho compound shows the greatest affinity for collagen, and if authors mentioned had acquainted themselves with the literature on the hydrogen bonding of diphenols, as given in Pauling's well-known treatise, they would have been avoided this error. Also, reference to Pfeiffer's paper on the existence of the hydrogen-bonded structure between sarcosine and catechol is informative (32). As an example of the lyotropic effect of the dihydric phenols in 2 M solutions on collagen, the decrease in shrinkage temperature of the treated skin is instructive (34). The ortho compound causes a decrease of 16 degrees, whereas the meta isomer causes a decrease of 8 degrees. Even at the concentration mentioned the diphenols do not degrade collagen into soluble products. The para isomer, the hydroquinone, in saturated solution (0.6 M) does not affect the shrinkage temperature of pelt.

6. Lyotropic Effects of Anions

Strong lyotropic effects are produced by the anions of many aromatic carboxylic or sulfonic acids, particularly those which also carry a hydroxy group, for instance sodium salicylate. They are most active in the form of the highly ionized salts of alkali metals. The action of the anions on collagen is probably connected with an indirect electrostatic interaction with the peptide bond, which leads to the subsequent breaking of intermolecular hydrogen bonds. Synthetic tannins of sulfonic acid type also show this effect in neutral solution, whereas as acids they stabilize collagen by irreversible fixation on its cationic groups. The ionic function of the acid preponderates in this instance. The stabilizing or labilizing effects of the same compound—according to its state in solution, as an acid or as a salt—are exemplified, indicating that the affinity of a given compound for collagen may result in tanning, or in its opposite effect, lyotropism, according to the condition of the reaction.

7. THE ACTION OF DETERGENTS AND SOME POLYACIDS

Detergents of the type of alcohol sulfonates, such as the sodium salt of dodecyl sulfuric acid, also show a specific anionic effect on proteins, which probably involves reactions similar to those described. The salt mentioned, when applied in solutions of 5% strength, swells hide and lowers its shrinkage temperature (36). This labilization of the fibrous structure is to some extent permanent, as proved by the increased fixation of coordination agents by the pretreated stock freed from the agent and made isoelectric (36). The interaction of sodium dodecyl sulfate with collagen may be conceived as the electrovalent reaction of the long chainlike anion of the salt with the cationic protein groups. The organic acid anion then tends to wedge apart the protein chains, thereby impairing the strength of the salt link. The disrupted protein chains with laterally attached anions of the detergent will then build up layers of negative charge in the form of micelles of the detergent, which tend to repel groups of equal charge on adjacent protein chains, causing rupture of hydrogen bond crosslinks by the contraction of the protein chains.

Two factors are involved in this interaction of dodecyl sulfate, according to Lundgren (37): (1) the ionic group of the detergent molecule, and (2) its specific affinity, which is related to the size and structure of the detergent, resulting in stabilization of the micelles by the mutual affinity of the hydrocarbon portions of adjacently bound detergent ions. Hence, the swelling and decrease in hydrothermal stability are secondary effects, similar to the disorganization of the collagen structure, produced by strong mineral acids, such as hydrochloric acid, at pH values 1 to 2, of maximum osmotic swelling not involving lyotropic action in itself. The important fact is that the dodecyl sulfate is unifunctional. Pankhurst's (38) investigations have contributed substantially to our knowledge of the reactions between detergents and collagen.

Theoretically interesting and of practical importance is the finding of Steinhardt and Fugitt (39) that anions possessing marked affinity for the cationic protein groups will accelerate the deamidation of the protein on subsequent treatment in weakly acidic solution. Application of detergents offers a method of catalyzing the deamidation during mild conditions of reaction and has been used for the analytical determination of the content of amide groups in proteins. However, Cassel and McKenna (40) have found that anions of high-molecular acids do not markedly increase the rate of deamidation of collagen.

The maximum degree of swelling of bovine skin by the detergents mentioned is approached under conditions that allow complete interaction of the detergent anions with the cationic protein groups. The dispergation and solubilization of codskin is obtained under similar conditions. Bovine skin is not degraded into water-soluble products by the corresponding treatment. The different behavior of the two types of collagen is in harmony with the view that mammalian collagen is stabilized by crosslinks of the hydrogen bond type mainly, supplemented by salt links. The latter type of cohesive forces contribute to the main organization and stability of collagen of fishskin (*Teleostei*). As mentioned earlier, the low hydroxyproline content of teleostean collagen may be one of the reasons for the scarcity of hydrogen bond crosslinks in fish collagen, if the view is correct that the hydroxy group of this residue forms a hydrogen bond with the keto-imide group.

Investigations of the behavior of skin collagens of mammals and fishes toward solutions of the high-molecular fraction of lignosulfonic acid, condensed naphthalene sulfonic acids, and mineral acids are of interest in this connection (36). Thus, solutions of decinormal hydrochloric acid swells and dispergates fish collagen much more easily and extensively than bovine collagen, 85% of the former going into solution, in comparison with 1 to 2% of the latter. The high-molecular lignosulfonic acid, which slightly dehydrates bovine collagen, induces a peculiar shrinkage and curling of the fishskin. In solutions of final pH values of 1.5 to 2.0, the sulfo acid completely inactivates the cationic protein groups by irreversible combination with them, leading to complete discharge of the ionic protein groups which form the salt links, and hence destroying them.

The curling action of lignosulfonic acid on fishskin is not of an osmotic nature, comparable to that of strong mineral acids, since the irreversible fixation of the anion of the sulfo acid excludes the participation of Donnan effects, which require completely reversible systems with free, charged basic protein groups. The curling and irreversible swelling of fish collagen is in this instance probably related to its weak intermolecular cohesion. By elimination of the charge on the ionic protein groups and hence the saltlike ionic crosslinks which they form, the intermolecular cohesion of fish collagen is practically destroyed. Since the dominant stabilizing forces of the lattice of bovine collagen are supplied by nonionic forces, probably hydrogen bonds, the elimination of the relatively unimportant ionic crosslinks by the irreversibly fixed sulfo acid is a question of secondary importance for the stability of bovine collagen and does not lead to radical changes in the cohesion of the structure (36).

This concept receives further experimental support from measurements of the shrinkage temperature and the tensile strength of calfskin and fishskin collagen (cod) containing basic groups completely inactivated by the lignosulfonic acid. The shrinkage temperature of calfskin is not changed by this interaction, whereas codskin is irreversibly shrunk, even in water of 10 to 15°C., which means a decrease of the shrinkage temperature of at least 30 degrees, from a temperature of 40 to 45°C. to one of 10°C. On prolonged treatment, codfish skin in solutions of lignosulfonic acid will swell, curl, contract, and gradually lose its structural characteristics and tensile strength, finally becoming a gluelike mass, whereas the correspondingly treated calfskin takes on a "leathery" appearance with its tensile strength and other mechanical properties intact. These examples are illuminating, for they show the importance of the nature of the crosslinking bridges of various collagens for their swelling and stability (36).

8. OPTICAL STUDIES OF SWELLING

As emphasized before, the osmotic swelling produced by dilute solutions of strong acids is reversible in contrast to the lyotropic swelling, which fact makes it probable that the main features of the structural alignment remain fairly intact in this type of swelling. It is interesting to note that the high-angle X-ray diffraction is lost in collagen of maximum acid swelling. The diffraction and electron-optical methods are difficult to employ on swelled proteins because of the large amount of water associated with the proteins. Nutting and Borasky (41) have studied the effect of swelling agents on collagen fibrils with the electron microscope. Pictures of the dispersion of cowhide fibrils by a concentrated solution of barium chloride show a remarkably localized attack on the fibrils by the lyotropic agent. The tendency of the swollen fibrils to loop and twist is characteristic, as is also the enormous swelling that takes place explosively. In the unaffected segments adjacent to the sites of swelling, the periodicity is practically normal, with spacings between 600 and 625 Å. Heat-shrunk fibers give pictures similar to the ones described.

Hydrochloric or acetic acid in 0.05 N solution gives similar pictures. The acid swelling produces longitudinal subdivision, but the striations are readily traceable across the groups of filaments. The distribution of the spacings broaden. The most frequently occurring interval is at 540 Å.

Prolonged liming—for two months in saturated lime—causes a marked degradation of the fibrils of cowhide. The most noteworthy feature of the overlimed fibril is its dissolution into a coiled filament.

In view of the low degree of internal cohesion and crosslinking of fishskin collagen, the electron-microscopic pictures of native sharkskin collagen taken by Nutting and Borasky (41) are of interest, since they are similar in appearance to the last-mentioned sample. The fibrils appear faint and indistinct and are markedly swollen by hydration only, showing spiriforms.

Striations are hardly noticeable. The indistinct pictures of fishskin collagen with a shrinkage temperature of 40°C., compared to 68°C. for the cowhide collagen, are not surprising in view of the weakly developed lateral cohesion of the fibrils of the teleostian collagen.

Similar electron micrographs (41) are given by the cowhide fibrils which have been contracted by shrinkage. These findings are discussed in this chapter, although they really belong to the following one, since the similarity of the processes of hydrothermal and lyotropic shrinkage is strikingly demonstrated. The smaller fibers began to shrink at 63°C., and the larger ones at 68°C. The 63°C. specimens strongly resembled the barium chloride-treated specimens. The main part of the fibrils were striated. However, at irregular intervals along the fibrils, particularly at the ends, they were enormously swollen. The distribution in periodicity was broadened and decreased, the lowest value observed being 450 Å. The heat-denatured collagen took the form of a thread, arranged as a loose, flattened spiral, embedded in a thin, transparent film much wider than the diameter of the spiral.

From the electron-microscopic evidence, Nutting and Borasky (41) conclude that shrinkage of collagen by swelling agents and by heat may be described as follows: Collagen is initially composed of orderly arrays of chains, the striated fibrils. In plasticizing by heat in the presence of water and by swelling agents, the cohesive forces maintaining the orderly structure are weakened. The inherent natural contractile tendency of the fibrils, due to the entropy, results in a less orderly arrangement, in which the fibril as a whole is shortened by contraction of the filaments.

In his lucid comments on the swelling of collagen, Bear (42) stresses two distinct types: (1) *osmotic* swelling, associated with the Donnan effects and (2) *lyotropic* swelling. In Bear's model of collagen, which has been described earlier, the electrovalent groups of collagen were placed together at fibrillar bands. Now, most of the information derived from electron optics concerns the interband structure, and unfortunately little can be determined regarding the details of the band organization. The present investigations of the swelling phenomena have not contributed much to our knowledge of the steric relationship of the salt links and the hydrogen bond-forming linkages, or side chains of the collagen fibrils. The existence of the former requires the location of the ionic groups at a close proximity in the same locality, e.g., in the bands.

Figure 14 shows a diagram of Bear's explanation of the changes in the shape of the dry fibril (shown at *a*) taking place on osmotic and lyotropic swelling. On swelling in water at neutrality, which may principally represent lyotropic swelling, the fibril takes the form shown at *b*. And finally, on acid swelling (osmotic swelling), the more profound changes are as represented by the structure at c. Only polar side chains are shown in these diagrams. The open-circled heads of the side chains denote uncharged R groups, and those with $+$ and $-$ signs represent correspondingly charged groups. The protons are designated H.

The picture of the dry fibril (a) shows that the large charged side chains in the band region distort the vertical main chain helices from a straight course. The diagram at b pictures the change of the protofibrillar spaces by the penetration of the isoelectric fibril by water. Both bands and interbands are involved in this hydration. The result is a widening of the distance between individual chains, which also are straightened out, because more room becomes available for the ionic side chains at the band level. A limit to the degree of swelling is set by the hydrogen bonds between the polar side chains at interbands. The bulky structure at c represents the acid-swollen fibril. By addition of acid, the negatively charged R groups are discharged by the protons, and an equal number of positively charged side chains are freed. By the repulsion of these free positive ions, the distance between the chains is markedly increased. This is not restricted to the bands, since by the contraction of the polypeptide chains, and also by the rupture of the hydrogen bonds, the interbands are partially ruptured or weakened indirectly. Although this osmotic swelling is initially located in the bands, the interbands will also be affected by the contraction of the main chains. Bear points out that it is fairly well agreed that salt links such as those shown in the bands are of minor importance in integrating fibrillar structures of fully hydrated collagen, and that the main cohesive forces are supplied by the hydrogen bonding of the chains at the interband level. The latter bonds are involved in the thermal contraction, the lyotropic swelling, and the dispersion of proteins. Such diagrams are very helpful in the study of collagen behavior.

REFERENCES

1. Balfe, M. P., J. Soc. Leather Trades Chem. **32**, 39 (1948); **34**, 30 (1950).
2. Braybrooks, W. E., McCandlish, D., and Atkin, W. R., J. Intern. Soc. Leather Trades Chem. **23**, 111, 135 (1939); Page, R. O., J. Soc. Leather Trades Chem. **37**, 183 (1953).
3. Thomas, A. W., and Foster, S. B., Ind. Eng. Chem. **17**, 1162 (1925); Thomas, A. W., and Kelly, M. W., ibid. **19**, 477 (1927).
4. Wilson, J. A., "The Chemistry of Leather Manufacture," Vol. 1, p. 232. Chemical Catalog Co., New York, 1928.
5. Gustavson, K. H., J. Am. Leather Chem. Assoc. **21**, 206 (1926).
6. Stiasny, E., Science **57**, 483 (1923); Z. angew. Chem. **33**, 456 (1920); Collegium **1920**, 255.
7. See Cohnheim, O., "Chemie der Eiweisskörper," 3rd ed., p. 77. Vieweg, Brunswick, 1911.
8. Bergmann, M., Collegium **1922**, 314; **1925**, 556; **1926**, 494; Abderhalden, E., Naturwissenschaften **12**, 719 (1924).

9. Waldschmidt-Leitz, E., and Schaeffner, A., *Ber.* **58**, 1356 (1925).

10. Bergmann, M., Miekeley, A., and Kann, E., *Z. physiol. Chem.* **140**, 128 (1924); **146**, 247 (1925); *Biochem. Z.* **177**, 1 (1926).

11. Meyer, K. H., and Mark, H., *Ber.* **61**, 1932 (1928).

12. Astbury, W. T., "Fundamentals of Fibre Structure," Oxford University Press, London, 1933.

13. Loeb, J., "Proteins and the Theory of Colloidal Behavior." McGraw-Hill, New York, 1922; Loeb, J., and Kunitz, M., *J. Gen. Physiol.* **5**, 693 (1923).

14. Pfeiffer, P., and Würgler, J., *Z. physiol. Chem.* **97**, 128 (1926); *Ber.* **48**, 1938 (1915).

15. Gustavson, K. H., *Colloid Symposium Monograph* **4**, 79 (1926).

16. Gustavson, K. H., *Svensk Kem. Tidskr.* **56**, 14 (1944); *J. Soc. Leather Trades Chem.* **30**, 264 (1946); *J. Colloid Sci.* **1**, 397 (1946).

17. Gustavson, K. H., unpublished investigation.

18. Gustavson, K. H., *in* "Handbuch der Gerbereichemie" (W. Grassmann, ed.), Vol. II, Part 2, p. 192. Springer, Vienna, 1939.

19. Grassmann, W., Janicki, J., and Schneider, F., *in* "Stiasny Festschrift," p. 74. Roether, Darmstadt, 1937.

20. Sizer, I. W., *Enzymologia* **13**, 293 (1949).

21. Batzer, H., and Weissenberger, G., *Makromol. Chem.* **7**, 320 (1952).

22. Gustavson, K. H., and Holm, B., *J. Am. Leather Chem. Assoc.* **47**, 700 (1952).

23. Gustavson, K. H., *Biochem. Z.* **311**, 347 (1942).

24. Burk, N. F., and Greenberg, D. M., *J. Biol. Chem.* **87**, 197 (1930).

25. Katchalsky, A., Eisenberg, H., and Lifson, S., *J. Am. Chem. Soc.* **73**, 5889 (1951).

26. Pauling, L., and Brockway, L. O., *Proc. Natl. Acad. Sci. U. S.* **20**, 336 (1934); Pauling, L., "The Nature of the Chemical Bond," pp. 306–308. Cornell University Press, Ithaca, N. Y., 1940.

27. Gustavson, K. H., *Svensk Kem. Tidskr.* **55**, 191 (1943).

28. Pauling, L., "The Nature of the Chemical Bond," pp. 320–327. Cornell University Press, Ithaca, N. Y., 1940.

29. Herzog, R. O., and Adler, J., *Collegium* **1908**, 178, 182.

30. Küntzel, A., and Schwank, M., *Collegium* **1940**, 489.

31. Vickerstaff, T., "Physical Chemistry of Dyeing," p. 168. Oliver and Boyd, London, 1950.

32. Pfeiffer, P., "Organische Molekülverbindungen," 2nd ed., pp. 21–22. Enke, Stuttgart, 1927.

33. Küntzel, A., *in* "Handbuch der Gerbereichemie" (W. Grassmann, ed.), Vol. I, Part 1, p. 519, Springer, Vienna, 1944; Küntzel, A., and Schwank, M., *Collegium* **1940**, 500.

34. Gustavson, K. H., *J. Soc. Leather Trades Chem.* **33**, 256 (1949).

35. Shuttleworth, S. G., and Cunningham, G. E., *J. Soc. Leather Trades Chem.* **32**, 183 (1948).

36. Gustavson, K. H., *Acta Chem. Scand.* **4**, 1171 (1950).

37. Lundgren, H. P., *Advances in Protein Chem.* **5**, 305 (1949).

38. Pankhurst, K. A. G., *J. Soc. Leather Trades Chem.* **37**, 312 (1953).

39. Steinhardt, J., and Fugitt, C. H., *J. Research Natl. Bur. Standards* **29**, 315 (1942).

40. Cassel, M., and McKenna, E., *J. Am. Leather Chem. Assoc.* **48**, 142 (1953).

41. Nutting, G. C., and Borasky, R., *J. Am. Leather Chem. Assoc.* **43**, 96 (1948); Borasky, R., and Rogers, J. S., *ibid.* **47**, 312 (1952).

42. Bear, R. S., *Advances in Protein Chem.* **7**, 69 (1952).

CHAPTER 9

The Contraction of Collagen, Particularly Hydrothermal Shrinkage and Crosslinking Reactions

1. Introduction

The contraction of the collagen fiber is generally considered to result from the weakening or dislocation of the interchain crosslinks of the collagen fibrils. This may be accomplished by various means, for instance, by the application of energy in the form of heat (thermal shrinkage), by means of agents which interfere with the crosslinks by direct competition with the valency forces, or by the creation of unfavorable steric conditions in the protein chains. The effect of lyotropic agents is of the first type. A stretched chain of a high-polymer molecule which is free to take on the most probable form of configuration will spontaneously revert to a state of the greatest freedom, the folded form of maximum entropy content. The behavior of the nonpolar chain molecules is of interest in a discussion of the behavior of molecular chains of collagen in the free folded state.

The contraction or extension of a threadlike molecule devoid of crosslinks, which does not carry electrical charge and which exists in the free coiled state, is to some extent influenced by the environment (1). Thus, if the chain is present in a melt, it will on setting to an elastic solid be restrained by the neighboring molecules. The application or release of tensional forces is of fundamental importance for the understanding of the behavior of collagen fiber in the native extended state in skin, as well as in the denatured contracted state, even if the collagen chains differ from the nonpolar chains in many fundamental respects because of the chemical and electrochemical differences between the two materials. In collagen the restraining effects of the fiber-bundle weave and the stabilizing forces of the interchain crosslinks must first be overcome before the simple treatment of a free chain can be applied (2).

It is to be noted that the original coiled state and the artificially produced extended state show identical contents of energy. The inherent tendency of the stretched coil to revert to its natural state has nothing to do with change in energy. This very important point for the theory of the elastic behavior of rubber, for instance, and also for the thermal shrinkage of tendon was first recognized by Meyer, who in collaboration with Ferri (1) experimentally proved his thesis by thermal investigations of the stretching of rubber. Experiments of a similar type have also been carried out by Küntzel (2) in his clarifying investigation of the shrinkage of collagen. The difference between the contracted and the extended states is the higher degree of probability for the disordered state and hence a question of the entropy content, if entropy is considered a statistical indication of the degree of order in a system. Thus, from the Boltzmann equation, connecting the probability, P, with the entropy, S, with $S = K \log P$, the following relation between stress and strain is obtained:

$$Z = nkT \left(\alpha - \frac{1}{\alpha^2} \right) = \rho \frac{RT}{M} \left(\alpha - \frac{1}{\alpha^2} \right)$$

Here Z is the tension per unit of cross-sectional area of the original fiber; n is the number of molecules per milliliter; and $\alpha = 1/l_o = $ the ratio of the stretched and unstretched length of the fiber; ρ is the density; and M is the molecular weight of the fiber between junction points.

This formula, which applies to both extension and counteraction, differs from Hooke's classical law, in which the stress, Z, is proportional to the strain, α. It predicts that the elastic behavior of a rubberlike solid is determined by only one molecular constant, M, the molecular weight between junction points, and is applicable to any chainlike molecule, irrespective of its structure and chemical composition. This equation has been applied to the stress-strain behavior of heat-shrunk tendon, native as well as formaldehyde-tanned, for an approximation of the segmental molecular weight of collagen between crosslinks, i.e., the estimation of the number of crosslinks formed by the interchain-reacting formaldehyde (3).

The crosslinking of the chains, typified by collagen, will have a marked effect, as will the charge of the molecule. With increasing number of crosslinks, the lengths of unaffected chain segments diminish, indicating that the intramolecular Brownian motion is seriously impeded. In native collagen a stage is reached where contraction involves dislocation of bonds and crosslinks, invalidating the above treatment and application of the equation. Energy effects instead of entropy changes will be the determining factor for the behavior of collagen on shrinkage. It is then obvious that the study of the contraction of native collagen fibers must first be directed toward the kind and amount of the stabilizing forces, the interchain links, which are acted upon in the shrinkage. In the first phase of the contraction of collagen fibers, the heat of activation dominates; the secondary process of folding runs its own course spontaneously. The reason is the aforementioned urge of the orderly arranged chains of collagen to revert to the state of greatest disorder, thereby increasing the entropy of the system. By supplying energy in the form of heat, as in thermal shrinkage (that is, by increasing the kinetic energy of the polypeptide chains), the crosslinks should be ruptured to an extent sufficient to allow the chains to be freed from their restraint. The fiber configuration will then be able to follow its natural course without change in energy, as described for the free nonpolar chains.

2. The Effect of Electrolytes and Nonelectrolytes on the Contraction of Collagen

As was pointed out in the discussion of the swelling of collagen, the transformation of the fiber into an axially contracted, radially swollen form takes place by the osmotic swelling of solutions of acids and alkalis. The contracted form can be brought back to its original length by applying an appropriate tension. Some organic solvents produce a similar shrinkage. This change of the fiber from the normal, slightly extensible form to the rubber-like form with long-range elasticity has been explained as due to the opening up of crosslinks which hold the chains in place and in parallel alignment in the extended form.

Lloyd and Garrod (4) have advanced the view that the passage of collagen from the normal form to the axially contracted form can be explained by the assumption that the fully extended chains are held in place by two or more chemically distinct types of lateral bonds, one of which is weakened under the condition leading to thermal shrinkage, while the other does not give way until the collagen passes into solution. They consider the salt link to be a more labile bond than the hydrogen bond type of crosslinks which are assumed to function between hydroxy and amide groups or between peptide bonds or both. However, present knowledge rather favors the view that the hydrogen bond crosslink is principally involved in the thermal shrinkage. The extent of the opening up of these crosslinks is expected to govern the degree of shrinkage, which varies according to the type, shrinkage by heat or by swelling differing only in degree, not in kind.

a. Effect of nonelectrolytes

The effect of nonelectrolytes on the shrinking process is best presented in an introductory discussion, since any complications due to electric charge of the solute will thus be avoided. Since the shrinkage concerned is hydrothermal, water must be present. The shrinkage of a moisture-free fiber taking place in an anhydrous medium is an entirely different problem. It must be re-emphasized that proteins are associated with water in their *natural* state and that a water-free protein is an artifact from the point of view of reactivity and general behavior. Nevertheless, the influence of the dielectric property of organic solvents on collagen with regard to its shrinkage is of some interest. The strength of the salt links may be expected to be affected by the dielectric constant of the medium; raising this constant facilitates discharge of the groups, and lowering the constant increases

TABLE 22

DIELECTRIC CONSTANT OF THE MEDIUM AND THE T_s OF COLLAGEN (4)

Medium	Dielectric Constant	T_s , °C.
Methanol	27	86
Ethanol	35	70
Glycerol	39	70
Water	81	60–65
Formamide	84	15

their strength. The effect of some solvents of very different dielectrical properties on the shrinkage temperature of collagen is illustrated in Table 22.

In a general way, these particular data support the claim that by raising the dielectric constant the T_s is lowered. However, on examination of additional experimental material, it is found that there is no simple relationship between these two quantities, from one group of compounds to another, although the degree of polarity of the solvent appears to be related to the T_s produced within a homologous group of substances. Constitutional differences among the compounds evidently may modify the influence of the polarity and cause variations in the effect on the nonionic crosslinks (hydrogen bonds), as illustrated by a comparison of glycerol and methanol, on the one hand, and water and formamide on the other.

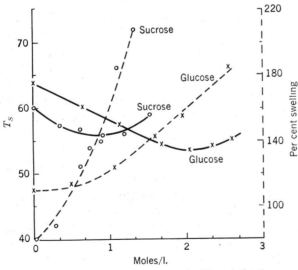

FIG. 31. The effect of sucrose and glucose on the T_s and the degree of swelling of skin as a function of the concentration of the sugars (4).

In Fig. 31, the shrinkage temperatures of collagen fibers treated in solutions of sugars are given as a function of the concentration of the solute. For comparison, the corresponding swelling curves are given, which on the whole bring out the close interrelationship of the two phenomena. Nevertheless some deviations exist, which indicate that other factors besides swelling are involved in controlling the T_s. In glucose, the marked swelling and the definite lowering of the T_s of the specimens treated in concentrated solutions of this sugar is of particular interest, since complications of electrical charges are eliminated. The presence of numerous hydroxy groups, functioning as hydrogen bonding sites, and their interaction with corresponding sites on collagen is probably the principal reason for the alterations observed. In all instances, the dehydrating effect of the very concentrated solutions appears to be involved, tending to elevate the T_s. This is particularly pronounced with ethanol. In connection with the effect of ethanol, the following interesting observation by Küntzel is worthy of mention (2). Collagen fibers which have been heat-shrunk in 80% ethanol, with T_s about 78°C., cannot only be restored to their original length by careful stretching of the fibers but can be elongated up to double the original fiber length by application of further tension. The X-ray diagram of the extended denatured fibers indicates the presence of chains aligned in parallel. This observation of the great extensibility of alcohol-treated collagen is especially interesting in view of the extensibility of collagen fibrils, which was first demonstrated by Schmitt (5, 6).

Another polyhydric nonelectrolyte of interest for its effect on the T_s is glycerol, which has been used as such or in admixture with water by Schiaparelli (7) and by Theis (8) as a medium for determination of the shrinkage temperature of leather, particularly chrome leather, which is stable to boiling water, in order to record T_s's exceeding 100°C. A solution of 75% glycerol and 25% water has even been sanctioned by the American Leather Chemists Association as a medium for determination of T_s generally in their provisional method (8). It has been pointed out (9) that glycerin lowers the T_s, in the concentration given by 10 to 11 degrees, and that it further may have secondary effects on the chromium complexes of chrome leather. Therefore it is not a suitable medium. The investigations of Weir and Carter (10) and of Balfe (11) point in the same direction. The use of water under pressure in a special apparatus has been tried with success on chrome leather with $T_s > 100$°C., as well as determinations in paraffin oil, by Bowes (11). The use of codskin with a spread of 60 degrees between the boiling point of water and the T_s of the skin has also been recommended in order to extend the temperature range of 35°C. obtainable by using the ordinary method for bovine collagen in chrome tanning tests (9). Weir and

Carter (10) point to the marked swelling of collagen taking place in glycerol solutions as an indication of the deterioration of collagen by glycerol.

Solvents, which evidently break the crosslinks completely cause dissolution of the fibers of proteins and of some polyamides, such as nylon. Examples are phenol, m-cresol, formic and lactic acids, and formamide. Since m-cresol dissolves nylon, its action should hence be directed toward rupture of the hydrogen bonds, the only stabilizing links present in this polyamide. The main effect of these agents on collagen is probably of the same nature. Organic solvents, such as the alcohols, do not contract the fiber, but only increase its width. The other solvents mentioned earlier decrease the length to about the same extent, one-fourth of the original length, as the thermal shrinkage does. The width may be increased three or four times. However, the most characteristic change is the rubberlike elasticity imparted to the collagen.

The role of water in the shrinkage process is strikingly shown by diverse observations. From an extreme point of view, the effect of the solutes generally, both electrolytes and nonelectrolytes, may in the final analysis be traced to the shift in the water equilibrium in the direction of depolymerization of aquo aggregates by breaking of hydrogen bonds, thus making reactive monomers of OH_2 molecules available for interaction with the hydrogen-bonding and other crosslinking protein groups. The importance of the water equilibrium for processes of peptization has been strongly and convincingly emphasized by Bancroft (12).

It is also quite clear that determination of the shrinkage temperature in organic solvents or in solutions of lyotropic agents tends to give lower values than those in water, since the effects of these agents on collagen are similar to that of heat. It seems to this author that the effect of any lyotropic agent on collagen should be appraised by the permanent alteration imparted to collagen. Thus, subsequent to the pretreatment, the agent should be removed, the treated protein brought back to the isoelectric state, and its T_s determined in water. This procedure has always been adhered to in the author's work, since it gives definite and significant results.

b. Effect of electrolytes

The effect of electrolytes on the hydrothermal stability of collagen is an exceedingly complicated problem. The effect of strong acids and bases in solutions of moderate concentration will not be treated, since the swelling of collagen produced in such solutions is similar to hydrothermal shrinkage, although reversible. Thus the fact that at high H ion and OH ion concentrations the T_s of collagen is lowered and a zone of maximum hydrothermal stability exists in the pH range 5 to 7 needs no further explanation. Neither will the lyotropic effect of strong acids in concentrated solutions, such as 2 M HCl solution, with complete shrinkage occurring at room temperature or lower, be discussed, since it is a consequence of the irreversible break- down of the intermolecular forces of the protein.

As to the neutral salts of lyotropic behavior, their action in solutions of low concentrations, such as 0.1 M, appears to be chiefly electrostatic, owing to the association of the ions of the salt with the charged groups of collagen. This type of interaction therefore mainly involves the salt link, which is weakened. However, on short interaction and after removal of the salt, the links are reformed, which is not the case with ruptured hydrogen bonds functioning as crosslinks.

The effect of 0.1 M solution of KCNS in lowering the T_s is rather slight. In high concentration, however, this salt will shrink and gelatinize collagen at temperatures of 15 to 20°C. (4), and in 8 M KCNS solution even at 2 to 3°C. (2). This effect is probably due to the molecules of KCNS, with an extensive rupture of nonionic crosslinks as the result, similar to the action of formamide. The relationship between the degree of swelling and the de- crease in thermal resistance of collagen is evident from comparison of the swelling and T_s curves. However, these effects are not always parallel. Thus, for the thiocyanate, the T_s decreases steadily with increasing salt concen- tration up to the saturation point of the solution, whereas maximum swelling is attained in a solution of 2 M strength. The chlorides of the alkali metals have only a slight effect on the T_s, decreasing it slightly in dilute solutions but increasing it in highly concentrated solutions, probably through their dehydrating effect, which creates favorable steric conditions for crosslinking. Attempts to explain the different effects of salts by the degree of hydration and the size of the ions has not met with success (13). It appears that the most important effects in the more concentrated solu- tions are connected with the action of the molecules themselves, as has been pointed out repeatedly.

A thermodynamic treatment of the effect of neutral salts and non-elec- trolytes of lyotropic nature on the thermal shrinkage of collagen (tendon) has recently been attempted by Weir and Carter (10), the former having earlier contributed a valuable investigation of the heat of activation of collagen in the shrinkage process along the same lines (14). This new approach to the problems involved shows great promise. Earlier thermo- dynamic considerations of the thermal shrinkage in the fundamental re- searches of the schools of Wöhlisch (15) and Meyer (16) should not be over- looked.

The effect of environment on the rate of shrinkage of tendon collagen was studied on aqueous solutions of neutral reaction containing organic solutes and lyotropic neutral salts (Weir and Carter, 10). Measurements of the rate of shrinkage were made at four different temperatures, spaced 2 to 3 degrees apart. The data of the length of the fiber and the time required for shrinkage were interpolated to obtain the time required for half shrinkage, $t_{1/2}$, which is defined as the time at which the length of the tendon, l, is one-half of the sum of the original length, l_o, and the final length, l_{60}. Experimental values of $t_{1/2}$, in seconds, and the reciprocal of the absolute temperature, $1/T$, were then introduced into the equation:

$$\log \frac{0.693h}{KTt_{1/2}} = \frac{-\Delta H}{2.303R} \cdot \frac{1}{T} + \frac{\Delta S}{2.303R}$$

where h is Planck's constant, K is Boltzmann's constant, ΔH is the heat of activation, and R is the gas constant. The equation is derived from the theory of absolute reaction rates, with $t_{1/2}$ in place of the reaction-velocity constant. A plot of the left term as the ordinate and $1/T$ as the abscissa yields a line having a slope proportional to the heat of activation, ΔH, and an intercept proportional to the entropy of the reaction, ΔS, as shown in Fig. 32. From the fundamental relationship $\Delta F = \Delta H - T \Delta S$, the free energy of reaction, ΔF, was determined. Since ΔF is directly related to the rate of shrinkage, the value of ΔF_{60} obtained at a shrinkage temperature of 60°C. may be taken as a measure of the temperature range in which

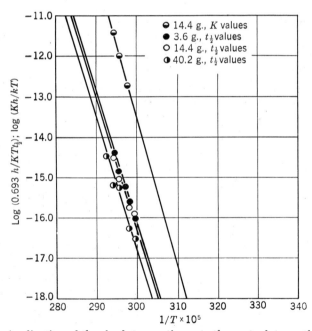

FIG. 32. Application of the absolute reaction rate theory to data on the shrinkage of collagen fibers (kangaroo tail tendon) at different loads of the fibers (Weir, 28).

shrinkage occurs at an experimentally measurable rate. In experiments with test media of various lyotropic agents, such as those of Weir and Carter (10), it is very difficult to compare the results with those of a standard environment, such as water, at pH 6 to 7, since the chemical potentials of solvent and solute are probably involved in the activation process. The data obtained also showed these effects. In the present connection, the effects of a strongly lyotropic salt, magnesium chloride, and a nonlyotropic salt, the corresponding sulfate, will be considered. The diametrically opposite effects of the chloride and the sulfate are strikingly brought out, the ΔF_{60} being 11 and 25 for the respective salts in 1.0 M solution, and the corresponding T_s values 41 and 67°. In 75% aqueous glycerol, the ΔF_{60} value was 18 and T_s was 53°, to mention an example of an organic nonelectrolyte which has been recommended as a medium for T_s determination.

In his early work, Weir (14) favored the view that the salt interacts principally with the ionic bonds of collagen and thus with the salt links. From the results of the work discussed, he had to reverse his concept that the hydrothermal shrinkage was due to the breaking of ionic crosslinks. If the salt links were mainly involved, it could be expected that ΔH would increase with the lowering of the dielectric constant of the medium, and increased cohesion would be the result. The reverse was found. Thus, ionic links apparently are not appreciably acted on in the shrinkage, and the effects produced by salts such as $CaCl_2$ are probably not the result of interaction of ions on the salt bond. The data were considered to be satisfactorily explained by the assumption that hydrogen bonds were involved, particularly from the following considerations.

The number of salt links is expected to be small because of the spatial restrictions inherent in collagen by virtue of its amino acid composition. On the basis of the latter, a rough estimate will show that the hydrogen bonds outnumber the ionic crosslinks by a factor of 7, according to the approximation of Weir and Carter. Further, the salt links existing in hydrated collagen, present in aqueous medium, are expected to be unstable. It is also pointed out that deamination of collagen does not produce the effect expected if salt links are involved in the contraction of collagen; that is, the T_s is not lowered but rather is slightly raised by the removal of the ϵ-amino group of lysine.

An additional argument against the rupture of salt links during shrinkage is the similarity of results obtained with various solutions containing inorganic and organic solutes, which indicates the common effects of the two types of solute, in spite of the fact that the organic substances do not interfere with the ionic forces involved in the salt links. The results obtained by Weir and Carter with the organic solutes in solution were the reverse of what might be expected if salt links were involved. Therefore, it appears that the results produced by solutions of electrolytes and by heat in the shrinkage of collagen are also to be ascribed to the effects of the solutes on the coordinate links or the hydrogen bonds, as was shown by the present author in 1926 and 1940, by means of the changed reactivity of denatured and neutral salt-treated collagen (17, 18).

Wright and Wiederhorn (19) in Highberger's laboratory have investigated the influence of the swelling medium on the shrinkage process in collagen, in this instance comparing water and the strongly lyotropic formamide. They have found that the measured heat of denaturation is a function of the interaction of the medium with collagen and that the heat of reaction decreases with increased lyotropic potency of the medium. In other words, the lyotropic agent and heat denaturation have the same effect.

3. The Thermal Shrinkage of Collagen

a. Alteration of collagen

The hydrothermal shrinkage of collagen fibers and tissue has long been recognized as an outstanding characteristic of the principal constituent of connective tissue, collagen. *Mammalian* collagen fiber, in the form of skin or tendon, in contact with water of 60 to 70°C. contracts sharply at a given temperature, the T_s, to about one-third to one-quarter of its initial length (20). The shrunken specimen feels like glue and shows rubberlike elasticity. The tensile strength of the fiber is greatly lowered. The original resistance of native collagen to trypsin is destroyed (21). Marked hydrolytic changes, in the form of splitting of peptide bonds, do not seem to occur (21). The elementary composition, including the nitrogen content, is unchanged (21). The maximum acid-binding capacity is not affected, and the water content remains the same (18, 21).

However, the optical properties of the fiber are changed by the denaturation. With regard to the high-angle X-ray diagram, shrinkage destroys the orientation of this pattern (22). However, as Astbury and Atkin (23) have shown, the original collagen pattern returns unaltered if the collagen (tendon) is re-elongated after shrinkage. The fundamental discovery of Katz and Gerngross (24) in their classical research on the stretching of gelatin films—that by stretching of an unoriented film of gelatin it becomes oriented, as proved by the formation of a regular collagen X-ray pattern—is of interest in this connection. The work of Wright and Wiederhorn (19) indicates that the low-angle diffraction method better reflects the marked changes which occur in the shrinkage of collagen. They stress the important fact that collagen can be completely in the unoriented state with respect to long-range crystallinity (low-angle refraction) and yet the short-range crystallinity, which is reflected in the high-angle pattern, remains unaltered.

Bear's researches with the low-angle diffraction method show that completely shrunken collagen loses its orderly structure. Although the denatured collagen can be re-extended to its original length, the low-angle pattern does not reappear (25). This indicates that the long-range structural alteration in the thermal shrinkage of collagen is an irreversible process. Wright and Wiederhorn (19) have shown that, when the shrunken collagen recrystallizes during drying, the long-range order present in native collagen does not reappear. Further, the conclusion was drawn from X-ray observation, and from the fact that denatured collagen absorbs more water than native collagen, that thermal shrinkage does not involve a shortening of the units in the crystalline material, but rather a fusion of crystalline regions. The disoriented collagen formed is in a low state of entropy and consequently tends to fold into a more random configuration, thereby gaining in entropy.

It should be noted that by intramicellar incorporation of certain tanning agents with collagen, e.g., formaldehyde, almost complete reversal of the shrinkage is attained when the shrunken fiber is cooled (Ewald reaction, 26), probably owing to the presence of aldehyde crosslinks. Thus, Bear (27) has carried a formaldehyde-tanned tendon through the shortening and spontaneous lengthening cycle, examining it at low-angle diffraction. A diagram was obtained which showed a periodicity of 550 Å.

The cyclic nature of the Ewald reaction (contraction–re-extension) illustrates clearly the facts that (1) in the cyclic changes protofibrillar properties are involved, the fibril stabilization being only the means by which the massive structure behaves as do the individual protofibrils; and that (2) the normal state of the protofibrils, for instance in water of pH 6 to 7 at room temperature, is not the contracted random form, but the extended configuration.

b. Rate of shrinkage

As an introduction to the discussion of the mechanism of shrinkage, an examination of the behavior of a tendon immersed in water on raising the temperature of the water is instructive. This has been schematically pictured by Weir (28) in Fig. 33. At a fixed temperature, about 60°C., the tendon becomes distorted at certain points, because of tiny nodules formed inside the tendon. Their appearance marks the onset of shrinkage. These nodules grow into lumps which form a gelatinous node, as the picture shows. Zones in the neighborhood of these nuclei are gradually acted on as the nodules grow. They coalesce, and shrinkage takes place. Reference is also given to the work of Nutting and Borasky (29).

Inasmuch as the collagen structure probably varies as to chain spacings and spatial orientation, it is likely that the crosslinks possess different energies and that some regions contain fewer bridges than others. A small region of the collagen lattice, containing few crosslinks of low energy, should offer the right conditions for initiating shrinkage, i.e., form a shrinkage nucleus. Even at low water temperature a certain degree of freedom is imparted to any adjacent chains by the breaking of a crosslink by the kinetic energy of thermal agitation and the kinetic impulses of the water molecules. Shrinkage of a pair of collagen chains that have been set free is not likely to occur because of the stabilization of the structure by neighboring crosslinked chains. However, as the temperature is raised, more energy is supplied and an additional number of crosslinks are ruptured, increasing the thermal movement of the chains. It may then be assumed that a point will be reached at which the structure is so weakened that it is most likely that the structure will take on a more stable configuration (the disordered state) by chain folding. This process probably involves many chains simultaneously. The region with a sufficient number of ruptured crosslinks is considered to be the activated complex.

Figure 34 shows the shrinkage curves of tendons immersed in water of three different temperatures, of which the highest, 62°C., is some degrees below the temperature of instantaneous shrinkage. The effect of a few degrees variation in temperature is large. In general, a 2-degree rise in temperature reduces the time required for shrinkage by half. For an ordinary chemical reaction every increase of 10 degrees doubles the speed of the reaction (28).

In the shrinkage curves of Fig. 34 two main parts are shown: (1) the induction period with highly accelerated rate of shrinkage, and (2) a branch

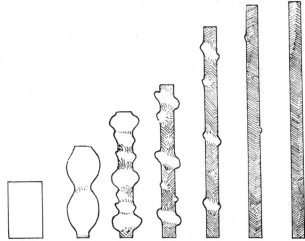

Fig. 33. Behavior of tendon during shrinkage (Weir, 28).

with lower rate of shrinkage (28). The curves indicate that the process of shrinkage is a *rate* phenomenon and that a true shrinkage temperature does not exist from the thermodynamic point of view. This does not detract from the importance of the T_s for characterization of the efficiency of tannages in imparting hydrothermal stability to skin, or from the value of determination of T_s, if the medium in which the test is made has a temperature only a few degrees below the finally obtained T_s. However, it should be realized that, for example, if pelt having an instantaneous shrinkage temperature of 65°C. is kept for a few hours in water of 55°C., a slight shrinkage will take place. This slowly occurring contraction and denatura-

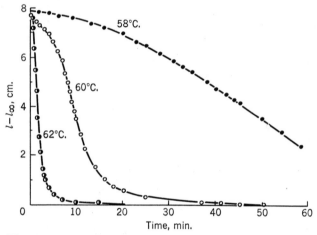

FIG. 34. The effect of the temperature on the shrinkage of tendon collagen (Weir, 28) kept at 58, 60, and 62°C. for various periods of time.

tion of collagen, long known, has been given the name "incipient shrinkage" by Pankhurst (30).

For microscopic determination of the T_s of collagen in the microshrinkmeter devised by Borasky and Nutting (29), suspended collagen or leather fibers are placed in a sealed capillary glass tube which is gradually heated by an electric heating element. The contraction of the fibers on gradual heating in water is observed at an optimum magnification of 75 diameters. This method has several advantages over the ordinary method for theoretical investigation of the nature of the shrinkage process of collagen. Among the more obvious improvements are: uniform temperature of the specimens and temperature equilibrium of the system are assured; the effects of the structure of the skin and tension are eliminated; the shrinkage process can be followed continuously; and, finally, estimations of the T_s can be made in water up to temperatures of 140°C. or higher. Usually the temperature

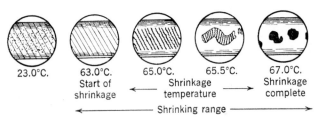

FIG. 35. Diagrammatic sketch of the shrinking reaction of cowhide collagen (29).

is noted when the bulk of the fibers begins to shrink, when marked shrinkage occurs, and when the fiber bundles are completely shrunk. The first and last temperatures constitute the T_s range. The temperature at which the marked shrinkage occurs is defined as the T_s . Figure 35 shows a diagram of the structural changes of bovine collagen fibers taking place during the determination of the T_s by this method.

That the *instantaneous* shrinkage occurring at a fixed temperature, T_s , has its counterpart in similar, although less drastic, changes induced in the collagen structure by prolonged heating in water of temperature considerably lower than that causing rapid denaturation, for example in water of 50°C., was recognized by Grassmann in 1936 (21). Pankhurst noticed the incipient shrinkage of pelt in water of 45°C. Such changes have practical importance and must be considered in the pretreatment of hide in tanning. It was found earlier (31) that prolonged treatment of skin in water of 40 to 45°C. leads to increased affinity of the treated collagen for coordinate agents, although this is less pronounced than the effect of complete shrinkage, as will be evident from the data to be presented.

c. Thermodynamics of shrinkage

The primary reaction in shrinkage is in all probability a melting of the hydrated crystallites, as assumed by Wöhlisch (15) and by Meyer (16). As was pointed out before, from the thermodynamic point of view, the fibrous state is artificial and labile, and the coiled globular state with a random distribution of the protein chains represents the more probable and stable state of the protein configuration. This important point was first emphasized by Mirsky and Pauling (32) and by Kuhn (33), who have shown that the change from an oriented structure to a random state of configuration of the protein units is a natural consequence of the tendency of the structure to increase its entropy. The entropy of activation, ΔS, which is identified with the degree of disorganization occurring in the activation process, is therefore an important figure, as is also the free energy of activation, ΔF, which is related to the T_s . Instantaneous shrinkage of collagen takes place at temperatures at which ΔF_T is about 25 kcal. per mole, which means that rapid shrinkage will take place only if the activation equilibrium has been displaced to a degree sufficient to provide the required number of activated molecules. From the equation $\Delta F = \Delta H - T \Delta S$, it follows that reactions which increase ΔS or decrease ΔH will decrease ΔF, and consequently the T_s of collagen. As examples of the magnitudes of these quantities, the values of the activation constants of tendon collagen, determined by Weir, are of interest: ΔH, 140 kcal.; ΔS, 350 cal. per degree; and ΔF_{60}, the free energy of activation at 60°C., 25 kcal.; the corresponding standard deviations are 15, 43, and 0.6. These figures apply to a "mole" or a "molecule" of collagen whose weight can only be approximated. This "molecule" represents the region or number of chains which are required to be activated at one time. Weir calculated this "molecular" weight to be about 11,300. Since the contraction process does not involve any change in ΔH, the value of ΔH given by Weir is the heat of the activation process, whose over-all heat has been determined to 25 cal. per gram (34).

The size of the values for ΔH and ΔS indicate the participation of chemical reactions involving large molecules and are of an order comparable with corresponding data for the denaturation of proteins. The term ΔH is associated with the rupture of bonds during the activation, and the entropy changes are identified with the marked disorientation of the structure induced by the activation process.

With regard to the thermodynamic data of the region of the protofibrillar segment (i.e., the "molecule" of a segmental molecular weight of about 11,300, recorded for tendon collagen at 60°C.), it is tempting to calculate the approximate number of bonds ruptured in the shrinkage. Since the information at hand favors the view that the hydrogen bond type of crosslink is the dominant stabilizing force of the collagen lattice, this type of crosslink will be considered. From the results of the thermodynamic approach of Weir, and with due consideration of the findings regarding the effect of the denaturation of collagen on its reactivity, it appears safe to conclude that the rupture of crosslinking bonds during heat denaturation mainly concerns the hydrogen bond crosslinks. Since the nucleus of the chains has a mean "molecular" weight of 11,300 and the mean residue weight of collagen is 93, it follows that the activation process of the nucleus should affect about 120 residues. On the basis of the value of 140 kcal. given for the activation energy, assuming it to be largely used for dislocation of hydrogen bonds, which have an energy content of about 5 kcal. per bond, the number of ruptured crosslinks will be 28. Since the total number of residues in the region of shrinkage is 120, then one hydrogen bond for every four to five residues is broken in thermal shrinkage. However, it is likely that a much greater number of crosslinks have to be broken before the structure is sufficiently labilized. It must also be remembered that, while some links are broken, other bonds are formed by hydration of broken bonds simultaneously. Hence, the value of ΔH represents the heat absorbed in breaking crosslinks as well as the heat given off in the hydration of the protein. It is a well-known fact that dehydration elevates the T_s of collagen, as was mentioned in the discussion of salt effects in pickling.

According to the view of Wöhlisch (15), whose early work on thermal contraction is in many ways outstanding, the contraction of tendons should be a reversible process between two states, collagen I and collagen II, corresponding to the crystalline state and the melted or dissolved condition of ordinary crystalloids. Meyer and his co-workers (16) consider that the first stage of the thermal contraction is a melting process. Collagen dissolves in the water, and the reaction is completely reversible. The irreversibility of the shrinkage may be caused by the secondary gelatinization. These investigators have also studied the shrinkage of elastoidin and ichthyocol, the collagenlike fiber proteins of teleostean origin which interesting structures have been methodically investigated by Fauré-Fremiet and his school (35). In the case of ichthyocol, the reversible melting can be studied separately from the irreversible hydrolysis. The irreversibility of the shrinkage has been strongly stressed by Küntzel in his important experimental contributions (2). It now appears that the process of shrinkage is most satisfactorily represented by the following scheme:

Collagen I $\rightleftarrows$ Collagen II $\rightarrow$ Collagen III

(inactive, native)   (activated, complex)   (heat-shrunk)

The heat, entropy, and free energies of activation apply to the equilibrium process (shown to the left), which is governed by ΔF. Its relation to the equilibrium constant of the activation process is given by the equation

$$\Delta F = -RT \ln K^1$$

which may be used for estimation of the thermodynamic constants, since there is a numerical relationship between K^1 and $T_{1/2}$.

d. Shrinkage of special collagens

Elastoidin is an excellent fiber protein for the study of the thermal contraction, because it represents the reversible reaction between collagen I and collagen II, without complications due to gelatinization. The following principal points, due mainly to the researches of Fauré-Fremiet and his co-workers (35), are of interest. At the outset, it should be noted that elastoidin, which contains more than 1 % sulfur, probably in part as a cystine bridge (36) gives the Ewald reaction. Thus in regard to the mechanism of shrinkage, it may not be directly comparable with mammalian collagen. Rather, its behavior is similar to formaldehyde-tanned tendon collagen in many respects. Shrinkage of elastoidin with transformation from state I to state II takes place in water of 62°C. Restraining tension, e.g., by applying a load, increases the T_s, which also applies to collagen, as the work of Wöhlisch (15) and of Grassmann (21) has demonstrated. The elastoidin II is contractible and rubberlike with a large thermoelastic coefficient. The contracted fibers are disoriented, as shown by an X-ray pattern characteristic of the amorphous state. The birefringence is changed from positive to negative, and the tryptic resistance is lowered. The coiled fiber of elastoidin II tends to revert to the original state, and it regains over half of the initial length spontaneously at 20°C. Simultaneously, the positive double refraction and the normal high-angle X-ray pattern are restored. All these observations form substantial support for the view postulating a reversible reaction between states I and II of collagen, in the initial stage.

e. Some aspects of the shrinkage reaction

As pointed out by Weir (14), a true T_s does not exist, since the thermal contraction is a rate process. The high heat of activation of the process greatly minimizes the errors in determining the T_s at a fixed point and is probably responsible for the fact that shrinkage was not generally recognized as a rate phenomenon earlier. The interpretation of shrinkage as an instantaneous process at a fixed temperature is not only subject to the errors inherent in treating a rate process as a fixed-temperature process but also involves a serious error due to the fact that the rate of shrinkage is an accelerated reaction. Too high values of T_s are obtained in the regular determination of T_s because of experimental shortcomings, primarily due to heating the specimen in water at a rate of 2 to 3 degrees per minute, since the strip will not heat up as quickly as the medium. Several other minor deficiencies contribute to the error. For precise work, Weir suggests that the shrinkage be defined as the temperature causing half-shrinkage in 1 minute, as mentioned earlier in connection with the discussion of his work. This necessitates rate measurements from which ΔF and the equilibrium constant of the activation process can be calculated, highly valuable thermodynamically. The importance of the rate at which the specimen is heated in T_s determinations on pelt and fibers was also brought out in the afore-mentioned microscopic investigation of the shrinkage process by Borasky and Nutting (29). For example, they report a T_s of 64.5°C. by heating at the rate of 2.5 degrees per minute, and a T_s of 67.5 at a temperature increase of 4 degrees per minute in the microshrinkmeter. By the ordinary macromethod on strips of pelt the corresponding T_s values were 68 and 72°C. Probably the constraint imposed on the weave structure of the skin is partially responsible for the high T_s values recorded by the ordinary method, although the micromethod tends to give lower values. The increase in the T_s of untanned collagen, which results when the rate of heating is increased, is probably due to failure to attain thermal equilibrium on rapid heating. With leather which contains instable complexes as tanning agents, subjected to protolytic changes and aggregation which improve the tanning potential, the rate of heating has the reverse effect on the T_s recorded, as has been pointed out earlier and will now be discussed more fully.

In the determination of the T_s of tanned skin, the possible changes in the valency distribution between tanning agent and collagen taking place during slow heating (periods of 20 minutes not being unusual for reaching 90 to 95°C. from an initial temperature of 40 to 50°C.) should not be overlooked. Thus, by slow heating, collagen in combination with hexathiocyanatochromiate shows a T_s increase of 10 to 15 degrees, whereas actually the shrinkage temperature of collagen is *decreased* a few degrees as a result of this combination (37). The reason is that hydroxy-chromium compounds are formed during the time required for reaching the temperature at which shrinkage sets in. The hydrolytic products formed have tanning power. In such instances, the T_s test should be carried out by means of the "shocking" method; i.e., the specimen should be brought into contact with water of a temperature of the final T_s or a few degrees below, which will cause *instantaneous shrinkage*. Then, the chromiated skin will shrink at a temperature 4 to 5 degrees below that of the pelt. For chromed leather of regular tannage (cationic chromium), the slow heating and the "shocking" methods give practically the same results (37).

A similar case was reported by Sykes (38), who found that the T_s of pelt tanned with mercuric acetate in the acid range, or at pH 2 to 3, is considerably raised by subsequent washing of the leather. Thus, by washing of the leather tanned at pH 2.8, the T_s was increased from 72°C. to 82°C. No change in T_s occurred in the specimens tanned at the higher pH values (pH > 4). It was suggested by Sykes that the T_s increase of the pelt tanned at pH < 4 is due to hydrolysis of the mercuric salt. A more basic compound of enhanced crosslinking ability is formed. The reason that subsequent washing had no effect on the T_s of leather tanned with mercuric acetate at pH > 4 is probably that the acetates already were aggregated in solutions of pH > 4, and thus that they possessed tanning potency. The tanning effect of the nonaggregated mercuric acetate in solutions of pH 2 to 3 is first obtained *in situ*, by protolysis and aggregation of the mercury complexes in the washing.

f. T_s of mammalian skin collagen

It has frequently been mentioned that the T_s of the collagen fiber and tendon is increased when tension is applied to the fiber. Thus, a freely suspended strip of skin will shrink at temperatures lower by 1 to 2 degrees than a strip fastened at both ends and lightly weighted (see Fig. 32). This fact also explains why the T_s of specimens from a compact part of skin is higher than that of looser sections of the same skin. The fiber bundles of a close-textured weave are subjected to strain from adjacent fibers, whereas no appreciable effect of neighboring fibers on the fiber bundles in the loosely interwoven specimens is apparent. The shrinkage temperatures of samples from various parts of the same skin generally do not differ more than 2 to 3 degrees. As for the T_s of skins of different specimens of mammals, the variations in T_s among skins of one species are often greater than the variations found between skins from entirely different species. Results from various laboratories are difficult to compare, since the spread of values is often wider than the actual differences between skins of different species. Hence, series of T_s values obtained by the same technique should preferably be compared. A number of T_s values obtained in the author's laboratory for mammalian skins is given in Table 23. A list of T_s values for fishskin will be given later (in Tables 25 and 26). In future determinations of the amino acid composition of various collagens, it will be important to ascertain if and how the chemical composition of collagen affects the T_s. The difference between mammalian and fishskin collagen appears to be due to the different composition of the side chains (hydroxyproline), particularly with regard to hydrogen-bonding potency, which will result in different degrees of cross-linking of the collagen chains, and accordingly be evident in the hydrothermal stability as expressed by T_s measurements.

4. NATURE OF THE BONDS SEVERED IN THERMAL SHRINKAGE

It was mentioned earlier in this chapter that the maximum binding capacity of collagen for ionic compounds, such as mineral acids, is not altered by heat shrinkage. However, the acid-binding curve (titration curve)

TABLE 23

T_s OF NATIVE SKINS FROM MAMMALS (39)

(T_s determined on freely suspended strips)

Type of Skin	T_s , °C.	Type of Skin	T_s , °C.
Calf	63–65	Dog	60–62
Cow	65–67	Moose	60–62
Sheep	58–62	Ground hog	58–60
Goat	64–66	Rabbit	60–61
Horse	62–64	Hare	59–60
Deer	60–62	Whale	61–63
Cat	60–62	Reindeer	60–62

shows that the contraction of the chains has made a part of the ionic protein groups, the carboxyl ions, more reactive in the pH range 2.5 to 5. This is probably due to the weakening of the electrostatic attraction between some of the oppositely charged ionic groups which form the salt links, induced by the unfavorable steric conditions created in the contracted protein chains (18).

The most convincing experimental contributions for ascertaining the type of groups principally involved in shrinkage have been supplied by comparative studies of the reactivity of collagen, on the one hand, and heat-contracted collagen, on the other. A brief outline of the results of these investigations will be given. They were begun several years ago, at a time when data on this problem were very scanty (18).

In his excellent review of the denaturation of globular proteins, Anson (40) points out that it is not possible at present to define denaturation by means of description of the change in the structure of the protein molecule. Anson remarks that the alterations in the reactivity of protein groups that occur when a protein is denatured must be explained by some general structural theory. The changes are probably connected in some way with the breaking of the bonds between polypeptide chains, although, as Anson emphasizes, our present limited knowledge does not justify further theorization. Collagen offers better possibilities for investigating the groups involved in its particular denaturation than the globular proteins. These investigations have been carried out along the same general lines as were followed in the study of the effect of lyotropic agents on the reactivity of collagen, already described. It was then of interest to find out, first, if the ionic reaction between simple cationic chromium salt and collagen is influenced by thermal shrinkage. This type of reaction is governed by the state and amount of the carboxylic ions of collagen. Further, this study included the corresponding reactions with coordination-active chromium compounds, represented by the extremely basic chlorides and sulfates of chromium and the sulfito-chromium sulfate, and tanning with vegetable tannins of the condensed type, mostly mimosa extract. The solutions of the chromium compounds contained large amounts of nonionic and aggregated complexes. Hide powder was used, since it is not possible to employ shrunken pelt in tanning with vegetable tannins and with the last-mentioned chromium compounds, because the diffusion of the large molecules and aggregates into the gelatinized hide structure is severely obstructed, and even prevented in many instances. The topochemical alterations induced in the collagen network by the shrinkage, such as twisting of chains, probably leads to a reduction of the interfibrillar spaces at some locations, thus impeding the diffusion of the tannins and the large complexes, such as those of the sulfito compounds. A macroscopic case-hardening takes place

TABLE 24

FIXATION OF CHROMIUM COMPOUNDS BY NATIVE AND HEAT-DENATURED HIDE
POWDER

(Chrome fixation in mg. equiv. of Cr fixed by 1 g. of collagen)

No.	Compound	Dominant Type of Complex	Hide Powder (blank)	Shrunken Hide Powder
1	67% acid chromium chloride	100% cationic	3.3	3.3
2	67% acid chromium sulfate	96% cationic	4.2	4.15
3	33% acid chromium chloride	70% nonionic	5.6	7.8
4	40% acid chromium sulfate	35% noncationic	6.4	8.0
5	Sulfito-chromium sulfate	80% nonionic	7.1	12.2

in many instances, and case-hardening involving microscopic and submicroscopic elements is very likely to occur. By means of finely subdivided, completely hydrated hide powder, these topochemical complications of the
macro type may be largely eliminated. Table 24 shows some characteristic
data from the series with various chromium compounds which were run at a
concentration of 1.0 equiv. of chromium per liter, with time of tanning of 72
hours. The hide powder was denatured by immersion in water of 70°C. for
2 minutes.

These data prove that by denaturation of collagen the reactivity of the
ionic groups is not altered. With regard to the carboxyl groups, solutions
1 and 2 of the table bring out that fact. The data from the irreversible fixation of condensed naphthalenesulfonic acid and the high-molecular fraction
of lignosulfonic acid, which figures are identical for the two types of collagen,
prove that the basic protein groups (18) have not been affected. On the
other hand, denatured collagen possesses considerably greater affinity and
binding power for solutions containing noncationic and aggregated chromium complexes. An exceptionally large effect is evident in the fixation of
the sulfito compound which, according to experimental information available, reacts mainly by means of coordinate valency forces probably with
the hydroxy groups of collagen.

These findings show the same trend as those of the chrome fixation by
hide powder after pretreatment with lyotropic agents, constituting evidence for the similarity of the changes produced by thermal shrinkage and
lyotropic swelling. The increased fixation of the coordinate type of compounds is evidently caused by structural alterations in the collagen during
shrinkage. Since agents predominantly fixed by collagen by means of its
anionic groups (carboxyl), such as the simple cationic chromium salts, or
by means of its cationic groups, such as the sulfo acids mentioned, are not
affected by denaturation of collagen, it follows that the increase in the fixa-

tion of the highly aggregated chromium compounds by denatured collagen is indicative of activation, or freeing, of nonionic valency forces in collagen by thermal shrinkage, caused by rupture of hydrogen bridges between keto-imide links and those crosslinking the $—CO \cdot NH—$ link and the OH group.

Confirming evidence is supplied by data showing the effect of the thermal contraction of collagen on its binding of vegetable tannins of the type which has been proved to be fixed mainly on the nonionic groups, in all probability by the $—CO—NH—$ bonds of collagen, i.e., the condensed type of tannins. Thus, to cite an example from solutions of mimosa tannins at pH 4.8, hide powder fixed 42 % tannin irreversibly, compared with 67 % fixed by denatured hide powder. The corresponding figures for sulfited quebracho extract at pH 5.5 were 46 and 71 % (18).

From these observations, the following conclusions were drawn, on the plausible assumption that the main cohesive forces in the collagen super-structure consist of (1) crosslinks in the form of coordinate valency forces

between $\overset{|}{CO} - - - \overset{|}{HN}$ groups in juxtaposition and (2) salt links between

oppositely charged acidic and basic groups on adjacent protein chains: The hydrothermal denaturation of collagen involves a folding of the collagen chains. By the distortion of the structure, the distance between the chains may at certain points be so greatly enlarged that the valency forces do not suffice for bridging the chains. Interlocking links located on the protein backbone (hydrogen bonds) are primarily affected and ruptured. The free valency forces on the liberated groups (hydrated), no longer internally compensated, will then be available for further reactions. The shrunken collagen will hence possess greater power of coordinate reactivity of its peptide bonds than the original collagen. The electrostatic intermolecular forces, the ionic groups, are not affected, or only slightly so, by the shrinkage of the chains. The widening of the gap between chains occurring in the coiling, and concomitantly the diminished internal compensation of the electrostatic forces or the groups affected by the steric changes, indicates easier discharge of the COO^- groups by the hydrogen ions, which will affect the titration curve in the acid range (pH 2.5 to 5.5). The evidence presented supports the view that, by hydrothermal denaturation of collagen, cross-links of the hydrogen bond type are ruptured, this being the main change.

From purely thermodynamic considerations, Weir and Carter (10) claim that the *only* bonds involved in the thermal shrinkage are the hydrogen bonds existing between laterally adjacent peptide linkages. They base their conclusion on data pointing to the nonparticipation of saltlike bonds, and not on direct evidence of the participation of hydrogen bonds. The experimental data provide both the positive and negative evidence.

5. THERMAL SHRINKAGE OF COLLAGEN OF FISHSKIN
(*Teleostei*)

It has long been known that fishskin is easily damaged if exposed to water of moderate temperatures, such as those in the range 35 to 40°C., which are normally applied in the bating process of bovine skin. It is also susceptible to degradation by many agents, including acidic and alkaline solutions. However, experimental information on the shrinkage temperature of fishskin collagen and on its behavior toward the action of proteinases, electrolytes, and tanning agents were first supplied by investigations begun several years ago (41–47). Table 25 contains some selected data on the T_s of native skins of various fishes from Swedish lakes and shores. These data were obtained on freely suspended strips of skin (39).

Takahashi (48) has studied the amino acid composition of collagens of skins of a great number of Japanese fishes, particularly the contents of hydroxyamino acids and methionine, in an attempt to ascertain whether the T_s is directly related to the amino acid composition of these collagens, particularly the hydroxyproline content. In Table 26 some figures have been selected from his unpublished investigations. The hydroxyproline content was determined by the Neuman-Logan method.

It is evident from Tables 25 and 26 that the T_s values of fishskin form two main groups, those of fishes living in cold (deep) water being in the range 35 to 45°C., and those of fishes living in warm (surface) water in the range 54 to 57°C., with a few species in the intermediate range between 45 and 55°C. This difference between cold- and warm-water fishes was first noted by Takahashi.

The large difference between the T_s of skins of deep-water (cold) fishes and skins of surface-water (warm) fishes, which is of the order of 15 to 20 degrees, is remarkable. It is probably connected with the difference in habi-

TABLE 25

T_s OF FISHSKIN (*Teleostei*) IN THE NATIVE STATE (39)

Common Name	Scientific Name	Habitat	T_s, °C.
Cod	*Gadus morrhua*	Salt water, cold	40–42
Halibut	*Hippoglossus vulgaris*	Salt water, cold	38–42
Wolf fish	*Anarhichas lupus*	Salt water, cold	37–40
Plaice	*Pleuronectes platessa*	Salt water, cold	40–42
Mackerel	*Scomber scombrus*	Salt water, cold	50–52
Pike	*Esox lucius*	Fresh water, warm	54–57
Eel	*Anguilla vulgaris*	Any water, warm	55–57
Perch	*Perca fluviatilis*	Fresh and brake water, warm	54–56
Young bream	*Abramis brama*	Fresh water, warm	54–56

TABLE 26

T_S AND HYDROXYPROLINE CONTENT OF COLLAGEN FROM JAPANESE TELEOSTS (48)

Common Name	Scientific Name	Habitat	Hydroxproline, g. in 100 g. Collagen	T_s, °C.
Rock cod	*Sebastodes baramenu*	Cold water	7.0	33–34
Dogfish	*Squalus suckleyi*	Cold water		34–38
Arrow-toothed halibut	*Atheresthes matsuurae*	Cold water		35
Alaska pollak	*Theregra chalcogramma*	Cold water	8.2	36–39
Rock trout	*Hexagrammos otakii*	Cold water		37
Cod	*Gadus macrocephalus*	Cold water	7.7	39–42
Flathead flounder	*Hippoglossoides dubius*	Cold water	8.6	40–42
Deep-sea shark	*Dalatias atromarginatus*	Cold water		40–42
Flounder	*Tanakius kitaharae*	Cold water	8.5	42–44
Porgy	*Evynnis japonicus*	Warm water		49–52
Mackerel	*Scomber japonicus*	Warm water	9.7	52–54
Common sea bass	*Lateolabrac japonicus*	Warm water		53–55
Japanese eel	*Anguilla japonica*	Warm water	9.8	54–55
Great blue shark	*Prionace glaucus*	Warm water	10.7	53–55
Carp	*Cyprinus carpis*	Warm water	11.0	56–58
Wild goldfish	*Carassius carassius*	Warm water	12.1	53–56
Cattle hide (control)	*Bos taurus*	—	12.6	64–66

tat and it may indicate the importance of the skin structure and its hydro-thermal stability for the vital functions. It is hoped that further data on the amino acid composition of species from deep- and surface-water habitats will extend our understanding of the structure of collagen and its properties and behavior. Even now it can be stated that an obvious correlation exists between the T_s and the content of hydroxyproline of different types of collagens.

In the early work (41–43) on fishskin collagen, at a time when information on the composition of mammalian collagen was far from quantitative, and no reliable analysis of the amino acid make-up of fish collagen was available, it was suggested that the marked difference in hydrothermal stability of bovine skin and ·codfish skin, the substrate mainly used, was probably not due to the different chemical composition (amino acids) but rather was a problem of the intermolecular stabilization of the two classes of collagen, and was thus a question of molecular architecture.

The following findings (41–47) point to a lower degree of crosslinking of the polypeptide chains of fish collagen by means of nonionic bonds (hydrogen bonds), compared to bovine collagen, the foremost representative of mammalian collagen of technical importance:

1. A lowering of the T_s by 25 to 30 degrees. It had earlier been proved that complete elimination of the salt links by the inactivation of the cationic and anionic protein groups forming this link, by means of naphthalene-β-sulfonic acid, lowered the T_s of collagen by 14 to 16 degrees. However, the difference in T_s between the two types of collagen is practically twice as much, and hence not only ionic crosslinks but also some of the nonionic ones must have been opened up. It was further pointed out that lyotropic agents such as thiocyanates and perchlorates, which specifically act on the nonionic links, decrease the T_s by more than 50 degrees.

2. Fish collagen is almost completely brought into solution by aqueous solutions of sodium dodecyl sulfate at pH 6; bovine collagen is only slightly attacked, after thermal shrinkage it is also made more soluble in the solution mentioned. The large anion of dodecyl sulfate combines with the cationic protein groups, severing the ionic crosslinks, which leaves insufficient internal cohesion of the collagen for maintaining the fibrillar structure. In other words, fish collagen goes into solution.

3. Naphthalene-β-sulfonic acid in solutions of final pH 1.4 to 1.5 shrinks fishskin collagen, the structural features and tensile strength of which are completely lost. Bovine collagen is not adversely affected in these respects, although its T_s is decreased by about 14 to 16 degrees.

4. Strong mineral acids, such as hydrochloric acid, at final pH values of 1.0 to 1.2, solubilized more than 80 % of fish collagen within 48 hours. The identical treatment of bovine skin resulted in a loss of only 6 % of the original collagen. By equilibrating collagen with hydrochloric acid at pH 1.0 to 1.2, complete discharge of the carboxyl ions of collagen takes place and complete elimination of the saltlike crosslinks is effected. The difference in behavior of the two classes of collagen indicates that little cohesion is left in fish collagen after the complete elimination of the ionic crosslinks.

5. Native bovine collagen of skin resists the action of proteinases (trypsin), whereas native codfish collagen is susceptible to this action (41). Collagen of fishskin and that of bovine skin possess identical combining power for ionic reactants, such as hydrogen ions and cationic chromium complexes (43). On the contrary, nonionic compounds and aggregated agents such as the vegetable tannins, which are attached to collagen by coordination on the peptide linkage, combine much more extensively with fish collagen than with bovine collagen.

It was pointed out in Chapter 2 that a close correlation of T_s values and the hydroxyproline content of collagens exists. Further, it appears that the most important interchain link of collagen is the one formed between the hydroxy group and the keto-imide oxygen. Also, by exhaustive acetylation of the hydroxy groups of bovine collagen, its T_s is decreased by about 25 degrees, or to the point of the T_s of collagen of cold-water fishes. One out of four hydroxy groups resists acetylation. It appears that this nonreactive group, perhaps inaccessible to the reagent, forms the "backbone" of collagens and participates in the formation of a strong intermolecular link. There is evidence in favor of the view that such a link, possibly of the ester type, is responsible for the marked stability of collagen (49).

It is interesting to note that collagen of earthworm cuticles shrinks and dissolves in water of 40 to 50°C., yielding a solution which does not gel on cooling, according to the findings of Reed and Rudall (50). It shows no sign of cross-striation. Dr. Rudall has kindly informed the present author that the teleostean collagen investigated by him was regularly cross-striated like the mammalian type. Of the collagenlike proteins, elastoidin with a T_s of about 62°C. resembles bovine collagen, from the point of view of hydrothermal stability. The probable presence of —S—S— bridges complicates its behavior, as was mentioned earlier in connection with the Ewald reaction. More akin to teleostean collagen is ichthyocol, as would be expected from a protein of the swim bladder of fish. Its T_s values are located in the vicinity of 40°C. The complete amino acid composition of these proteins has not yet been established.

6. THE EFFECT OF TANNING AGENTS ON THE SHRINKAGE TEMPERATURE OF COLLAGEN

One of the most widely used and most practical determinations of this effect is that of the shrinkage temperature of the leather (T_s), which measures the hydrothermal stability of the leather. The first T_s determinations were carried out some forty years ago. In 1910 Powarnin, and some ten years later, Powarnin and Aggeew (51), pointed out that the T_s of leather is an indication or measure of the tanning effect. The measurement of the hydrothermal stability of chrome leather by immersion of a piece of leather in boiling water, the well-known "boiling test" for chrome leather, has long been a standard tannery routine. In certain respects, the T_s measurements are more important than the amount of tanning agent which is contained in the leather.

It is generally the rule that tanning of collagen increases its T_s. The T_s values are therefore important in controlling tanning processes, and also as a means of establishing the qualities of the leather. However, the degree of hydrothermal stability should not be used as the sole criterion. It is advisable to combine it with other criteria, such as "leatherlike drying-out," fullness, softness, resistance to water and to microorganisms, and, from a practical point of view, to consider also the mechanical properties of the

TABLE 27

INCREASE IN SHRINKAGE TEMPERATURE OF COLLAGEN ON TANNING

Tannage	Laboratory Conditions	Commercial Leather	Source
Basic chromium sulfate	+30->35	+20->35	Hobbs (53)
Basic chromium chloride	+17->35	—	—
Oxalatodiolchromiate	+17-22	—	—
Two-bath chrome tannage	+25->35	—	—
Vegetable tannins	−2-+24	+5-20	Hobbs (53)
Formaldehyde	+15-20	+3-10	Balfe (54)
Quinone	+20-28	+25	Theis (55)
Zirconyl sulfate	+20-25	—	—
Mercuric acetate	+20-30	—	Sykes (56)
Aluminum sulfate	−10-0	−13-0	Hobbs (53)
Basic aluminum sulfate	+10-20	+10-21	Balfe (54)
Synthetic tannins	0-22	—	—
Lignosulfonic acids	−2-+2	—	—
Polymetaphosphoric acid	0-+5	—	—
Oil (chamois)	−5-+2	−10-+5	Hobbs (53) Chambard and Michallet (57)
Resin leather	0-+30	—	— Balfe (54)

grain and the behavior of the leather on general handling. Thus, the T_s is *one* of the many properties useful in the evaluation of leather.

A discussion of all the aspects of hydrothermal stabilization of collagen by tanning agents will not be attempted. For a general orientation, some data on the increase of the shrinkage temperature, T_s, of collagen effected by a full tannage with some principal tanning agents presented in Table 27. These results pertain to leather samples prepared in the author's laboratory. Values for specimens of commercial leathers, recorded in the literature and by the present author, are included.

A pioneer in the application of measurements of the shrinkage temperature to rawhide and to leather in its various stages of manufacture, including the finished product, is Chater (52), whose numerous papers are still worthy of study. A simple construction of a T_s meter is shown in Fig. 36 (Sykes, 38).

A number of factors are involved in the hydrothermal stabilization of leather; for chrome leather tanned by means of a basic sulfate of a certain basicity, these factors include the neutral salt content and the kind of salt added in tanning, the extent of pickle, the temperature of the tanning bath, and the stability of the sulfate groups of the complexes. Furthermore, the degree of neutralization and the possible displacement of acido groups in the neutralization, the dyeing, or the fat-liquoring, or in the subsequent processes, are contributory factors. The upper limits given in the column "Laboratory conditions" may be taken as the optimal values, obtained under the most favorable conditions. In some types of leather, such as the

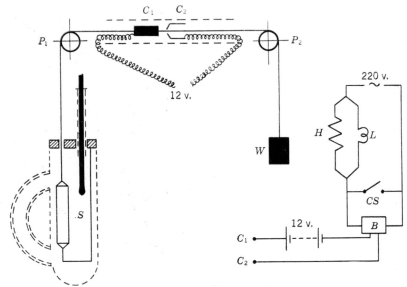

FIG. 36. Self-recording apparatus for the determination of the shrinkage tempera-ture, T_s (Sykes): a, arrangement of apparatus; b, circuit diagram. This apparatus works on the principle that when shrinkage occurs the supply of heat is cut off. The highest temperature attained is recorded on a maximum thermometer. The sample, S, is attached to two spring clips, the lower of which is fixed rigidly to the apparatus, and the other to a light nylon cord which passes over two frictionless pulleys, P_1 and P_2, and is maintained under tension by the weight W. A metal contact, C_1, is attached to the cord which passes freely through a second contact, C_2. Both contacts are cylindrical in shape and arranged so that they can move freely in a horizontal glass tube, indicated by the dotted lines. The sample is placed in the side-arm tube which is electrically heated. To commence the test, C_2 is pushed along the glass car-rier until it is in contact with C_1. This closes the 12-volt circuit, which through the relay R operates the mains heating tape (175 watts). A warning lamp, L, indicates that the circuits are closed. During the initial expansion of the sample, the circuit is maintained as C_1, which is fixed to the cord, moves along the tube, pushing C_2, which is free to slide, in front of it. When shrinkage commences, C_1, being attached to the cord, moves away from C_2, which remains stationary, thus causing the circuit to be broken. Through the relay, the mains circuit is also broken and consequently the supply of heat is discontinued. The temperature is read from the thermometer; and as this is of the maximum reading type, there is no need to read it immediately. The switch CS is introduced to cut out the relay system, thus enabling heating to be continued after shrinkage commences, when it is required to measure the extent of shrinkage.

vegetable-tanned, the removal of certain loosely held constituents will improve the T_s of the leather (53, 58–60). This applies also to the washing out or neutralization of acid or acidic constituents present (58). The T_s determinations should be carried out at the neutral pH of the leather; for instance, a leather tanned by means of chestnut wood extract, which shows a pH of about 3.5, should be determined in *water* (pH ∼6) in the natural condition and also after adjustment of the leather to pH 5 in water, since the T_s of collagen has its optimal value in the pH range 5 to 7 Determination of T_s of leathers by equilibrating with buffer solutions, and using these solutions as media for the test is not recommended.

7. THE EFFECT OF CROSSLINKING OF COLLAGEN BY TANNING AGENTS ON ITS T_s

a. General aspects

The degree of the stability of fibrous proteins is governed by the amino acid pattern, with reference to the groups supplying the chemical and sterical possibilities of interaction between adjacent polypeptide chains, and the number and the strength of the crosslinking bridges formed. The low degree of hydrothermal stability of fish collagen and the relatively high degree of stability of the protein chains in keratin may be conceived to be related to the small number of rather weak crosslinks of the former protein, and to the strong —S—S— bridge and the large number of interchain hydrogen bonds of great strength of the keratin. By severing the cystine crosslinks of the wool protein, the general stability of the protein is drastically lowered. Hence, the importance of the crosslinking of protein chains for the hydrothermal stability is apparently an established fact. Accordingly, the ability of tanning agents to increase the T_s of collagen has been explained on similar lines. Meyer (61), who was the first proponent of the present conception of fibrous proteins as parallelly aligned long peptide chains, suggested in 1929 that in tanning of proteins crosslinking of protein chains takes place by means of the tanning agent introduced in the protein lattice. This idea has been further elaborated by many investigators since then. However, very few workers have shown a critical attitude toward this concept.

The following evidence is presented in support of the crosslinking hypothesis. The first condition requisite for crosslinking lies in the polyfunctional nature of the tanning agent; i.e., its molecule must possess at least two groups functioning as sites for the formation of a crosslink. This fact is best illustrated by an example. Naphthalenesulfonic acid, which has only one functional group in its molecule, does not cause swelling and disorganization of the polypeptide chains when combined with collagen, and does not possess coordinative groups, will decrease the T_s of collagen by about 14 to 16 degrees (62). This labilization is ascribed to the discharge of the carboxyl ions of the collagen by means of the hydrogen ion of the acid and the simultaneous attachment of the univalent anion to the cationic protein groups, the final result being breaking of the saltlike crosslinks. By joining two naphthalenesulfonic acid rings by means of the —CH₂— groups (condensation with formaldehyde), a bifunctional acid is formed. The number of naphthalene rings can be further increased by extending the condensation. The polynuclear structures formed contain two terminal rings, each possessing one sulfonic acid group. These compounds are bifunctional and possess sufficient length of the molecule to be able to react with cationic protein groups on different chains at some points, forming a weak crosslink with the polynaphthalene chain as the center. The T_s of collagen in combination with the maximum amount of these condensed acids, satisfying the acid-binding capacity of collagen, will be about the same as that of the original collagen (62). The bifunctional agent will then make up for the 14- to 16-degree decrease of the T_s caused by the breaking of the salt links, as effected by the unifunctional compounds, and actually elevate the T_s by 14 to 16 degrees (62).

A similar case, involving coordination valency forces, is exemplified by the effect of phenols and polyphenols on collagen (63). The unifunctional phenol is directed toward interaction with hydrogen bonds and hence tends to break crosslinks of that type present in the collagen lattice. It will gelatinize collagen if applied in moderately concentrated solutions (63), whereas a multifunctional polyphenol (natural tannins), the molecule of which is chemically and sterically able to form a number of stable crosslinks with adjacent protein chains and their molecules, increases the T_s of collagen by 10 to 20 degrees.

Another example offers an interesting anionic chromium compound, hexathiocyanate chromate. It associates itself with the cationic protein groups, probably unifunctionally rupturing salt links mainly. The molecule of this chromium compound is evidently not large enough to enable it to function as a bridge for the protein chains. As a result of this combination, the T_s of collagen is decreased by about 5 degrees, as determined by the "shocking" method (direct immersion of the test specimen in water of a temperature very near that of the real T_s). By determining the T_s by the slow heating method generally practiced, at an increase of 2° degrees per minute, the labile chromium compound originally present in collagen has ample time to stabilize itself by hydrolytic changes, enabling the enlarged and chemically more potent secondary products to enter into a more stable combination with collagen, probably crosslinking the chains, since the T_s is increased by 10 to 15 degrees. An actual increase of the T_s of 15 to 20 degrees is obtained. Sykes (56) has found similar conditions in pelt treated with mercuric acetate in a slightly acidic solution.

b. Evidence for the crosslinking of globular proteins

The examples given support, but do not prove, the crosslinking concept. The first experimental evidence for crosslinking taking place in the tanning of proteins was supplied by Fraenkel-Conrat and Mecham (64), who found that the molecular weight of globular proteins is increased after treatment with formaldehyde. At an earlier stage of their fundamental work on form-aldehyde tanning of globular proteins, Fraenkel-Conrat et al. (65) pointed out that the insolubility and the marked resistance to swelling of proteins and synthetic polypeptides tanned by formaldehyde may indicate the formation of methylene crosslinks between the amino group, on the one hand, and the amide, guanidyl or imidazole groups, on the other. Later Fraenkel-Conrat and Mecham (64) were able to demonstrate intermolecular crosslinking of proteins on treatment with formaldehyde through the marked increase of the average molecular weight of the treated proteins, evaluated by osmotic pressure measurement. The series for bovine serum albumin is given in Table 28. The reaction between formaldehyde and the aqueous solutions of the albumin was permitted to proceed for 10 to 15 days at room temperature. The molecular weight of serum albumin was 62,000,

TABLE 28

MOLECULAR WEIGHTS OF SOLUBLE PREPARATIONS OF FORMALDEHYDE-TREATED SERUM ALBUMIN (64)

Protein, %	Concentration of Formalde-hyde, %	Final pH	Molecular Weight	Ratio of $\frac{\text{F. albumin M.W.}}{\text{albumin M.W.}}$
10	4.4	3.5	330,000	8:1
10	5	3.5	262,000	6.5:1
10	1	3.5	78,000	2:1
10	0.4	3.8	95,000	2.3:1
5	10	3.5	80,000	2:1
1	5	3.5	61,000	1.5:1
1	0.5	3.5	53,000	1.3:1
10	5	7.5	150,000	2.5:1
10	1	7.5	90,000	1.5:1
10	0.4	7.3	200,000	3.2:1
5	10	7.5	162,000	2.6:1
1	0.5	7.5	55,000	0.9:1
10 (blank)	None	3.5	41,000	—
10 (blank)	None	7.5	62,000	—

determined osmotically. Results of a similar trend were obtained with form-aldehyde-treated egg albumin also.

A very important point in this research is the crucial factor of protein concentration. With 10% protein solutions, crosslinking was effected at formaldehyde concentrations of 0.4 to 10%, at pH 3.5 and 7.5. *No cross-linking* occurred in the 1% protein solution. In the former instance the *molecular weight* of the protein has *increased six- to eight-fold* in high concentrations of formaldehyde. The effect of the concentration of the protein solution is evident, an increase in protein content facilitating an increase in molecular weight (crosslinking). This trend is not surprising in view of the fact that in concentrated solution the molecules of the protein are more closely packed, providing better opportunity for colliding molecules to be joined by methylene bridges.

The crosslinking faculty of vegetable tannins has been proved by experiments in which tannic acid was reacted with globulins and albumins. By means of the ultracentrifuge, Danielsson (66) measured the sedimentation constants of the precipitates formed at pH values <8. These were washed free from occluded tannin and dissolved at pH 9.4. Prior to the determination of the molecular weight, the solutions were adjusted to the lower pH values of the original precipitates. The sedimentation constant of the tannin-protein complex which was formed at pH 6 to 7 was about 25% higher than that of the pure albumin. The increase of the molecular weight of a water-soluble protein resulting from its combination with tannic acid is the second experimental proof of the crosslinking function of tannins.

The third experimental proof of the postulate that crosslinking occurs in the tanning process pertains to the effect of basic chromium sulfates on gelatin solutions, presented in an interesting contribution of Pouradier and his associates (67). From osmotic pressure measurements on a 10% solution of gelatin, with a mean molecular weight of 65,000, at 38°C. and pH 4.75, it was found that the addition of 1.5% Cr_2O_3 in the form of chrome alum, based on the weight of dry gelatin, increased the mean molecular weight of the chromed gelatin to 88,000–95,000. It is noteworthy that as little as 1% Cr_2O_3, which was the amount of chrome fixed by the gelatin, suffices for the crosslinking of the gelatin molecules. Pouradier and his co-workers found also that the crosslinking does not take place in dilute solutions of gelatin, an observation that confirms the finding of Fraenkel-Conrat and Olcott in their formaldehyde researches. In such dilute solutions, the chromium complexes are fixed and attached to one molecular chain. Thus the reaction is of the *intramolecular* type. In concentrated solutions of gelatin, the steric conditions favor intermolecular reactions of chromium, which is shown by both the increased molecular weight and the properties of the solution, and of the gel formed, with respect to viscosity, jelly strength, and melting point. Also the pH of the solution has a marked effect on the crosslinking reaction, as is evident from Fig. 37, which presents a schematic illustration of the governing importance of the form of the protein chains on the interaction of gelatin molecules with chromium complexes. Intrachain crosslinking dominates in the contracted gelatin chains at the isoelectric point, whereas interchain crosslinks are mainly formed at a pH on the acid side of the pH of the isoelectric point, when the gelatin molecule is extended by repulsion of its positively charged groups. In view of the facts presented, it appears that the theory that crosslinking takes place in tanning is not merely a speculation, as appears to be the belief in certain quarters.

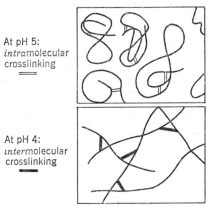

At pH 5:
*intra*molecular
crosslinking

At pH 4:
*inter*molecular
crosslinking

FIG. 37. Schematic diagrams of the fixation of chromium salts by gelatin in 1% solution, according to Pouradier *et al.* (67).

This concept is by now an experimentally established fact, based on data bearing on a variety of proteins and a number of tanning agents.

c. Steric factors

Two other questions which may be raised as to the steric possibilities in the collagen lattice for establishing such crosslinks, and the number of links required for imparting stability to collagen, are not so easy to answer, because they are intimately connected with the arrangement of the amino acid residues taking part in the crosslinking reaction, including the distance between the active sites on adjacent protein chains and the distance between the active groups in the molecule of the tanning agent, its size, and its orientation in the lattice. Nothing definite can be stated concerning the first question, the distance between active sites on different protein chains which will have to be bridged, but some possibilities may be presented. Bowes (68) has considered the steric possibilities for crosslinking in formaldehyde and chrome tannages. The distance bridged by one formaldehyde molecule —N—C—N— is 2.9 Å.; for two molecules of formaldehyde the bridge —N—C—O—C—N would be twice the value. If the methylene bridge were established between two ϵ-amino lysine groups of adjacent chains, there would not be much chance for such a bridging, since the distance is calculated to be of the order of 70 Å., on the assumption that the lysine residue, which occurs only in every twenty-five amino acid residues, is equally spaced throughout the whole molecule. The possibility that the lysine residues in adjacent chains are spaced intermediately between these extremes makes the prospect more favorable. Further, in formaldehyde tannage it is possible for crosslinking to take place between an ϵ-amino group of lysine, which group is an absolute requisite for this tannage, and some other group, such as the NH— group of an adjacent peptide bond, or an amide group. The same considerations of the crosslinking of collagen by means of cationic chromium complexes, in which reaction the charged carboxylic groups of collagen are the binding sites, show that a bridge of the simplest type, Cr—O—Cr, representing the smallest model of the basic salts of average basicity as used in practical tanning, will be about 6 Å. in length. Since about every sixth residue in collagen consists of a carboxyl group, it is not unlikely that a few strong bridges of the type $\uparrow$ COO·Cr—O—Cr·COO $\uparrow$ can be formed on chains containing a few hundred amino acid residues. The formation of longer chains of basic chromium complexes, such as Cr—O—Cr—O—Cr—O—Cr with a length of 12 to 18 Å., as secondary hydrolysis products in the collagen lattice would provide still better facilities for crosslinking. Complexes with four chromium atoms are present in large amounts in solutions of 50% basic chromium sulfates. It has been emphasized by Elöd (69) and by the author (70) that probably only a small part of the amount of chromium introduced into the collagen structure takes part in the stabilization of collagen, the main part being the dead weight required for introducing the small amount of chromium necessary for the formation of the effective crosslinks in the few intermolecular spaces available for crosslinking. This also seems to apply to the chroming of gelatin gels, amounts of 0.3% Cr_2O_3 being ample to secure films resistant to boiling water, provided that the film is made from chromed solution of gelatin (69). By thermodynamic treatment, Weir (14) finds that only small amounts of chromium, less than 1% Cr_2O_3, on the basis of collagen, are sufficient for maximum increase of the entropy of activation and the heat of reaction, i.e., optimal stabilization. These observations point in the same direction. It has further been pointed out by the author (71), that the fixation of the main part of formaldehyde by the basic protein groups does not have any direct effect on the rigidity of collagen. A comparatively large fixation of formaldehyde is required for the inactivation of all reactive basic groups, to enable only a few of them to react with formaldehyde, to form connecting links for strengthening of the supermolecular structure. The stabilization of the collagen chains results from a few bridges formed by the tanning agent. This points to the marked alteration in the properties of the linear polymers of polystyrenes caused by the copolymerization of such a minute amount as 0.003% divinylbenzene with the polystyrene, which effects crosslinking, turning the benzene-soluble product into a gel of highly developed structural restraint (72).

d. Evidence for the crosslinking of collagen

Wiederhorn and his co-workers (3, 73) have made use of the fact that thermally contracted collagen (tendon) obeys the kinetic theory of rubber elasticity. From the stress-strain behavior of the shrunken tendon, the molecular weight between points of crosslinking can be determined. Formaldehyde-tanned collagen, which gives the Ewald reaction, also shows this property. Wiederhorn et al. (3) found the segmental molecular weight of native collagen to be 55,000. By formaldehyde tannage this value is lowered to approximately 11,000, which indicates that new crosslinks have been formed between the collagen chains. Formaldehyde introduces a maximum of two to four crosslinks per fundamental structural unit of collagen. The data indicate that only one out of eight side-chain amino groups of collagen takes part in the crosslinking reaction and that the increase in hydrothermal stability is a direct consequence of the crosslinking reaction.

The earlier discussion of the distance of the groups to be bridged by the crosslinking agent was based on an arrangement of the residues of amino acids in the simplest statistical manner, uniformly over the polypeptide chain, according to their frequency. A number of findings on the reactivity of collagen are difficult to reconcile with this view of a uniform spacing of the residues over the chains. Bear suggested (see Fig. 14) that the bulky polar side chains are mainly present in the band region of the protofibrils and that the hydroxyamino acid and similar residues in the interband region will furnish spatial conditions between reactive side chains, for instance the carboxyl groups, more favorable for crosslinking. An unsymmetrical distribution of the amino acid residues in collagen appears to be essential for the interpretation of the reactivity of collagen. This point of view is supported indirectly by Sanger's findings that insulin consists of two different types of polypeptide chains, one of which contains all the basic and hydroxy-amino acid residues. The results of a recent investigation by Zahn and Wegerle (74) constitute convincing proof of the soundness of the Bear model. By interaction of the bifunctional reagent, difluorodinitrodiphenylsulfone,

$$F\underset{}{\overset{NO_2}{\diagdown}}\diagup SO_2\underset{}{\overset{NO_2}{\diagdown}}\diagup F,$$ according to Zahn and Zuber (75), with tendon

collagen, the T_s was elevated by 10 degrees, evidence of crosslinking. According to Zahn, the difluorodinitro compounds react with about 60% of the ϵ-amino groups of the lysine residues and about 80% of the hydroxylysine groups. The reaction of the sulfone with collagen is bifunctional to a large extent (T_s increase). By chromatographic examination of the acid hydrolyzate of the sulfone-treated collagen, the presence of considerable amounts of sulfone bislysine was established. Also the formation of the bishydroxylysine compound and the sulfone lysine- hydroxylysine was shown.

Zahn and Wegerle stress the point that the isolation of the bis compounds and the presence of the compound of lysine and hydroxylysine residues crosslinked by the sulfone molecule are evidence for the occurrence of the residues of these two basic amino acids in close proximity on adjacent polypeptide chains. It is considered to be an experimental proof of the Bear concept that the bulky polar side chains are confined to the open-structured band section of the collagen fibrils. This important investigation also supplies the first direct isolation of the condensation products formed by a crosslinking agent and the residues of amino acids which have partaken in the tanning reaction. The bisamido methylene compounds had been previously isolated by the Peacock group (76) in the enzymatic hydrolyzates of vegetable protein fibers (Ardil) tanned with formaldehyde in acidic solution, demonstrating the presence of glutamine and asparagine residues in close proximity, as is required for crosslinking by the methylene residue of formaldehyde.

8. Some Reactions in the Crosslinking of Keratin

a. General aspects

The molecular pattern of keratin is typical for a fibrous protein already crosslinked by Nature (—S—S— links). Although keratin (wool) shows a high degree of stability compared to collagen, a further improvement of its tensile strength and other properties is occasionally desirable. A great many organic compounds have been claimed to affect crosslinking of wool. Several of these are out of the question for collagen, because of the severe conditions of application.

On the other hand, in its low degree of hydrothermal stability collagen has a decided advantage over keratin for detecting the formation of crosslinks and for measuring the degree of stabilization effected by the crosslinking agent. The temperature of instantaneous shrinkage of the collagen fibers provides a simple and sensitive measure of the degree of stabilization of the structure by crosslinking and by tanning agents.

Various techniques for the crosslinking of the wool fiber are of practical importance, since the reactivity and properties of the wool may be altered, and its resistance to various agents including proteinases (the cloth moth) is improved. As for the altered properties, the felting power of the wool is reduced and its resistance to wear is increased. Measurement of the degree of crosslinking is carried out by two independent methods mainly: (1) the Speakman load-extension method and, (2) the Zahn test of estimating the temperature at the point of softening of the fiber. According to Speakman (77), the load-extension curve up to 30% extension is determined on the untreated fiber and on the treated fiber. By the crosslinking of the protein chains, the resistance of the fiber to extension is increased. The change in resistance to deformation may reach values of 25%, for instance by quinone tannage. This method is affected by the ionization of the keratin (pH), however, and it is not very sensitive. The Zahn test (77a) is based on the contraction of the wool fibers brought about by its treatment in a 50% w/v solution of phenol in water on heating for 20 minutes. The point of softening is defined as the temperature at which 20% contraction of the fiber takes place. The phenol ruptures the crosslinks of the hydrogen bond type mainly. A classical method is the treatment of wool in a boiling solution of sodium bisulfite which results in supercontraction of the fiber, probably by splitting of the —S—S— bridge. This method is too severe for most crosslinking agents. Another method on the same basis is the peracetic acid method (78), which appears to be more suitable because it is applied in cold solution.

b. Crosslinking by alkylation agents

Apart from the ordinary tanning agents, chromium salts (surprisingly, mainly the acetate of questionable tanning potency), benzoquinone, and formaldehyde, and a number of aliphatic and aromatic compounds have been tried for the crosslinking of wool. Only a few of these show promise of gaining practical importance. Many of these agents consist of alkylating agents, with the molecule containing epoxide groups, such as $O\underset{\diagdown CH_2}{\overset{\diagup CHR}{|}}$,

or ethylenimine, $R \cdot N\underset{\diagdown CH_2}{\overset{\diagup CH_2}{|}}$. In the latter instance, polymerization and crosslinking take place concurrently. The most active agents are nucleophilic. Thus, they possess great affinity for groups with heavy accumulation of electrons, such as carboxyl ions and the amino groups of proteins

(79). They do not react with the un-ionized carboxyl group or with the charged amino group. The alkylating agents are generally applied in aqueous solution buffered with bicarbonates. The solvent and the protein compete for the agent, the protein gaining the upper hand mostly. According to Alexander (79), the monofunctional dinitrofluorobenzene (Sanger reagent) crosslinks wool. The corresponding difluoro compound, and particularly the difluorodinitrodiphenylsulfone, $F\langle\rangle SO_2\langle\rangle F$, with the NO_2 substituents, introduced by Zahn (74), are also excellent crosslinking agents for collagen. The effect of the Sanger reagent is apparently due to the participation of weak dipoles on the aromatic ring (π electrons), a parallel to the Otto concept of the fixation of aromatic compounds by proteins (80). These auxiliary forces make the monofunctional agent into a bifunctional one. (Compare the Novolak monosulfonic acid in tanning) (81).

Potent crosslinking agents (79) are the epichlorohydrins, such as $Cl \cdot CH_2 \cdot CH\text{——}CH_2$ with the epoxide O and the diepoxides, for instance,

$$O$$
$$CH_2 \cdot CH\text{——}CH_2$$
$$O$$
$$CH_2 \cdot CH\text{——}CH_2$$
$$O$$

which preferentially react with the carboxyl group at pH 6 to 7 and temperatures of about 50°C. Among the ethylenimines, the following compound is especially effective:

$$CH_2\text{——}CH_2$$
$$N$$
$$C$$
$$CH_2 \quad N \quad N \quad CH_2$$
$$N \cdot C \qquad C \cdot N$$
$$CH_2 \quad N \quad CH_2$$

Another group of valuable crosslinking agents are the methanesulfonyloxy compounds, particularly the following two compounds:

$$X(CH_2 \cdot C \equiv C \cdot CH_2) \cdot X \quad \text{and} \quad X \cdot CH_2 \cdot \underset{\underset{CH_3}{|}}{\overset{\overset{NO_2}{|}}{C}} \cdot CH_2 \cdot X$$

where $X = CH_3 \cdot SO_2 \cdot O$—.

Speakman and his school (77, 82) have studied the diepoxy compound: 3,4-isopropylidine-1,2,5-dianhydromannitol,

$$CH_2 \overset{}{—} CH \cdot CH \overset{}{——} CH \cdot CH \overset{}{——} CH_2$$

which is applied in a water solution of 50°C. at pH values of 5 to 7. This compound stabilizes completely deaminated keratin as effectively as it does intact keratin. This and other evidence indicates that the carboxyl group of keratin is mainly involved. Fraenkel-Conrat has proved such a reaction mechanism for simple epoxides with globular proteins. A simple but unequivocal proof is the fact that the reaction is forestalled by the addition of carboxylates, the reason being the preferred reaction of the epoxide with the carboxyl group of the added agent, e.g., phthalate, applied as a buffer. Speakman suggests a combination of crosslinking the carboxyl groups of the keratin by biepoxide and the basic groups by formaldehyde.

Pondering over the problem of how to overcome unfavorable steric conditions in the keratin structure, Lipson and Speakman (82) reasoned that by polymerization of a monomer in the fiber any free reactive group in the deposited polymer would occur with such a frequency that there must always be one within the range of every reactive protein side chain. This would facilitate crosslinking on introduction of the second agent. Thus, methacrylamide was polymerized in the wool. By applying formaldehyde, crosslinks were set up between the amide group of the polymer and the amino group of keratin. This method of introducing new reactive groups, e.g., the guanidyl, by means of formaldehyde tanning is due to Fraenkel-Conrat. Lipson and Speakman (82) found that by polymerization of methacrylamide in wool fibers, the resistance of the fibers was raised by 22%. The subsequent treatment with 4% formaldehyde solution at pH 5 increased the resistance to extension to 47% above that of the untreated fibers.

An interesting example of *in situ* polymerization is given by Lipson and

Speakman (82). The wool is first impregnated with a 0.2 M solution of ferrous ammonium sulfate, followed by the application of an aqueous solution of hydrogen peroxide and a monomer, e.g., methacrylic acid, at 50°C. The hydrogen peroxide reacts with the ferrous ion within the fibers. Hydroxyl radicals are formed

$$Fe^{++} + H_2O_2 \rightarrow Fe^{+++} + OH^- + HO^+$$

Polymerization is thus initiated:

$$HO^+ + CH_2{=}C \cdot CH_3 \cdot COOH + CH_2{=}C \cdot CH_3 \cdot COOH \rightarrow$$

$$HO \cdot CH_2 \cdot CH \cdot CH_3 \cdot COO \cdot CH_2 \cdot CH \cdot CH_3 \cdot COOH$$

Large amounts of polymers of different properties, acidic or basic, hydrophilic or hydrophobic, may be formed within the fibers, with amounts up to 80% of the weight of the wool, allowing variation of certain properties within wide limits.

9. THERMODYNAMIC CONSTANTS

To finish with a brief outline of the thermodynamic approach to the effect of tanning agents on the T_s of collagen, introduced by Weir, the conclusions drawn from the purely chemical aspects may be compared with those derived from considerations of thermodynamic potentials and their relation to the T_s and crosslinking reactions. The effect of some tanning agents on the thermodynamic quantities of collagen in tendons is illustrated by the data in Table 29 (83). The determinations and calculations were carried out as described earlier in this chapter.

Looking over these data, it is striking to find the unique position of the chromium salts as tanning agents, effecting large increases of all three fundamental thermodynamic quantities. Three other tannages show a similar behavior, although less pronounced—quinone, glyoxal, and cyclohexane disulfonyl chloride, the latter a *bifunctional* agent. Attention must be called to the fact that the *unifunctional* monosulfonyl compound has no effect on collagen. In this instance, no crosslinking is possible, since the general reaction scheme is:

$$R \cdot SO_c Cl + H_2N \cdot P \rightarrow R \cdot SO_2 \cdot HN \cdot P + HCl$$

where R = cyclohexane and P = protein. With the disulfonyl chloride, crosslinking of two chains can take place according to the simplified equation

$$P \cdot NH_2 + Cl \cdot SO_2 R \cdot SO_2 Cl + H_2 NP \rightarrow P \cdot NH \cdot SO_2 \cdot R \cdot SO_2 \cdot HN \cdot P + 2HCl$$

TABLE 29

EFFECT OF TANNING AGENTS ON THE THERMODYNAMIC CONSTANTS OF COLLAGEN
(TENDON) (83)

Treatment	ΔH, kcal./ mole	ΔS, cal./ mole/ deg.	ΔF_{60}, kcal./ mole
Cyclohexane monosulfonyl chloride	145	361	24.9
Cyclohexane disulfonyl chloride	217	573	26.4
Glyoxal, pH 5.2	288	760	34.6
Quinone, pH 4.0	271	710	35.9
Chromium sulfate (1.0% fixed Cr_2O_3 on collagen)	390	1040	44.1
Chromium sulfate (1.1% fixed Cr_2O_3 on deaminated collagen)	456	1225	48.4
No treatment (blank)	141	349	24.7
Deaminated collagen	191	493	26.5

A marked increase of the thermodynamic quantities is also recorded in this instance. Deamination of collagen increases the thermodynamic quantities not unexpectedly, since by removal of the ϵ-amino groups of the lysine residues the T_s of collagen is increased a few degrees (84). The loss of these amino groups does not detrimentally affect chrome tannage, as far as the stabilization of the protein is concerned, as is evidenced by the augmented thermodynamic quantities of the deaminated collagen. This finding adds support to the view that the amino group of lysine is not essential for the stabilization of collagen by means of cationic chromium compounds. The data of the thermodynamic characteristics given are decidedly in favor of the crosslinking concept of tanning processes.

REFERENCES

1. Meyer, K. H., and Ferri, C., *Helv. Chim. Acta* **18**, 570 (1935); *Pflügers Arch. ges. Physiol.* **238**, 78 (1936); Meyer, K. H., von Susich, G., and Valko, E., *Kolloid-Z.* **59**, 208 (1925).
2. Küntzel, A., in "Stiasny Festschrift," p. 191. Roether, Darmstadt, 1937.
3. Wiederhorn, N. W., Reardon, G. V., and Browne, A. R., *J. Am. Leather Chem. Assoc.* **48**, 7 (1953).
4. Lloyd, D. J., and Garrod, M., *Trans. Faraday Soc.*, **64**, 441 (1948).
5. Schmitt, F. O., Hall, C. E., and Jakus, M. A., *J. Cellular Comp. Physiol.* **20**, 11 (1942).
6. Schmitt, F. O., *Advances in Protein Chem.* **1**, 53 (1944).
7. Schiaparelli, C., and Careggio, L., *Cuir tech.* **14**, 68 (1925); Schiaparelli, C., and Busino, G., *J. Intern. Soc. Leather Trades Chem.* **11**, 53 (1927).
8. Theis, E. R., *J. Am. Leather Chem. Assoc.* **36**, 682 (1941).
9. Gustavson, K. H., *Advances in Protein Chem.* **5**, 392 (1949).

10. Weir, C. E., and Carter, J., *J. Research Natl. Bur. Standards* **44**, 599 (1950).
11. Balfe, M. P., *in* "Progress in Leather Science," Vol. 2, p. 417. BLMRA, London, 1947.
12. Bancroft, W. D., *Colloid Symposium Monograph* **4**, 29 (1926).
13. Meyer, K. H., and Dunkel, M., *Z. physik. Chem.* Bodensteinfestband, p. 553 (1931).
14. Weir, C. E., *J. Am. Leather Chem. Assoc.*, **44**, 142 (1949).
15. Wöhlisch, E., *Ergeb. Physiol.* **34**, 405 (1932); *Biochem. Z.* **247**, 329 (1932); Wöhlisch, E., and Du Mesnil de Rochemont, R., *Z. Biol.* **85**, 406 (1927).
16. Meyer, K. H., and Ferri, C., *Pflügers Arch. ges. Physiol.* **238**, 78 (1936); Cherbuliez, E., Jeannerat, J., and Meyer, K. H., *Z. physiol. Chem.* **254**, 241 (1938); see also Meyer, K. H., "Die Hochpolymeren Verbindungen," pp. 428–433. Akademische Verlagsgesellschaft, Leipzig, 1940.
17. Gustavson, K. H., *Colloid Symposium Monograph* **4**, 77 (1926).
18. Gustavson, K. H., *Biochem. Z.* **311**, 347 (1942); *Acta Chem. Scand.* **1**, 581 (1947); *J. Am. Leather Chem. Assoc.* **41**, 47 (1946).
19. Wright, B. A., and Wiederhorn, N. W., *J. Polymer Sci.* **7**, 105 (1951); Wiederhorn, N. M., and Reardon, G. V., *ibid.* **9**, 315 (1952).
20. See, e.g., Ewald, A., *Z. physiol. Chem.* **105**, 115, 135 (1919); for the early history see ref. 15.
21. Grassmann, W., *Kolloid-Z.* **77**, 205 (1936).
22. Herzog, R. O., and Gonell, H. W., *Naturwissenschaften* **12**, 1153 (1925); *Collegium* **1926**, 189; Gerngross, O., and Katz, J. R., *Kolloid Beihefte* **23**, 368 (1926).
23. Astbury, W. T., and Atkin, W. R., *Nature* **132**, 348 (1933).
24. Katz, J. R., and Gerngross, O., *Naturwissenschaften* **13**, 900 (1925).
25. Bear, R. S., *J. Am. Chem. Soc.* **66**, 1297 (1944); *Advances in Protein Chem.* **7**, 69 (1951).
26. Ewald, A., *Z. physiol. Chem.* **105**, 115, 135 (1919).
27. Bear, R. S., *J. Am. Chem. Soc.* **64**, 727 (1942); **66**, 1297 (1944).
28. Weir, C. E., *J. Am. Leather Chem. Assoc.* **44**, 108 (1949).
29. Nutting, G. C., and Borasky, R., *J. Am. Leather Chem. Assoc.* **43**, 96 (1948); Borasky, R., and Nutting, G. C., *J. Am. Leather Chem. Assoc.* **44**, 830 (1949).
30. Pankhurst, K. G. A., *Nature* **159**, 538 (1947).
31. Gustavson, K. H., *J. Am. Leather Chem. Assoc.* **41**, 47 (1946).
32. Mirsky, A. E., and Pauling, L., *Proc. Natl. Acad. Sci. U.S.* **22**, 439 (1936).
33. Kuhn, W., *Kolloid-Z.* **68**, 2 (1934).
34. Küntzel, A., and Doehner, K., *Kolloid-Beih.* **51**, 277 (1940). Küntzel, A., *in* "Stiasny Festschrift," p. 191. Roether, Darmstadt, 1937.
35. Fauré-Frémiet, E., *J. chim. phys.* **34**, 125 (1937); *Arch. anat. microscop.* **33**, 81 (1937); Champetier, G., and Fauré-Frémiet, E., *J. chim. phys.* **34**, 197 (1937); Fauré-Frémiet, E., and Woelfflin, R., *ibid.* **33**, 801 (1936).
36. Krukenberg, C. F. W., *Mitt. zool. Station Neapel* **4**, 286 (1885).
37. Gustavson, K. H., *Svensk Kem. Tidskr.* **62**, 165 (1950).
38. Sykes, R. L., *J. Soc. Leather Trades Chem.* **37**, 294 (1953).
39. Gustavson, K. H., *Svensk Kem. Tidskr.* **65**, 70 (1953).
40. Anson, M. L., *Advances in Protein Chem.* **2**, 361 (1945).
41. Gustavson, K. H., *Svensk Kem. Tidskr.* **54**, 74 (1942).
42. Gustavson, K. H., *Svensk Kem. Tidskr.* **54**, 249 (1942).
43. Gustavson, K. H., *Biochem. Z.* **311**, 347 (1942).

44. Gustavson, K. H., *J. Soc. Leather Trades Chem.* **33**, 332 (1949).
45. Gustavson, K. H., *J. Am. Leather Chem. Assoc.* **45**, 789 (1950).
46. Gustavson, K. H., *Acta Chem. Scand.* **4**, 1171 (1950).
47. Gustavson, K. H., *Ing. Vetenskaps Akad. Handl.* No. 177 (1944).
48. Takahashi, T., private communication.
49. Gustavson, K. H., *Acta Chem. Scand.* **8**, 1299 (1954); *Nature* **175**, 70 (1955).
50. Reed, R., and Rudall, K. M., *Biochim. et Biophys. Acta* **2**, 7 (1948).
51. Powarnin, G., *Collegium* **1914**, 658; Powarnin, G., and Aggeew, N., *Collegium* **1924**, 198; see also Schiaparelli, C., and Careggio, L., *Cuir tech.* **13**, 70, 134 (1924).
52. Chater, W. J., *J. Intern. Soc. Leather Trades Chem.* **13**, 24, 427 (1929); **14**, 28, 133 (1930).
53. Hobbs, R. B., *J. Am. Leather Chem. Assoc.* **35**, 272 (1940).
54. Balfe, M. P., and Humphrey, F. E., "Progress in Leather Science," *Vol.* **2**, p. 417. BLMRA, London, 1947.
55. Theis, E. R., and Lams, M., cited in "The Chemistry of Leather Manufacture," (G. D. McLaughlin and E. R. Theis, eds.), pp. 405–406. Reinhold, New York, 1945.
56. Sykes, R. L., *J. Soc. Leather Trades Chem.* **37**, 294 (1953).
57. Chambard, P., and Michallet, L., *Cuir tech.* **16**, 520 (1927).
58. Chater, W. J., *J. Intern. Soc. Leather Trades Chem.* **14**, 28 (1930).
59. Gustavson, K. H., *J. Am. Leather Chem. Assoc.* **42**, 13, 313 (1947).
60. Page, R. O., *J. Intern. Soc. Leather Trades Chem.* **28**, 156 (1944).
61. Meyer, K. H., *Biochem. Z.* **208**, 23 (1929); Meyer, K. H., and Mark, H., "Der Aufbau der hochpolymeren Organischen Naturstoffe," pp. 186–187. Akademische Verlagsgesellschaft, Leipzig, 1930.
62. Gustavson, K. H., *Ing. Vetenskaps Akad. Handl.* No. 177 (1944).
63. Küntzel, A., and Schwank, M., *Collegium* **1940**, 489.
64. Fraenkel-Conrat, H., and Mecham, D. K., *J. Biol. Chem.* **177**, 477 (1949).
65. Fraenkel-Conrat, H., Cooper, M., and Olcott, H. S., *J. Am. Chem. Soc.* **67**, 950 (1945); Fraenkel-Conrat, H., and Olcott, H. S., *ibid.* **68**, 34 (1946); **70**, 2673 (1948).
66. Danielsson, C. E., *Svensk Kem. Tidskr.* **60**, 142 (1948).
67. Pouradier, J., Roman, J., Venet, A., Chateau, H., and Accary, A., *Bull. soc. chim. France* **19**, 928 (1952).
68. Bowes, J. H., "Progress in Leather Science," Vol. 3, pp. 541–542. BLMRA, London, 1948.
69. Elöd, E., and Schachowskoy, T., *Collegium* **1933**, 701; **1934**, 281; *Kolloid-Z.* **72**, 221 (1935); *Kolloid Beihefte* **51**, 1 (1939); Elöd, E., Schachowskoy, T., and Weber-Schaefer, E., *Collegium* **1935**, 406.
70. Gustavson, K. H., *Svensk Kem. Tidskr.* **52**, 75 (1940); "Handbuch der Gerbereichemie" (W. Grassmann, ed.), Vol. I, Part 2, p. 27. Springer, Vienna, 1939; *J. Am. Leather Chem. Assoc.* **48**, 559 (1953).
71. Gustavson, K. H., *J. Intern. Soc. Leather Trades Chem.* **24**, 377 (1940).
72. Staudinger, H., "Zur Entwicklung der Chemie der Hochpolymeren," p. 152. Verlag Chemie, Berlin, 1937.
73. Wright, B. A., and Wiederhorn, N. W., *J. Polymer Sci.* **7**, 105 (1951).
74. Zahn, H., and Wegerle, D., *Das Leder* **5**, 121 (1954).
75. Zahn, H., and Zuber, H., *Ber.* **86**, 172 (1953).
76. Haworth, R. D., MacGillioray, R., and Peacock, D. H., *J. Chem. Soc.* **1952**, 298.
77. Speakman, J. B., *J. Soc. Leather Trades Chem.* **37**, 37 (1953).
77a. Zahn, H., *Kolloid-Z.* **113**, 157 (1949).

78. Alexander, P., Fox, M., Stacey, K. A., and Smith, L. F., *Biochem. J.* **52,** 177 (1952).
79. Alexander, P., *Melliand Textilber.* **35,** 3 (1954).
80. Otto, G., *Das Leder* **4,** 1 (1953).
81. Gustavson, K. H., *Discussions Faraday Soc.* **No. 16,** 109 (1954).
82. Lipson, A., and Speakman, J. B., *J. Soc. Dyers Colourists* **65,** 390 (1949).
83. Weir, C. E., *J. Soc. Leather Trades Chem.* **36,** 155 (1952).
84. Kremen, S. S., and Lollar, R. M., *J. Am. Leather Chem. Assoc.* **43,** 542 (1948); Lipsitz, P., Kremen, S. S., and Lollar, R. M., *ibid.* **44,** 371 (1949); Page, R. O., *J. Soc. Leather Trades Chem.* **37,** 183 (1953); Weir, C. E., and Carter, J., *J. Research Natl. Bur. Standards* **44,** 599 (1950).

CHAPTER 10

Inactivation of Specific Groups of Collagen for the Study of Its Reactivity

It is possible to inactivate or remove specific protein groups, for instance the ϵ-amino group of the lysine residue (to mention a classical example), without interfering with other groups or the general properties of the protein. In many respects collagen is an excellent substrate for such structural alterations, particularly because of its high degree of stability. It is also apparently the first protein on which such modifications have been made in order to investigate the role any particular protein group plays in the fixation of reactants and for studies of the general reactivity. In collagen, the chief reactants are the various tanning agents. Excellent general reviews on methods of modifying proteins, more particularly on the aspects of the inactivation of specific groups of proteins, have been given by Herriott (1), Olcott and Fraenkel-Conrat (2), and Putnam (3). In this chapter an outline of the methods generally employed for the modification of collagen will be given and also some suggestions regarding new methods not generally applied to collagen.

1. Removal and Inactivation of the ϵ-Amino Group of the Lysine Residue

a. Diazotization (deamination)

By diazotization of collagen with nitrous acid, the basis for the Van Slyke method for determination of the protein group mentioned, the first modifying reaction was introduced for the study of the reactivity of collagen by Thomas and Foster (4) more than thirty years ago. The ideal reaction scheme is

$$P \cdot NH_2 + HONO \rightarrow P \cdot OH + N_2 + H_2O$$

Hence, the hydroxyl group takes the place of the primary amino group. If diazotization is carried out at a pH of about 4, in a solution of sodium nitrite acidified with acetic acid, the reaction appears to run according to the equation given above. The protein groups which are most easily attacked by nitrous acid, apart from the amino groups, are the phenolic and sulfhydryl groups; fortunately, the latter are absent, or practically so, in collagen. Therefore gelatin and collagen offer the best possibilities for selective removal of the ϵ-amino groups by this technique.

The main difficulty is presented by the guanidyl group of collagen. By the Thomas and Foster method, almost complete removal of the lysine amino group is generally obtained on prolonged interaction of nitrous acid at the moderately acid conditions employed. Nevertheless, even when some of these amino groups are left intact after standard deamination, it is often found that a small part of the guanidyl groups are attacked by the nitrous acid. Thus, Bowes and Kenten (5) report not only nearly complete removal of the ϵ-amino groups by the standard procedure of deamination but also a decrease in the arginine content by about 20%. They stress the fact that little attention has apparently been given to the reaction with the guanidyl groups. For complete removal of this group a very low pH value of the diazotization bath is required, the procedure being to employ a solution of sodium nitrite acidified with a strong mineral acid to reach acidities of the order of pH 1 to 2 (6). An extensive deamidation will then also occur (7).

The rather inert nature of the guanidyl group of collagen has been stressed on a number of occasions, the probable reason being its function as the site of strong crosslinks and its interlinking with other protein groups. Thus, in the Sakaguchi reaction, which involves treatment with hypochlorite in a strongly alkaline solution, less than half of the arginine residues are attacked. This reaction is markedly retarded by the presence of compounds containing aliphatic hydroxyl groups, only about 10% of the total number of arginine residues being reacted upon. The fact that extremely high pH values are required for the titration of the guanidyl group points in the same direction. Also, the low pH value at which the diazotization of the arginine residue of collagen must be carried out to yield results is understandable from the point of view of this group's being strongly interlinked with some other protein groups.

An additional complication is introduced by the secondary interaction of the arginine residues with nitrous acid through the occurrence of a peculiar side reaction, with cyanamide and ammonia as the final products. These reactions are known to occur with the arginine molecule and its simple derivatives (8). If the same reaction takes place with the arginine residue of collagen, which is indicated to be the case (5), it introduces certain difficulties in assaying and interpretating the analytical data. This reaction follows the equation:

$$-CH_2NH \cdot C \overset{NH_2}{\underset{NH}{\diagup\diagdown}} \xrightarrow{HONO} -CH_2 \cdot NH \cdot CN + NH_3$$

Bowes and Kenten (5) have found that the value of amide nitrogen of their deaminated collagen was higher than that of the original collagen. The additional ammonia may have come from the —NH·CN— group formed in the reaction given above, in the course of determining the amide nitrogen. The increase in amide nitrogen was about equal to the decrease in arginine residues. The formation of the cyanamide compound also explains the fact that the decrease in the nitrogen content of the deaminated collagen, expressed in milligram equivalents per gram of collagen, occasionally is less than the corresponding decrease in milligram equivalents of acid bound per gram of collagen. In view of the fact that some deamidation of collagen takes place on diazotization, an additional complication is introduced in the estimation of the amount of ε-amino groups removed in the deamination, from the estimation of nitrogen.

The golden yellow color characteristic for deaminated proteins is probably caused by the intermediate formation of nitroso compounds with residues of aromatic amino acids (9) in the case of collagen, the phenylalanine. These compounds are then converted into deep-colored azo compounds, which change explains the marked darkening of color that takes place when deaminated pelt is stored, particularly on exposure to daylight. It is interesting to note that the T_s of freshly deaminated collagen is about the same as that of the original collagen. However, the T_s increases on storage (10), and also the thermodynamic quantities, as found by Weir and Carter (10a).

The method of deaminating collagen originally devised by Thomas and Foster (4) has been used by many workers with great satisfaction (11). An outline of the method follows. One hundred grams of hide powder is soaked in 1 l. of distilled water for a few hours. A quantity of 500 ml. of 20% solution of sodium nitrite is then added. The contents are stirred and allowed to stand overnight. Glacial acetic acid in a quantity of 70 g. is then added slowly with constant stirring which is continued throughout the day. After 24 hours, the excess of liquid is squeezed off through a cheesecloth (hide powder cloth, for instance). The deaminated hide powder, now of a bright yellow color, is washed several times with a 10% solution of sodium chloride and finally very exhaustively with distilled water. It is then dehydrated with three changes of acetone and dried in the open air, care being taken to have the deaminated collagen spread out on a large filter paper. It is finally dried in vacuum at 50°C. for a few hours and transferred to a dark bottle. In order to eliminate side reactions as far as possible, it is advisable to keep the diazotization bath at a low temperature, 2 to 4°C., extending the time of diazotization to 48 to 72 hours.

In an investigation of the effect of different degrees of deamination of collagen (carried out at different pH values) on its fixation of formaldehyde, collagen specimens of three different degrees of deamidation were used (12).

The deamination at pH 2 was carried out as follows: An amount of delimed calfskin pelt collagen equal to 100 g. of collagen was treated for 24 hours in 1 l. of solution containing 50 g. of sodium sulfate and 4.5 g. of sulfuric acid (pickle). The pelt removed about 4 g. of sulfuric acid. The pickled pelt was pressed to remove superfluous solution and transferred into 500 ml. of a 5 % solution of sodium nitrite. After 30 minutes of shaking, 18 g. of sulfuric acid in 10 % solution was added drop by drop. After 4 hours, 25 g. of sodium nitrite in 25 % solution was added, followed by 18 g. of sulfuric acid in 20 % solution. The stock was kept in this solution with intermittent shaking for 24 hours. The pelt was then pressed and treated for an additional 24 hours in a new solution of 50 g. of sodium nitrite (10 % solution) to which 36 g. of sulfuric acid in 500 ml. of water was added gradually. This procedure was repeated twice during the next two days. The deaminated pelt was then washed and treated in acetate buffer of pH 4.0 to remove the acid and to make it isoelectric. Further treatments were the same as described for the regular deaminated collagen. Data on the nitrogen content and the decrease in acid-binding capacity of collagen caused by deamination are given in Table 30.

Since the lysine content of collagen is 0.31 mg. equiv. per gram of protein, it is found that diazotization in acetic acid solution removes about 85 % of the ε-amino groups, provided that there is no interference with other protein groups. By diazotization at pH 2, with complete removal of the lysine-amino groups assumed, the figure on acid binding indicates that about two-thirds of the arginine residues have been attacked. Processing at pH 2.5 gives the corresponding figure of one-third of the arginine groups as altered and inactivated, with regard to acid-binding capacity.

In a method recommended for globular proteins (9) and claimed to be specific for the ε-amino groups of the lysine residues, the protein is first equilibrated in a 0.5 M solution of sodium acetate adjusted to pH 4.0, and 20 % of sodium nitrite, based on the weight of the protein, is added. The

TABLE 30

DEAMINATED COLLAGEN (CALF SKIN PELT) (12)

Type	N, %	NH$_2$ Removed, mg. Equiv.	Decrease in Uptake of HCl, mg. Equiv./g. Collagen	T_s
Pelt (collagen) (blank)	17.85	0	0	66
Pelt deaminated at pH ∼ 4	17.48	0.26	0.25	66
Pelt deaminated at pH ∼ 2.5	17.25	0.43	0.48	66
Pelt deaminated at pH ∼ 2	17.04	0.60	0.65	65

temperature of the bath is kept at 0°C. The duration of the treatment is varied according to the degree of deamination desired.

The use of the deaminated collagen for elucidation of various tanning processes will be discussed under their respective headings in the chapters on tanning in "The Chemistry of Tanning Processes."

b. The Sanger Reagent (Dinitrofluorobenzene, DNFB)

This remarkable compound has become very important as a reagent for the determination of N-terminal groups of proteins and the ϵ-amino groups of lysine residues in the hands of Sanger (13) and the Cambridge school. The great advantage of the DNP derivatives formed with proteins containing free amino groups is that the resulting bond is completely resistant to acid hydrolysis, enabling the opening up of the end-standing peptide bond and isolation of the DNP-amino acid compound. These compounds are brightly colored and are easily separated by ordinary chromatographic methods. The reaction takes place under mild conditions of pH and temperature, in 1% solution of sodium bicarbonate. The reaction follows the scheme

$$NO_2\!\!\left\langle \right\rangle\!\!F + H_2N \cdot P \rightarrow NO_2\!\!\left\langle \right\rangle\!\!HN \cdot P + HF$$
$$NO_2 NO_2$$

Bowes and Moss (14) have employed this method for estimating the N-terminal groups of collagen, as was mentioned earlier. More recently Sykes (15) has inactivated the lysine-amino groups by the Sanger reagent. The following procedure was employed: 1 g. of collagen was wet back in 150 ml. of distilled water containing 5 g. of sodium bicarbonate, in a stoppered bottle, and 5 g. of DNFB dissolved in 300 ml. of ethanol was added. The flask was stoppered and the reaction allowed to proceed. On completion of the reaction, the collagen was quantitatively transferred to a sintered glass filter and thoroughly washed with water, then with ethanol, and finally with ether to remove by-products of the reaction. Sykes found 0.24 mg. equiv. of NH₂— groups to be irreversibly inactivated by the Sanger reagent in tests carried out at room temperature for 7 days or at 35°C. for 2 days. Since the collagen originally contained 0.31 mg. equiv. of primary amino groups of lysine residues, it follows that about 80% of these groups are accessible to the large DNFB molecule. Porter (16) had earlier found that not all the ϵ-amino groups of certain globular proteins react with the Sanger reagent. Bowes and Moss (14) could recover only 55% of the lysine as the DNP derivative from collagen treated with DNFB.

c. Acetylation

Acetyl derivatives of proteins are obtained by treatment with ketene, $CH_2=C=O$, which is rather specific for the amino group of lysine in the absence of phenolic groups, as the case is with collagen (17). The amino-acetyl compounds are stable in acid and alkaline solution, whereas other acetyl compounds are split. Only a part of the ϵ-amino groups are reacted on, however. A more complete, selective acetylation of the amino groups of collagen is obtained by the use of acetic anhydride in aqueous solution at pH 7 to 8 at low temperatures. It is the preferred agent where acetylation of the amino groups of collagen is desired.

The following method has been found useful (18): 10 g. of collagen in the form of hide powder is suspended in 200 ml. of a half to fully saturated sodium acetate solution, cooled in an ice bath, for 1 hour. Then 12.0 ml. of acetic anhydride is added, with stirring, in several portions in about 1 hour's time. After the odor of the reagent has disappeared, the acetylated hide powder is washed in ice-cold water, treated in sodium acetate buffer of pH 4, and finally washed thoroughly and acetone-dehydrated. A more recent method of acetylating collagen (19) will be considered below.

Carbon suboxide, $O=C=C=C=O$, has been used on globular proteins (20). Its reaction is similar to that of the ketene. It is more specific for ϵ-amino groups than the latter and does not react with guanidyl, imidazol, or aliphatic hydroxy groups. It has not been used on collagen, as far as the author knows.

A new acetylating agent is 2-acethylthioethylacetamide, $CH_3CO \cdot NH \cdot CH_2 \cdot CH_2S \cdot CO \cdot CH_3$ introduced by Baddiley, Kekwick, and Thain (21). Conditions are chosen to ensure a reasonable proportion of the amino groups in the $—NH_2$ form, as distinct from the $—NH_3^+$, in order to facilitate the acetylation. Therefore, a borate buffer of pH 10 was used. A 2 % solution of serum albumin in borate buffer of pH 10, to which had been added 1.5 % of the reagent, was kept at room temperature for 3 days. Van Slyke determination of free amino groups showed that 34 to 39 amino groups per mole (70,000) had been acetylated of the 64 groups present in native serum albumin. After exhaustive acetylation at pH 10, the product still appeared to have 25 to 30 free amino groups per mole. This indicates that, of the 59 lysine residues present in the molecule, about half are inaccessible to acetylation under the conditions of reaction employed, assuming that all end α-amino groups, (9 groups per mole) are acetylated.

Phenylisocyanate has been used for inactivation of amino groups of gelatin, the reaction being carried out in aqueous solution buffered at pH 8, at 0 to 25°C. (22). Hopkins and Wormall (23) report the content of bromine introduced into gelatin by means of β-bromophenylisocyanate to be equal to the equivalent of the ε-amino groups of this protein.

Collagen with inactivated primary amino groups is mainly used for investigation of tannages which involve these groups, such as tannages by aldehydes, synthetic tannins, polysulfonic acids, and vegetable tannins. These will be discussed under their appropriate headings in the monograph on "The Chemistry of Tanning Processes."

Since this chapter was prepared, a paper on the acetylation of collagen has appeared which is of sufficient importance to be included here. Green, Ang, and Lam (19) have used an acetylation method similar to the one described (18), which is recommended by Fraenkel-Conrat as a specific method for N-acetylation. They have reported satisfactory results in studies of the influence of inactivation of the amino group of collagen on the fixation of several tanning agents, such as chromium salt, vegetable tannins, formaldehyde, and quinone. They have also devised a technique for complete acetylation of the amino and hydroxyl groups of collagen, employing N- and O-acetylated collagen for their investigation of the tanning systems mentioned.

N-ACETYLATION. Collagen in the form of hide powder was soaked for 24 hours in half-saturated sodium acetate solution at a temperature below 10°C. It was then stirred vigorously for 1 hour, while 10 % by weight of acetic anhydride was added gradually. The pH was held near 8.0 by addition of NaOH solution, and the temperature was kept below 10°. The product was then filtered and freed from sodium acetate by washing with frequent changes of distilled water for one week. Thorough washing is essential, since any residual acetate will cause trouble in the subsequent acetyl estimation. The washed product was dehydrated with several changes of acetone and then dried at room temperature. It was found that prolonging the reaction beyond 1 hour did not increase the degree of acetylation. One re-acetylation increased it considerably and is obligatory (preferably two re-acetylations), as shown by the data in Table 31.

Again, in order to attain the maximum degree of N-acetylation, it is necessary to repeat the treatment, since prolonging the time of interaction or increasing the amount of acetic anhydrides added in a single acetylation is not sufficient. As the data of the table show, the number of N-acetyl groups introduced in three consecutive acetylations is equal to the total number of lysine and hydroxylysine residues found by analysis (0.38 mmol. per gram of collagen).

N- AND O-ACETYLATION. Completely dry collagen cannot be acetylated with cold acetic anhydride. However, acetylation takes place if acetic acid is present. By using equal parts of acetic anhydride and acetic acid with a ratio of acetylating agent to collagen of 6:1, and 8 days' interaction, the

TABLE 31

ACTION OF ACETIC ANHYDRIDE ON COLLAGEN IN AQUEOUS SOLUTION
(In millimolar per gram of collagen)

Nature of suspension	O-acetyl	N-acetyl	Amino N (Van Slyke)
N Acetic acid	0.0	0.05	0.31
Water	0.15	0.05	0.31
Sodium acetate (pH 8)			
First acetylation	0	0.24	0.12
Second acetylation	0	0.36	0.01
Third acetylation	0	0.38	0.00
Fourth acetylation	0	0.38	0.00

maximum amount of acetyl groups was introduced into collagen. (1.76 mmol. per gram of collagen). After acetylation the product was washed and extracted with acetone and finally dried. The completely acetylated specimens swelled during the reaction, and after drying they resembled heat-shrunken collagen in appearance. Apart from this, the completely acetylated hide powder retained its fibrous nature and the color was not impaired.

By the method outlined, the acetylated product contained: 16.6% N, 0.40 mmol. N-acetyl, and 1.33 mmol. O-acetyl per gram of collagen. Hence, the lysine and hydrolysine amino groups have reacted completely, and about 80% of the total number of hydroxy groups, which amount to 1.68 mmol. per gram of collagen (serine, threonine, hydroproline, hydroxylysine, and tyrosine).

It is evident from the investigations of Green et al. that acetylation in an aqueous alkaline suspension rapidly introduces alkali-stable acetyl groups to the extent of 0.40 mmol. per gram of collagen. Simultaneously the amino nitrogen falls to zero. The number of groups introduced is nearly equivalent to the sum of the lysine and hydroxylysine residues. Therefore this reaction is apparently specific for the amino groups.

The maximum number of alkali-labile acetyl groups introduced in the nonaqueous medium is 1.33 mmol. per gram of collagen. Since these groups are easily removed by 0.05 N sodium hydroxide, and in view of other observations, the authors consider it almost certain that these acetyl groups are present as esters of hydroxyl groups.

A number of other agents with selective affinity for the basic groups have been tried. Thus, for instance, Sykes (15) has experimented with carboxymethylation by means of sodium bromoacetate, which apparently does not offer any advantages over the specific agents already described. Sodium glyoxalate is of some theoretical interest from the point of view of oil tannage; as an aldehyde, it will combine with the amino groups and at the same time introduce carboxylic groups into the collagen. Its main use will probably be for addition of carboxyls to proteins.

2. INACTIVATION OF THE GUANIDYL GROUP

As mentioned earlier, there is no satisfactory method available for modifying the guanidyl group quantitatively. The Sakaguchi reaction, which avails itself of the oxidative and chlorinating power of hypochlorite, has been applied to collagen by Highberger and Salcedo (24). They found that more than half of the arginine groups were not acted on. The probable reason for this inertness of the arginine group has already been mentioned. A brief description of the method applied by Highberger and Salcedo (24) to collagen follows.

To 100 g. of collagen (hide powder), contained in a large flask in an ice bath, 750 ml. of water is added. After 15 minutes of stirring, 260 ml. of a sodium hypochlorite solution, containing 5 % available chlorine, is added. After a further 15 minutes of stirring, 750 ml. of N sodium hydroxide is added in portions over a period of 15 minutes. Stirring is continued until a temperature of about 2°C. is reached. Then 1000 ml. of a chilled solution of sodium hypochlorite of the afore-mentioned concentration is added in portions over a period of 4 hours, at a temperature close to 0°C., with vigorous stirring. After all the hypochlorite has been added, the stirring is continued for an additional 45 minutes. The hide powder is then strained through a cloth, soaked in 0.5 N solution of acetic acid for a few minutes, restrained, and soaked in 0.5 N acetic acid overnight in the icebox. It is then exhaustively washed in cold water and dehydrated with acetone. The yield is about 33 %. The product differs in appearance from ordinary hide powder only in its light straw color. Only about 43 % of the arginine of collagen is inactivated (cf. ref. 12).

For the study of the free guanidyl group, a modified collagen in which the reactive amino groups are transformed into guanidyl groups by reacting collagen with S-methylisothiourea, or o-methylisourea, seems promising (25). This reaction is comparatively simple, and other protein groups are not affected. Such substituted collagen preparations should be of interest in studies of the fixation of formaldehyde by collagen.

3. INACTIVATION OF THE CARBOXYL GROUP

Inactivation of the carboxyl group is carried out primarily by esterification. Dimethyl sulfate, diazomethane, methyl iodide and bromide, and 1,2-epoxides have been used on globular proteins and also on wool and collagen (5, 26). The reagents mentioned require a great number of consecutive treatments for complete esterification, which leads to considerable degradation of the collagen. Moreover, these reagents are nonspecific for the carboxyl group and react with many different protein groups. In the special case of collagen, guanidyl and lysine residues are largely affected. The best method available is methylation by means of methanol made 0.1 N in hydrochloric acid, according to the procedure of Fraenkel-Conrat and Olcott (27). Amino and amide groups are not affected. For globular proteins, it was found that the carboxyl group was almost quantitatively esterified by one treatment, the number of the methoxyl groups being in good agreement with the number of carboxyl groups present in the original protein.

The method has been used by the author (28) on collagen with very satisfactory results. Burton *et al.* (29) have independently verified these findings. Applied to collagen (hide powder and pelt), the following procedure has been found useful: 20 g. of collagen in the form of acetone-dehydrated hide powder is shaken intermittently for 7 days in 2.0 l. of methanol, made 0.1 N with respect to hydrochloric acid (15 ml. of concentrated acid). After the reaction is complete an equivalent amount of sodium hydroxide is added and the suspended hide powder shaken for 30 minutes. The methylated stock is freed from the solution by suction filtering and then shaken two consecutive times with 2 l. of water, 10 minutes each time. It is then dehydrated in acetone twice and dried at a starting temperature of 40°C., finishing at 60°C. The yield is of the order of 80 to 85 %. The esterified collagen, which resembles the intact collagen, has a great swelling tendency, and for its use in experiments the presence of swelling-depressing neutral salts in the systems is recommended.

The following analytical data on its composition are of interest. The nitrogen content was 17.2 to 17.3 %, on ash-free dry substance; the ash content was 0.1 to 0.3 % (NaCl); and the combined chloride was 2.4 to 2.6 % as Cl (0.7 to 0.75 mg. equiv. of Cl per gram of collagen), present as hydrochloric acid fixed by the cationic protein groups. The isoelectric point corresponded to a pH of about 9. The degree of esterification is given by the content of methoxyl groups, which amounted to 2.55 to 2.70 % OCH_3, on ash-free dry substance. After correction for the CH_3O content of the original hide powder (0.03 mg. equiv. of methionine), the amounts of methoxyl groups given correspond to 0.80 to 0.85 mg. equiv. of esterified carboxyl groups per gram of collagen, which is about 85 to 90 % of the total amount of carboxyl groups of the original collagen. The acid-binding capacity (0.05 N HCl) was 0.10 to 0.12 mg. equiv. per gram of collagen. Since the intact collagen possesses an acid-binding capacity (0.1 N HCl) of 0.92 mg. equiv. per gram of collagen, the degree of inactivation of the carboxyl groups is 80 to 90 %. The close agreement between the figures of methoxyl and non-acid-binding carboxyl groups indicates that the methylation does not go far outside the carboxylic groups. The methylated hide powder did not fix chromium from solutions of 67 % acid chlorides and sulfates of chromium, 0.6 equiv. per liter of chromium, containing cationic chromium complexes solely. The shrinkage temperature of the esterified collagen (pelt) was 30 degrees lower than that of the original pelt. This drastic lowering of the hydrothermal stability as well as the great swelling tendency of the methylated collagen is probably due to the breaking of ester crosslinks and hydrogen bonds in the process of methylation.

Bowes and Kenten (5) had earlier studied various tanning systems employing collagen methylated by means of dimethyl sulfate and methyl bromide. Since a great number of consecutive severe treatments were required to achieve complete esterification of the carboxyl groups, the resulting product apparently was highly degraded, as the figures of the original paper bring out. The data obtained on the various tanning systems appear to be of doubtful value for elucidating the role of the carboxyl group.

Apart from the use of esterified collagen for investigation of the processes of chrome tanning, it should prove helpful for the study of tanning processes generally. It seems especially promising for the study of the nature of the fixation of polyacids such as lignosulfonic acid, polysulfonic acids of dyestuffs, and polymetaphosphoric acids. The particularly interesting point is the fact that only one-tenth of the carboxyl groups of collagen are available for the hydrogen ions of the polyacid, whereas the *polyvalent* anion is irreversibly fixed by the cationic protein groups, which all can function as cationic sites of reaction for the numerous anionic groups of the fixed polyvalent anion. The degree of displacement of the chloride groups associated with the basic protein groups and the effect of steric hindrance are problems involved in such reactions of esterified collagen.

It should also be noted that war gases of the type of mustard gas, $Cl \cdot CH_2 \cdot CH_2 \cdot S \cdot CH_2 \cdot CH_2 \cdot Cl$, and N-mustards, have been used as an esterifying agent for the carboxyl group (30). Since collagen of the skin is the protein first involved in the attack of such gases on the organism, the reaction of these combatting chemical agents with collagen is of more than academic interest.

Epoxides have also been tried for the esterification of carboxyl groups of globular proteins in aqueous solution at room temperature. Thus, Fraenkel-Conrat (31) obtained almost complete esterification of the carboxyl groups by means of epoxides. The isoelectric point of the treated protein was shifted 3 pH units toward the alkaline side. The amino group is not affected, but phenolic and sulfhydryl groups are interacting. Sykes (32) has used epoxides to block the carboxyl groups of collagen. The bifunctional epoxides, such as epichlorohydrin, and particularly 4-vinyl-1-cyclohexene dioxide, proved to crosslink the carboxyl groups very effectively. The last-mentioned agent increased the T_s of collagen by about 20 degrees. Its tanning power was pH independent in the range of pH 6 to 10.

4. THE AMIDE GROUP

The amide group is relatively inert. Even if hydrolysis of this group occurs more rapidly than that of the peptide bond, no acceptable methods are available for quantitative removal of amide groups without some splitting of the peptide bonds. In the case of collagen and gelatin, it is important to ascertain the content of amide groups, i.e., the degree of inactivation of the carboxylic groups of the residues of glutamic and aspartic acids.

An important point in that respect is the finding of Steinhardt and Fugitt (32a) that acids with anions of high affinity for wool will catalyze the hydrolysis of the amide group more strongly than that of the peptide links. By keeping the concentration of the most favorable anion within the stoichiometric limit of the amide groups present in the protein, the latter groups may be rapidly hydrolyzed without extensive general hydrolysis of the protein. Dodecyl sulfate is an excellent agent, when used at low concentration. Collagen does not show this effect appreciably, according to the statement of Cassel and McKenna (33).

5. THE HYDROXY GROUP

The free hydroxy groups of collagen are those belonging to the residues of serine, threonine, hydroxyproline, and hydroxylysine. An interesting method of sulfation of globular proteins for the inactivation of the hydroxy groups has been proposed and tried by Fraenkel-Conrat and his associates (34). At low temperature, concentrated sulfuric acid reacts rapidly with proteins to form acid sulfate esters of the hydroxy groups. Since amino and other polar groups of the proteins do not react, sulfuric acid appears to be more selective in this respect, than other agents so far investigated. This method should be of interest for inactivation of the large amount of hydroxy groups present in collagen (hydroxyproline and serine). It has been tried in the author's laboratory, without much success. The reaction is performed by mixing the dry protein with concentrated sulfuric acid at temperatures below 0°C. The mixture is allowed to warm up to the room temperature, poured over ice, neutralized with sodium hydroxide, washed to remove inorganic sulfate and freeze-dried. Another sulfating agent, the addition product of pyridine and chlorosulfonic acid, reacts with most types of polar groups of proteins. The sulfate esters of gelatin are stable in the acid range down to pH 2 but are hydrolyzed in alkaline solutions of pH > 11. The hydroxy group is almost completely esterified. The acetylation of the hydroxy groups of the amino acid residues in collagen by the method of Green *et al.* has already been described.

REFERENCES

1. Herriott, R. M., *Advances in Protein Chem.* **3**, 169 (1947).
2. Olcott, H. S., and Fraenkel-Conrat, H., *Chem. Revs.* **41**, 151 (1947).
3. Putnam, F. W., *in* "The Proteins" (H. Neurath and K. Bailey, eds.), Vol. 1, Part B, pp. 893–972. Academic Press, New York, 1953.
4. Thomas, A. W., and Foster, S. B., *J. Am. Chem. Soc.* **48**, 489 (1926); see also Hitchcock, D. J., *J. Gen. Physiol.* **6**, 95 (1923); Thomas, A. W., *J. Am. Leather Chem. Assoc.* **21**, 487 (1926).
5. Bowes, J. H., and Kenten, R. H., *Biochem. J.* **44**, 142 (1949).
6. Speakman, J. B., and Stott, E., *J. Soc. Dyers Colourists* **50**, 341 (1934).
7. Fraenkel-Conrat, H., Cooper, M., and Olcott, H. S., *J. Am. Chem. Soc.* **67**, 314 (1945); Plimmer, R. H. A., *J. Chem. Soc.* **127**, 2651 (1925).
8. Bancroft, W. D., and Belden, B. C., *J. Phys. Chem.* **35**, 2685 (1931); Bancroft, W. D., and Ridgway, S. L., *ibid.* **35**, 2950 (1931); see also ref. 5, and Kanagy, J. R., and Harris, M., *J. Research Natl. Bur. Standards* **14**, 563 (1935).
9. See Philpot, J. S. L., and Small, P. A., *Biochem. J.* **32**, 542 (1938).
10. Lollar, R. M., and Kremen, S. S., *J. Am. Leather Chem. Assoc.* **43**, 542 (1948); Page, R. O., *J. Soc. Leather Trades Chem.* **37**, 183 (1953).
10a. Weir, C. E., and Carter, J., *J. Research Natl. Bur. Standards*, **44**, 599 (1950).
11. See Atkin, W. R., *in* "Stiasny Festschrift," p. 13. Roether, Darmstadt, 1937.
12. Gustavson, K. H., *Svensk Kem. Tidskr.* **52**, 261 (1940); *Kolloid-Z.* **103**, 43 (1943).
13. Sanger, F., *Biochem. J.* **39**, 507 (1945); **40**, 261 (1946); see also *Advances in Protein Chem.* **7**, 1 (1952).
14. Bowes, J. H., and Moss, J. A., *Nature* **168**, 114 (1951).
15. Sykes, R. L., *J. Soc. Leather Trades Chem.* **36**, 267 (1952).
16. Porter, R. R., *Biochem. et Biophys. Acta* **2**, 105 (1948).
17. Neuberger, A., *Biochem. J.* **32**, 1452 (1938); see also ref. 2, p. 177.
18. Fraenkel-Conrat, H., *in* "Amino Acids and Proteins," (D. M. Greenberg, ed.), pp. 532–585. Thomas, Springfield, Ill., 1951.
19. Green, R. W., Ang, K. P., and Lam, L. C., *Biochem. J.* **54**, 181 (1953).
20. Tracy, A. H., and Ross, W. F., *J. Biol. Chem.* **142**, 871 (1942); see also Fraenkel-Conrat, H., *J. Biol. Chem.* **152**, 385 (1944).
21. Baddiley, J., Kekwick, R. A., and Thain, E. M., *Nature* **170**, 968 (1952).
22. See Putnam, F. W., ref. 3, pp. 926–928; also Edman, P., *Acta Chem. Scand.* **4**, 277, 283 (1950).
23. Hopkins, S. J., and Wormall, A., *Biochem. J.* **27**, 740, 1706 (1933); **28**, 2125 (1934).
24. Highberger, J. H., and Salcedo, J. S., *J. Am. Leather Chem. Assoc.* **35**, 11 (1940).
25. Hughes, W. L., Jr., Saroff, H. A., and Carney, A. L., *J. Am. Chem. Soc.* **71**, 2476 (1949); Greenstein, J. P., *J. Biol. Chem.* **28**, 452 (1950).
26. Blackburn, S., Carter, E., and Phillips, H., *Biochem. J.* **35**, 627 (1941); **38**, 171 (1944); see also ref. 5.
27. Fraenkel-Conrat, H., and Olcott, H. S., *J. Biol. Chem.* **161**, 259 (1945).
28. Gustavson, K. H., *J. Am. Chem. Soc.* **74**, 4608 (1952); *Acta Chem. Scand.* **6**, 1443 (1952).
29. Burton, D., Danby, J. P., and Sykes, R. L., *J. Soc. Leather Trades Chem.* **37**, 219 (1953).

30. Kinsey, V. E., and Grant, N. M., *Arch. Biochem.* **10**, 303 (1946); Fruton, J. S., Stein, W. H., and Bergmann, M., *J. Org. Chem.* **11**, 559 (1946).
31. Fraenkel-Conrat, H., *J. Biol. Chem.* **154**, 227 (1949).
32. Sykes, R. L., *J. Soc. Leather Trades Chem.* **37**, 294 (1953).
32a. Steinhardt, J., and Fugitt, H. C., *J. Research Natl. Bur. Standards* **29**, 315 (1942).
33. Cassel, M., and McKenna, E., *J. Am. Leather Chem. Assoc.* **48**, 142 (1953).
34. Reitz, H. C., Ferrel, R. E., Fraenkel-Conrat, H., and Olcott, H. S., *J. Am. Chem. Soc.*, **68**, 1024 (1946).

CHAPTER 11

Some Aspects of the Action of Proteolytic Enzymes on Collagen and Leather

1. GENERAL ISSUES

The splitting of proteins into simpler units, peptones, polypeptides, and amino acids by proteolytic enzymes is a vital process for the utilization of proteins in the alimentary functions. It is also an important reaction in the decomposition of proteins undergoing putrefaction. The enzymes which are mainly concerned in the former process are pepsin and trypsin, which act on cationic and anionic proteins, respectively, with optimum activity in the pH-range 1 to 2 for pepsin and 7 to 9 for trypsin. The enzymes of major interest for tanning are the trypsin group (proteinases). A complex mixture of the trypsins is employed in leather manufacture in the form of a synthetic bate containing pancreatin.

Proteinases belonging to the cathepsin class are responsible for the changes occurring in collagen under storage. Cathepsin has its optimum action at a pH of about 5. It is inactive in its natural environment in the tissue, since the pH of the living tissue is too high. After death the post-mortem changes in the tissue, particularly the formation of lactic acid, lowers the pH value of the tissue to a point favorable for the autolysis of the proteins. The proteinases which are specifically involved in the destruction of collagen *in vivo* are grouped under the name collagenase.

The tenderizing of beef on aging is due largely to the proteolytic break-down of collagen, elastin, and connective tissue, generally by autolysis, cathepsin and similar proteinases being the active agents. Commercial preparations for the tenderizing of beef rely on the proteolytic action of papain, a proteinase present in the vegetable kingdom.

The behavior of collagen in the untreated (native) and treated (including the tanned) states toward proteinases involves questions of theoretical as well as of practical importance. Among the theoretical issues pertaining to collagen itself are the influence of the state of the skin, including the effect of various pretreatments on the degree of susceptibility to proteinases, the mode of attack of the proteinases, the alterations produced in collagen by the proteinases, particularly with regard to any changes of its reactivity, and the nature of the split products. Pancreatin (trypsinogen), which contains the group of tryptic enzymes, including trypsin, is usually chosen for investigations of collagen and leather, partly because it is traditionally used as a constituent of bates, but primarily because it is readily obtained in concentrated form and easy to handle. It also offers the most favorable possibilities among the protein-splitting enzymes. The influence of the tanning agents on the resistance of the collagen present in the leather substance toward proteinases is of interest, for the development of tanning processes as well as for the practical applications of leather, including the determination of the resistance of collagen in the tanned state (as leather) toward destructive enzymatic processes. An excellent presentation of the modern views on the specificity and mode of action of proteolytic enzymes is given in Crook's article (1).

A drawback of trypsin as a means of measuring the stability of leather toward proteinases is the location of its optimum effect at rather high pH values, which are unsuitable for many leathers, as detanning takes place in alkaline solution. Cathepsin II would be the ideal proteinase for this special purpose, its optimal action being at pH 5, at which point all leather show their maximum stability. Standardized preparations of cathepsin II are not readily obtainable, however, and, since the strength and purity of the proteolytic agent are primary requisites, it cannot be used. Papain has also a suitable pH optimum. Its drawback is the necessity of activation by reducing agents, which, particularly sulfites, introduce further complications.

Table 32A presents a general classification of the most common types of proteolytic enzymes. A more recent scheme of classification (2) is based on the location of the peptide group which is split in the proteolysis and the nature of the adjacent side group, as shown in Table 32B. The splitting of the substrate occurs at the —CO·NH— group and results in the formation of additional acid and basic groups. For the splitting action of the proteinases, the presence of a noncompensated peptide bond (not intermolecularly hydrogen bonded) and a side chain with specificity for the particular proteinase is required. For the part of trypsin, the lysine residue or the guanidyl group functions as the necessary side chain, according to Bergmann's last classification (2). The key function of side groups adjacent to the reactive portion of the molecule, the peptide bonds, such as the side chains formed by lysine and arginine residues, is a very important point which has emerged from the striking advances made possible by Bergmann's brilliant researches. The crucial importance of the side chains for the action of proteinases of the type of trypsin and pepsin has been demonstrated by Neurath and Schwert (3), who find these enzymes to be indifferent to the presence of a second peptide link, provided that the carboxyl group is not free.

Chymotrypsin, which is present in pancreatin, attacks proteins containing the keto-imide group adjacent to an aromatic side chain (phenylala-

TABLE 32

A. GENERAL CLASSIFICATION OF PROTEOLYTIC ENZYMES (NOT CONSIDERING THE
NATURE OF THE SIDE CHAINS) (Bergmann, 2)

Enzyme	Substrate	Specificity
Peptidases		
Dipeptidases	Dipeptides	$NH_2 \cdot CHR \cdot CO — NH \cdot CHR \cdot COOH$
Aminopolypeptidases	Polypeptides	$NH_2 \cdot CHR \cdot CO \quad NH$ - - -
Carboxypolypepti-dases		- - - $CO \cdot NH \cdot CHR \cdot COOH$
Proteinases		
Pepsin	High-molecular	Cations
Trypsin	proteins and	Anions
Cathepsin	peptones	
Papain		Zwitterions

B. CLASSIFICATION CONSIDERING THE NATURE OF THE SIDE CHAINS (Bergmann, 2)

Enzyme Group	Requisite Groups in Main Chain	Typical Side-chain Specificities, R=
Peptidases (exopeptidases).		
Aminopepti-dase from intestine	$NH_2 \cdot CHR \cdot CO \cdot NH \cdots$	$\begin{matrix} CH_3 \\ \diagdown \\ \quad\quad CH—CH_2— \\ \diagup \\ CH_3 \end{matrix}$
Carboxypepti-dase from pancreas	$\cdots CO—NH \cdot CHR \cdot COOH$	$C_6H_5 \cdot CH_2—$ or $HO \cdot C_6H_4 \cdot CH_2—$
Proteinases (Endopeptidases).		
Pepsin	$\cdots NH—CHR \cdot CO—NH—CHR—CO$	$C_6H_5 \cdot CH_2—$ or $HO—C_6H_4 \cdot CH_2—$
Cathepsin I Trypsin Cathepsin II	$\cdots CO—NH—CHR \cdot CO—NH—$	$NH_2—(CH_2)_4—$ or $\begin{matrix} NH_2 \\ \diagdown \\ \quad\quad C—NH \cdot (CH_2)_2— \\ \diagup\diagup \\ NH \end{matrix}$
Chymotrypsin	$\cdots CO—NH—CHR \cdot CO—NH$	$C_6H_5—CH_2—$ or $HO—C_6H_4—CH_2—$

nine or tyrosine). Since such aromatic residues are very scarce in collagen, it is not split by chymotrypsin. On the other hand, cathepsin II, like trypsin, will be satisfied with a guanidyl residue as the side-chain complement (4). Accordingly, it is able to split collagen. It is interesting to note that Anderson (5) has employed a pure grade of chymotrypsin for the bating of skins, with positive results. Provided that the chymotrypsin preparation was not contaminated with trypsin, it should imply that the specific effect of bating is not due to the modifying of collagen by the splitting action of the proteinases on the keto-imide groups of collagen. This observation is of sufficient importance for our understanding of the nature of bating to merit careful verification with chymotrypsin of established purity.

Denatured proteins, particularly collagen, are generally more susceptible to splitting by proteinases than are native proteins. Native collagen is practically inert to proteolytic enzymes under conditions that do not produce swelling of the protein. This has been considered as an indication that the native protein must undergo an initial reaction in order to make it susceptible to the proteolytic fission, a view stressed by Linderstrøm-Lang (5a) for globular proteins generally. This initial reaction may be a denaturation, or it may involve the splitting of a few strategically located peptide bonds (5b). There are indications that certain changes brought about by proteinases are similar to those caused by denaturation with urea. Thus, the large initial decrease in volume of the protein observed in the tryptic attack cannot be accounted for by the electrostriction of the ionic groups formed. This decrease is actually of the order of that produced by urea denaturation. Furthermore, the initial increase in optical rotation on the urea treatment of β-lactoglobulin is also shown on tryptic treatment of this protein in the *native* state, but the change is not associated with the tryptic digestion of the denatured lactoglobulin. These observations are in harmony with the view that the first change attributed to the proteinases is a denaturation of the native protein, similar to the denaturation effected by urea (5a). Linderstrøm-Lang assumes that trypsin catalyzes a process of this type. Presumably, the factor of steric hindrance enters prominently.

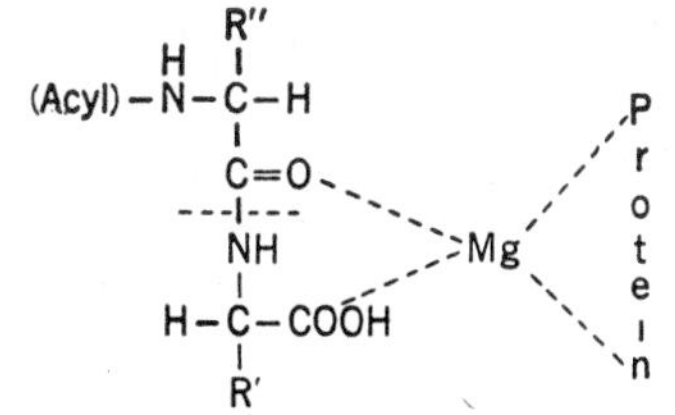

FIG. 38. Schematic drawing of suggested complex formed between the substrate, Mg ion, and carboxypeptidase (Smith, 6).

Lundgren and Williams (5c), also consider an intermediate unfolded form of the protein to be involved in this reaction.

Fig. 38 gives a schematic diagram of the splitting of a protein by proteinase. The action is far more complicated than the idea conveyed by the picture. Recent researches by Smith (6) indicate the vital role played by metals in the action of proteinases. The formation of chelate compounds between the substrate and the proteinase by means of ions of heavy metals in the proteinase (Mg, Mn, Zn, Co) is considered to take place in the initial stage. This leads to an electronic shift. A rearrangement of the electrons at the sensitive peptide bond is believed to occur, which results in a weakening of the C—N— links. Thus, the actual hydrolysis of the peptide bond takes place through a conventional acid-base catalysis. The lowered free energy of activation brought about by the chelating mechanism then explains why hydrolysis readily takes place under such mild conditions of pH and temperature (6).

For a long time biochemists had wondered why proteinases are not able to split peptides. The explanation was finally given by Max Bergmann (7). His researches showed that the chief difference between the proteinases and the peptidases is that the former are able to catalyze the hydrolysis of a peptide bond remote from a free α-amino or α-carboxyl group, whereas the peptidases require the close proximity of either or both of these groups. The proteinase is therefore able to attack and break up the long peptide chains of a protein at several points, i.e., where there is a linkage suited to its specificity requirements. It can then reduce the large molecule rapidly to smaller fragments. Most of these are immune from further attack, since they lack the particular type of link susceptible to the proteinase, as is clear from the schematic drawing in Fig. 39. Peptidases working from the free end groups are able to split these primary hydrolysis products. The different mode of attack of the various proteolytic enzymes led Bergmann to classify them as *endo*peptidases, represented by the great majority of proteinases, and *exo*peptidases, represented by the peptidases. The reason that trypsin, for instance, cannot split polypeptides is the presence of a charged side chain in close proximity to the peptide bond to be hydrolyzed. It was thus shown that by inactivation of the free amino group adjacent to a peptide bond in a tripeptide the latter bond is readily cleaved by an ordinary proteinase, pepsin (7).

The interaction of a proteinase such as trypsin, consisting of a rather large molecule of molecular weight about 40,000, with the insoluble substrate collagen, involves numerous factors such as the rate of diffusion of the enzyme molecule and the degree of accessibility of the peptide bonds susceptible to cleavage. Therefore the degree of swelling and disorganization of the collagen structure should be a prominent factor in determining the

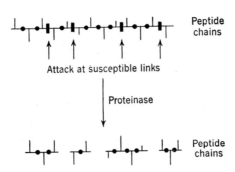

FIG. 39. Cessation of hydrolysis of protein by proteinase caused by hydrolysis of links which satisfy the stereochemical requirements of the enzyme, leaving peptide fragments, which no longer contain links to which the enzyme is specific (Crook, 1).

rate and extent of diffusion and hence also the extent of proteolysis. This has been demonstrated by Bergmann (8) and by Grassmann (9) particularly.

2. EFFECTS ON COLLAGEN

The reaction of collagen to trypsin will be outlined after a brief discussion of the effect of pepsin and the specific collagen-destructive enzymes classed as collagenase, as well as the peptidases specific for the peptides, in which the prolines enter as partners.

In the early stages of enzyme chemistry, it was believed that pepsin does not cause the breakdown of proteins as far as trypsin does. The action of pepsin was considered to affect the forces of secondary valency mainly, leading to peptones, whereas the cleavage of peptide bonds was characteristic for trypsin. This view was given up long ago. However, there is some truth in it. Thus, Sizer's experiments (10) indicate that the dissolving action of pepsin on collagen, present in the form of sutures, is partly due to the rupture of the forces which hold the fibrils together. It was established that on peptic hydrolysis the tensile strength of the fibers decreases much more rapidly than the loss of weight. It is also worthy of note that the viscosity change induced by pepsin in collagen gels has a very high temperature coefficient (activation energy, 277 kcal. per mole), whereas that produced by acids is considerably lower (109 kcal. per mole). As to the action of pepsin, this enzyme is not suitable as an agent for the determination of the resistance of collagen to proteolytic agents, since it requires too acid an environment, or pH values in the neighborhood of 1 to 2. At such low pH values, the collagen has been denatured and disarranged. It is interesting to note that the addition of salt to the hydrochloric acid solution of pepsin prevents its attack on collagen, as was shown by Grassmann (9). Accordingly, the high degree of swelling induced by the strong solutions of hydrochloric acid is necessary for creating suitable conditions of reaction and for cleavage of the collagen molecule to take place. In acid-salt mixtures, i.e. pickle solution, no swelling occurs, nor any hydrolysis of collagen. On the other hand, gelatin is attacked by pepsin, even in the presence of salt. Since gelatin exists in a disorganized state with a part of its keto-imide groups noncompensated internally, this is not surprising. Furthermore, it has been indicated by Northrop (11) that a special gelatin-liquefying enzyme, gelatinase, present in commercial preparations of pepsin, is probably partly responsible for the hydrolytic action. The gelatinase could be separated from the pepsin as a gelatin-liquefying agent.

Great interest on the part of the physiologist and the pathologist has been shown in the enzyme or enzyme complex called elastase, which is claimed (11a) to split elastin. This enzyme is present in beef pancreas and apparently is held in the inactivated state in the organism by an inhibitor present in sera of healthy persons. It appears that this inhibitor is absent in persons with vascular degeneration. Investigations (11a) suggest that elastase is not a true proteinase, splitting the keto-imide link, but a mucase which splits the mucoids associated with elastin. Elastase is particularly interesting in connection with problems related to arteriosclerosis and the degeneration of human elastic tissue. Its eventual role in the bating process is not known.

The name collagenase has been given to a mixture of enzymes produced by bacteria which split native collagen *in vivo*. It is not available in a pure state. The most effective preparations of collagenase are obtained from *Clostridium histolyticum* (12), which completely dissolve collagen in a few days. Less active enzymes mixtures are prepared from *Clostridium welchii*.

Most investigations of the collagenases have been carried out on unsuitable substrates, such as denatured or reconstituted collagen preparations. Thus, Nageotte's "collagéne-A" paper (paper impregnated with acid-extracted collagen) and "Azo-coll" (hide powder coupled with certain azo dyestuff) have been used in the majority of investigations. The activity of the collagenase on the azo dyestuff–hide powder preparation is measured by the amount of dyestuff released through the action of the enzyme. Jennison (12a) and Neuman and Tytell (13) were the first to point out the importance of using *native* collagen which has not been swelled in preparation, or otherwise denatured, as the substrate for this specific enzyme which is unique in that it splits and breaks down native collagen. Neuman and Tytell used Highberger's native bovine hide for their investigations. They emphasize that hide powder, or any denatured collagens, invalidates its use as a substrate for measuring collagenase activity. This view is upheld by Robb-Smith (14), who has made the interesting discovery that collagenases release polysaccharides from the skin.

The action of collagenase *in vivo* is of practical interest, since damage of stored skins is occasionally due to the presence of collagenase-producing bacteria. According to unpublished investigations of E. Lienert and W. Thorsell (private communication), the larva of the warble fly (*Hypoderma*), which penetrates the corium in order to molt in the adipose layer of the skin, avails itself of collagenase for digesting the corium. The problem of collagenase also enters the realm of medicine because gas gangrene and "collagenous diseases" are believed to be intimately connected with destruction of collagenous tissue by collagenases (14).

Because of its high content of proline and hydroxyproline, collagen offers quite different conditions from those offered by the natural proteins for the action of proteolytic enzymes, since every fourth residue of the collagen backbone consists of these amino acids. The $CO \cdot N=$ bond formed instead of the regular $CO \cdot NH-$ bond is not split by any proteinase known. Neither are polypeptides containing such a peptide bond lacking in the hydrogen atom susceptible to the action of the usual type of polypeptidases. It is not known if the specific collagenolytic enzyme collagenase is able to hydrolyze the bonds of the protein backbone to which the prolines contribute their NH— group. However, with regard to the splitting of synthetic substrates of polypeptides containing prolines with the —CO—N= bond, Bergmann and Fruton (15) have demonstrated that the intestinal mucosa contains an enzyme named *prolidase*, which is able to split the CO—N= bond. Hence, it will hydrolyze glycyl-L-proline:

$$
\begin{array}{c}
H_2C\!-\!\!\!-\!\!\!-\!CH_2 \\
|\qquad\qquad| \\
H_2C\qquad CH \cdot COOH \\
\diagdown\quad\diagup \\
N \\
\overline{\cdot} \\
CO \cdot CH_2NH_2
\end{array}
$$

Furthermore, back in 1929 Grassmann *et al.* (16) had found a new type of peptidase named *prolinase*, which possesses the faculty of splitting peptides of the type of prolylglycine or proline-containing polypeptides that do not carry a primary amino group in close proximity to the ordinary peptide bond. These enzymes, specific for polypeptides containing the residues of the prolines, are little known. This applies also to the collagenases.

As for the action of trypsin on collagen, the principal points are as follows. Native collagen, in the form of tendons or skin tissue which are mechanically intact and not swelled, resists the action of trypsin in the pH range 7 to 8, which is close to the optimal range (8, 9, 13, 17). At the pI mentioned, no swelling of collagen takes place. However, according t Bergmann *et al.* (8), it suffices to cut the fibers, freeing the ends of fiber: or to remove the grain layer, thus exposing the ends of the fiber bundles to make collagen susceptible to the attack of trypsin. At least two factor are at work in the tryptic digestion of native collagen: (1) the resistance o the trypsin molecule to diffusion into the fiber bundles offered by the net work structure; (2) the presence of noncompensated peptide bonds. I: native collagen such bonds are present, since the CO·NH— bond locate laterally to the CO—N= bond must contain free valency sites. By swelling additional sites are formed by rupture of hydrogen bonds bridging th adjacent regular peptide bonds. The slight mechanical deformation neede to make native collagen susceptible to trypsin probably is a matter of th enzyme's gaining admission to the fiber and a chance to diffuse into th fibrous structure. Then, the effect of the degree of swelling probably ma: be conceived in a similar manner, although here the disarrangement of th fibers and the dislocation of the hydrogen bonds, resulting in additiona sites of valency, is a potent factor in the attack of trypsin on collagen. Th following example will illustrate this point. Grassmann *et al.* (9) use simple fiber bundles from a bull hide, in the native state (*not* alkali-treated) Intact fiber bundles were resistant to trypsin after treatments in 0.1 % trypsin of the highest obtainable strength at 35°C. for 24 hours at pH 7.? (saturated solution of calcium carbonate). By making the wet hide tissu into a paste, the tryptic resistance was not lost, since only about 1 % of th total nitrogen was found in the solution after several days' digestion. Th solubilized nitrogenous matter consisted mainly of accessory proteins of th skin. After liming and deliming of the same specimen of hide tissue, marked hydrolytic breakdown was found. Swelling had the same effect. I was also found that after wet treatment of collagen at low temperature i: a "beater," with local heating of the stock avoided, the collagen was stil resistant. However, an important point was brought out. When heat wa: generated by grinding the dry hide in a mill, the resulting finely divide powder was to a large extent degraded and markedly dissolved by the sub sequent tryptic digestion. Some data are given in Table 33.

These figures show that the degree of subdivision does not determine th rate and extent of tryptic hydrolysis of collagen. The effect of heat or collagen during the process of grinding seems to be a governing factor fo its enzymatic susceptibility. The fact is that heat-denatured collagen i: very easily digested by trypsin. When the skin tissue is made into hid powder, part of the collagen evidently is denatured if no precaution is taken to prevent heating, as is shown by the fact that 83 % of collagen goe: into solution. If the wet split is minced at low temperature, no denaturation

TABLE 33

REATMENT OF COLLAGEN OF NATIVE HIDE (SPLIT) IN SOLUTIONS OF TRYPSIN (9)

Type of Collagen	N Dissolved, % of Total Collagen N
Middle split of corium (native)	1.1
Dry split, ground in mill	8.3
Dry split, ground in mill under cooling	2.7
Wet split, minced in the "beater"	2.3
Original split (blank)	1.1

ccurs, and the resulting powder resists the hydrolytic action of trypsin. s mentioned earlier, standard hide powder contains fractions of different egrees of fineness and with markedly different reactivity toward coordi- ation compounds, the trend of the reactivity being similar to that pro- uced by heat denaturation (shrinkage) of skin collagen. The conclusion eems appropriate, as stressed by Grassmann, that hide powder is not a uitable substrate for enzymatic investigations.

In general, it may be stated that the different degree of digestibility of roteins by trypsin is a function of their molecular structure and organi- ation. Native collagen of mammals is not attacked by trypsin, or only with lifficulty, owing to secondary alterations after prolonged treatment (hydro- hermal effects at the elevated temperature used, 35 to 40°C., tending to n incipient denaturation). On the other hand, collagen which has been welled by pretreatment in solutions of acids, bases, and lyotropic agents, r thermally shrunken, is easily digested by trypsin. The secondary product f collagen, gelatin, which is composed of unoriented chains, is easily and ompletely digested. These comments concern collagen of mammalian rigin.

Collagen of fishskin, cod being chiefly investigated, even in its native tate is attacked and solubilized by trypsin at such moderate temperatures s to eliminate secondary effects of hydrothermal denaturation largely (18). t is, of course, difficult to eliminate the incipient denaturation of fishskin ollagen completely, even on digestion at rather moderate temperatures nd in neutral solution—for example, about 25°C. with the pH of digestion ear 7. Hence a certain caution is necessary when ascribing tryptic suscep- ibility to native fishskin collagen. Ichthyocol is not markedly attacked by rypsin, but papain breaks it down easily (19). Fishskin in the tanned state nay advantageously be used for evaluation of the stabilizing effect of various tanning agents on collagen.

Another interesting aspect of the action of trypsin on collagen concerns the effect of the tryptic treatment on the properties and behavior of treated collagen, for instance pelt (limed skin brought to the isoelectric state). The nature of the bating process is directly related to this problem. Thaureaux (20) showed that bovine tendon pretreated with a solution of trypsin (0.25 %, buffered at pH 7.8), on subsequent removal of the proteinase, is easily soluble in water when kept at the temperature of shrinkage (68°C.). However, it is possible that the induced water solubility of trypsin-treated collagen is due to traces of trypsin left on the free surface of the native collagen. This trypsin will then act on the collagen, which is denatured in the heat treatment. This possibility was discounted by Thaureaux, since precautions were taken to remove trypsin completely. From Bergmann's work (8) this is known to be very difficult, because traces of trypsin are tenaciously held on free valency sites of the protein. This easy solubilization of the native collagen, after it has undergone tryptic pretreatment, evidently indicates that it is modified profoundly by trypsin in some other way than by digestion.

By pretreatment of pelt with solutions of trypsin, it was found (21) that the hide substrate, subsequently freed from trypsin and then shrunk in water at 70°C., is easily and to a great extent made soluble in water of 70°C. Thus, by treating calfskin pelt for 24 hours at 37°C. and pH 7.6 with a solution of 1 % trypsin (40,000 Fuld-Gross units), the resulting pelt, thoroughly washed to removed trypsin, was dissolved to about 90 % by treatment in water of 70°C. for 2 hours. Only about 10 % of the collagen which had been treated in an identical manner with heat-inactivated trypsin was dissolved.

Nevertheless the crucial point is the presence of trypsin in the treated pelt and the difficulty of inactivating any residual trypsin without interfering with the collagen. Further experiments have yielded results indicating a labilization of the collagen by the tryptic pretreatment, although no proof has yet been offered.

In a subsequent investigation, Neuman and Tytell (13) found that alkali and dodecyl sulfate practically eliminate the solubilization effect. This is ascribed to the effect of the remaining traces of trypsin on the collagen, on its denaturation in the hot-water treatment. In a recent paper, Eling and Lollar (22) report on the effect of bating (trypsin and other proteolytic enzymes) on collagen, particularly the alteration of the hydroxyproline content of the bated collagen. They followed the procedure by a hydroxyproline assay, and their results indicated that in the enzymatic treatment of collagen a fraction rich in hydroxyproline was removed. They found that the extensively bated collagen showed a trend toward a lower collagen purity from the hydroxyproline assay values. Those observations are consistent with the interpretation that the collagen is being modified, with the removal of a hydroxyproline-containing component. As was pointed out in another connection, the possibility that trypsin treatment may result in the hydrolysis of some small polypeptides from the huge collagen molecule should be seriously considered. It would be a reaction similar to that of the formation of plakalbumin. The amount of nitrogen passing into the solution at such a slight hydrolysis of native collagen would be difficult to detect and estimate. Nevertheless, in spite of the analytical findings that trypsin has no effect on collagen, such a modification of collagen by the splitting off of some polypeptide fractions may profoundly alter its properties. This problem deserves careful study.

Before leaving the problem of proteolysis, the reaction of keratin to trypsin merits a brief mention. Keratin, in the form of hair and wool, resists the action of trypsin and similar proteinases, probably because of the exceedingly stable sulfur bridge and the presence of the main part of the keto-imide groups in the compensated state. By prolonged swelling of wool, its tryptic resistance is lowered, and by breaking up the —S—S crosslink, the resulting products, the keratoses, are easily split by trypsin. The breaking of the cystine crosslinks of keratin is a vital factor for the clothes moth larva, as has been demonstrated by Linderstrøm-Lang and Duspiva (23) in their brilliant histochemical researches on the intestinal content of the larva of *Tineola biselliella*, the common clothes moth. The intestinal secretion contains a proteinase, and a reductase in a rather alkaline solution (pH 9 to 10). The reductase and the hydroxyl ions are jointly able to convert the cystine into cysteine, and the labilized keratins, the keratoses, are then easily split by the proteinase. The breakdown products furnish the food for the larva.

3. Effects on Tanned Collagen (Leather)

The behavior of leather toward proteinases, especially trypsin, has many interesting aspects. Leather consists of collagen in irreversible combination with certain substances of quite different chemical composition, collectively classified as tanning agents. Leather formation leads to increased stability of the protein lattice and a higher degree of organization of collagen. As already mentioned, information concerning the action of trypsin on collagen in the tanned state should be of practical value in as much as the action of proteinases is one of the main reactions in putrefaction. It may also serve as a method of evaluating leather. The problem also has wide theoretical ramifications, and it is expected to provide information on the nature of tanning processes and the behavior of proteins generally.

The action of trypsin on tanned hide powder—the tanning agents being basic chromium sulfate, formaldehyde, quinone, and tannic acid—was first studied by Thomas and Seymour-Jones (24) in the early 1920's. Experi-

mentally tanned leathers and commercial leathers were investigated by
Bergmann and Thiele (25), who studied their stability to trypsin. Great
advances have since been made in our knowledge of proteins and the pro
teinases and mechanism of tannages, and many details which were ther
puzzling, or even not recognized are now explained, or at least better known
The findings of these early investigators will be discussed in connection
with the more recent research.

In view of the fact that hide powder is not a suitable agent for investi
gation of proteinase action, being a mixture of native and heat-denatured
collagen, and further that limed skin tissue (pelt) used in the isoelectric
state is too resistant, the use of fishskin offers many advantages (26). The
degree of digestion of fish collagen is considerably greater than that of
bovine pelt (limed skin), which makes any effect of the tanning agent in
diminishing the hydrolysis of collagen more specific and more easily meas
ured and expressed. Thus, for testing the effect of the most important tan
nages on the tryptic resistance of collagen in combination with such agents
fishskin collagen enables a wider and more satisfactory recording of tanning
efficiency than does the bovine type of collagen. In view of the lower hydro
thermal stability of fishskin, however, the temperature of digestion, the
length of treatment, and the alkalinity of the bath must be adjusted.

Skins of cod (*Gadus morrhua*) with a T_s of about 40°C. and skins of eel
(*Anguilla vulgaris*), T_s 57°C., have been employed in such investigations
both in the natural state, after mechanical cleaning, and after a short
liming, followed by deliming and extraction of the fat in the case of the
eel skin. The digestions of the skin in the untanned and tanned condition
were carried out by treating portions equal to 1.0 g. of collagen in 50 ml
of 0.2% solution of trypsin (40,000 Fuld-Gross units), buffered at pH 7.8
with 0.2 g. of calcium carbonate at 25°C. (and 30°C.) for various lengths of
time, up to 20 hours. Blanks were run with heat-inactivated trypsin for
each series. This gives the hydrothermal digestion. Time of digestion was
20 hours. Table 34 gives some data on the composition, the change in T_s
and the degree of thermal and tryptic digestion of eel skin.

In experiments of this kind, it is imperative to carry out the treatment
under conditions not detrimental to the leather. Thus, by selecting pH
values too high for tryptic digestion, detanning of vegetable and chrome
tanned leather as well as of the syntan leather will be induced. The pH
should be about 7. The degree and the rate of digestion of the substrate car
obviously be controlled by varying the time, the temperature, and the pH
value of the treatment.

By chrome tanning collagen is made completely resistant to tryptic hy
drolysis. Tanning collagen by means of mimosa extract to an average degree
and by formaldehyde causes it to resist the hydrolytic action of trypsin

TABLE 34 (26)

THE EFFECT OF TANNING OF COLLAGEN ON ITS TRYPTIC RESISTANCE

Collagen Treated with:	Tanning Agent. Fixed by Collagen, %	ΔT_s	Collagen Digested, %		
			Total	Hydro-thermal	Tryptic
one (blank)	0	0	19	4	15
6% acid chromium sulfate, 0.8 equiv./l. Cr	8.8(Cr_2O_3)	+42	0	0	0
6% acid chromium chloride, 0.8 equiv./l. Cr	6.4(Cr_2O_3)	+34	0	0	0
ulfito-chromium sulfate (3Na_2SO_3:1Cr_2O_3) 0.8 equiv./l. Cr	8.5(Cr_2O_3)	+41	1	0	1
Iimosa extract, pH 4.5	57	+23	3	1	2
annic acid, pH 3.0	65	+14	15	4	11
umac extract	32	+16	8	2	6
yntan (condensed phenolsulfonic acid)	31	+4	12	1	11
yntan (condensed naphthalene-sulfonic acid)	31	0	24	5	19
ignosulfonic acid	37	0	54	29	25
ormaldehyde, pH 8	1.5	+30	4	0	4

Condensed tannins are far better stabilizers with respect to proteinase resistance than the hydrolyzable type, as is evident from the figures. The same tendency is shown with regard to the T_s of leather tanned by the two groups of tannins. The syntan based on phenol, containing sulfonic acid groups, gives some degree of protection to collagen. This is not the case with the corresponding syntan based on naphthalene, and still less with the lignosulfonic acids. They show a tendency to decrease the ordinary stability of collagen. On the whole, it appears that those agents which are multifunctional and possess the property of functioning as crosslinking agents impart increased stability of collagen toward trypsin by their combination with the hide protein. Tryptic resistance and increased hydro-hermal stability are phenomena indicating the same trend of the tanning effect in the great majority of cases (27).

No complications resulting from the slight alkalinity (pH 8) of the digestion bath, such as hydrolysis and removal of tanning agents, and no secondary action of the fixed tanning agents on the trypsin, such as consequent poisoning action, were found in the specimens tanned by means of chrome and formaldehyde (26). However, the vegetable-tanned stock was partly stripped of the tanning agent. By examination of the residual solutions of the digest from the vegetable-tanned leather, losses in the strength of the trypsin amounting to 60 to 80% of the original strength were estimated (26). Hence, in testing vegetable-tanned leather, this poisoning of the enzyme by the liberated tannins would tend to give too low values of the degree of the tryptic digestion. The stability shown by chrome- and formaldehyde-tanned collagen is not connected with any inactivation of trypsin by these tanning agents (26).

Thomas and Seymour-Jones (24) were particularly impressed by the finding that hide powder tanned with basic chromium sulfate was practically inert toward trypsin. The hide powder tanned with quinone possessed a marked stability, and formaldehyde tannage also improved the resistance of collagen to trypsin. Vegetable tannins, represented in this instance by tannic acid, were not very effective stabilizers. As mentioned earlier, the hydrolyzable tannins, to which class tannic acid belongs, are less effective than the condensed type of tannins.

In order to explain the unique effect of chromium salts, these authors drew attention to the possibility that peptide groups are involved in chrome fixation. From our present knowledge of the structure of fibrous proteins and the mechanism of chrome tanning, an explanation of tryptic resistance does not require the assumption of direct inactivation of peptide groups by the tanning agent. It seems that a certain stability of the protein lattice and an orderly arrangement of protein chains allowing interchain compensation of peptide bonds are the main reasons for the tryptic resistance of the native collagen. By incorporation of a small number of strong crosslinks in the form of the tanning agent into the lattice, the collagen chains are riveted together, thus providing an adequate explanation of the stabilization imparted to collagen. The effect of formaldehyde, quinone, and vegetable tannins on the tryptic resistance of collagen may be conceived on a similar principle. The lowered tryptic resistance of collagen in combination with the naphthalene and lignosulfonic acids is probably due to the weakly developed crosslinking and the impaired hydrothermal stability resulting from their interaction with collagen (26, 27).

In a recent paper, Lennox and Forss (28) have reported their investigations of the stability of various leathers to papain. These results are in line with the discussion given above. They used solutions of 1% papain made 3 M in urea and 0.1 M in sodium bisulfite for activating the papain in the digestion at temperatures of 50° and 35°C. The use of such a highly hydrotropic agent as urea in a rather concentrated solution, and such a powerful complexing agent as bisulfite, is open to serious criticism, since both of these agents interfere with the two main classes of tanning agents. Urea is a powerful detanning agent for vegetable-tanned leather and will as a denaturant detrimentally affect the leather characteristics, even on short digestion at 50°C. (29). The bisulfite anion interacts with the chromium complexes of the chrome leather, and the rather large digestion of chrome leather (12% of the original weight) found by the Australian workers is probably due mainly to alterations in the chromium complexes incurred during digestion. Their series were apparently also performed without controls, with solutions containing inactivated papain. From the analytical point of view, the use of concentrated solutions of urea makes the regular Kjeldahl method inapplicable, and the difficulty of removing sorbed urea from the substrate is likely to introduce an error in the weight of the remaining substrate, as the extent of digestion is obtained by the difference in weight of the original substrate and the digested substrate. The amount of tanning agent which goes into the solution of the digest, which in itself has nothing to do with the tryptic resistance, will be included in the figure. It seems that the amount of nitrogenous matter gone into solution should be used as a measure of the extent of hydrolysis of collagen, expressed as the percentage of the original nitrogen.

REFERENCES

1. Crook, E. M., J. Soc. Leather Trades Chem. **35**, 257 (1951).
2. Bergmann, M., Advances in Enzymol. **2**, 49 (1942).
3. Neurath, H., and Schwert, G. W., Chem. Revs. **46**, 69 (1950).
4. Bergmann, M., and Fruton, J. S., J. Biol. Chem. **117**, 189 (1937); **118**, 405 (1937).
5. Anderson, H., J. Intern. Soc. Leather Trades Chem. **29**, 209 (1945).
5a. Linderstrøm-Lang, K., Cold Spring Harbor Symposia Quant. Biol. **14**, 117 (1950); Linderstrøm-Lang, K., Hotchkiss, R. D., and Johanson, G., Nature **142**, 996 (1938).
5b. Linderstrøm-Lang, K., and Ottesen, M., Nature **159**, 807 (1947); Arch. Biochem. **19**, 340 (1948); Compt. rend. lab. trav. Carlsberg **26**, 403, 443 (1949); **27**, 1 (1949).
5c. Lundgren, H. P., J. Biol. Chem. **138**, 293 (1941); Williams, J. W., and Lundgren, H. P., J. Phys. Chem. **43**, 989 (1939).
6. Smith, E. L., J. Biol. Chem. **173**, 553 (1948); **176**, 9 (1948); Ann. Rev. Biochem. **18**, 35 (1949); Proc. Natl. Acad. Sci. U.S. **35**, 80 (1949); Smith, E. L., and Bergmann, M., J. Biol. Chem. **153**, 627 (1944); Smith, E. L., and Lumrey, R., Cold Spring Harbor Symposia Quant. Biol. **14**, 168 (1949); Hanson, H. T., and Smith, E. L., J. Biol. Chem. **175**, 833 (1948); 789 (1949); Johnson, N. J., Johnson, G. H., and Peterson, W. H., ibid. **116**, 515 (1936).
7. Bergmann, M., and Fruton, J. S., J. Biol. Chem. **127**, 627, 643 (1939); **118**, 405 (1937); Bergmann, M., Fruton, J. S., and Fraenkel-Conrat, H., ibid. **119**, 35 (1937).
8. Bergmann, M., Pojarlieff, G., and Thiele, H., Collegium **1933**, 581.
9. Grassmann, W., Janicki, J., and Schneider, F., in "Stiasny Festschrift," p. 74. Roether, Darmstadt, 1937.
10. Sizer, I. W., Enzymologia **13**, 288 (1949).
11. Northrop, J. H., J. Gen. Physiol. **13**, 739, 767 (1930).
11a. Banga, I., and Balo, J., Nature **164**, 491 (1949); **171**, 44 (1953); cf. Hall, D. A., Reed, R., and Tunbridge, R. E., Nature **170**, 264 (1952).
12. Maschmann, E., Biochem. Z. **297**, 284 (1938); Macfarlane, R. G., and MacLennan,

J. D., *Lancet* **249**, 1328 (1945); Oakley, C. L., Warrack, H., and van Heyningen, W. E., *J. Pathol. Bacteriol.* **58**, 229 (1946).

12a. Jennison, M. W., *J. Bacteriol.* **50**, 369 (1945); **54**, 55 (1947).

13. Neuman, R. E., and Tytell, A. A., *Proc. Soc. Exptl. Biol. Med.* **73**, 409 (1950).

14. Robb-Smith, A. H. T., *in* "Nature and Structure of Collagen" (J. T. Randall, ed.), pp. 14–26. Butterworths, London, 1953.

15. Bergmann, M., and Fruton, J. S., *J. Biol. Chem.* **117**, 189 (1937); *Science* **83**, 306 (1936).

16. Grassmann, W., Dyckerhoff, H., and von Schoenbeck, O., *Ber.* **62**, 1307 (1929).

17. Sizer, I. W., *Enzymologia* **13**, 293 (1949).

18. Gustavson, K. H., *Svensk Kem. Tidskr.* **54**, 74 (1942).

19. See Fauré-Fremiet, E., "Proprietes physique des Scleroproteines," Hermann, Paris, 1944; Fauré-Fremiet, E., and Cougny, A., *Bull. muséum natl. hist. nat.* (*Paris*) **9**, 188 (1937); Cherbuliez, E., Jeannerat, J., and Meyer, K. H., *Z. physiol. Chem.* **255**, 241 (1938).

20. Thaureaux, J., *Bull. soc. chim. biol.* **27**, 493 (1945).

21. Gustavson, K. H., *J. Intern. Soc. Leather Trades Chem.* **31**, 362 (1947); *J. Am. Leather Chem. Assoc.*, **44**, 392 (1949).

22. Eling, R., and Lollar, R. M., *J. Am. Leather Chem. Assoc.* **48**, 135 (1953).

23. Linderstrøm-Lang, K., and Duspiva, F., *Z. physiol. Chem.* **237**, 131 (1935).

24. Thomas, A. W., and Seymour-Jones, F. L., *Ind. Eng. Chem.* **16**, 157 (1924).

25. Thiele, H., Dissertation, Dresden, pp. 47–53, 1933; see also ref. 8.

26. Gustavson, K. H., *Svensk Kem. Tidskr.* **55**, 249 (1943).

27. Gustavson, K. H., *J. Intern. Soc. Leather Trades Chem.* **21**, 4 (1937).

28. Lennox, F. G., and Forss, H. M., *J. Soc. Leather Trades Chem* **36**, 322 (1952).

29. Gustavson, K. H., *J. Am. Leather Chem. Assoc.* **42**, 13 (1947).

CHAPTER 12

Unhairing and Gelatin

1. Unhairing and Keratolysis

a. Introduction

The problem of unhairing actually lies outside the scope of this book. However, in view of the importance of this process in leather manufacture, a brief outline of the main theoretical principles will be given.

The removal of hair and epidermal matter from the hide in order to obtain the leather-forming part, the corium, free from non-leather-forming constituents, is accomplished primarily by the liming process, which also brings the unhaired hide, the pelt, into a suitable state for tanning. Some outstanding functions of the alkaline pretreatment (liming) are: activating certain protein groups, plumping the hide by water uptake, "opening up" of fiber bundles, bringing about lateral splitting of the individual fibers, saponifying fats, and modifying or removing the accessory proteins, such as those present as interfibrillary matter, and reticulin.

Unhairing may be accomplished by means of two fundamentally different reactions: (1) dissolution of the epidermal proteins of the mucous layer, i.e., disintegration of the *stratum mucosum*; (2) destruction of the keratin, i.e., keratolysis.

b. Mild types of unhairing

The importance of the degree of keratinization of the epidermal constituents, from the mucous membrane deep down in the epidermis to the hair at the top, for the unhairing process has not yet been fully realized. Recent publications of Burton and Reed (1) show some emphasis on this type of unhairing, which actually is Nature's own. Hard keratins with cystine bridges are not present in large amounts in the mucous layers. Young keratins, with the sulfur mainly in the sulfhydryl form, are the predominating constituents. The usual keratolytic reactions on the disulfide links therefore do not apply to this type of depilation, which depends on the disintegration of the mucous layer. Hence, it is principally a reaction *not* involving the breaking of primary valency bonds, in contradistinction to keratolysis based on the cleavage of covalent bonds in the keratin molecule. The lucid contributions by Rudall (2) on the behavior of the epidermal proteins, the *epidermin*, illustrate the relationship between the chemical composition and the physicochemical properties of various proteins of the α-type structure present. The epidermin, which can be extracted from the skin by 50% urea solution, contains little sulfur compared to that in the hard keratins of the hair. The lower layers of the *stratum mucosum* show the relative absence of cystine, the sulfur present being mainly in the SH form. By dispergating these proteins, which may be accomplished by a lyotropic agent, the undamaged hair and epidermis can be detached from the corium. Concentrated solutions of urea are fairly effective unhairing agents by virtue of their solubilizing effect on the soft keratins (3). After 2 to 3 days' treatment of calfskin in a 6 *M* solution of urea at 20°C. (covered with toluene), the hair commenced to slip, the epidermal matter being loosened from the corium by the action of urea. Only about 1% of the corium (collagen) was lost in a treatment lasting 3 to 4 days. This lyotropic unhairing takes advantage of the different chemical compositions of the various strata of the epidermis, attacking the more reactive and soluble proteins forming the boundary layer between the corium and the epidermis.

Kritzinger (4) has stressed the importance of the solvent and dispersive effects of the mild unhairing agents on the globular proteins of the epidermis, demonstrating the depilatory action of 2 *M* solutions of sodium chloride on fresh skins. Even immersion of raw skin in water at a temperature just below the shrinkage temperature of collagen for a short while produced unhairing. The globular proteins are probably synonymous with the mucoids of the epidermis, in the light of Reed's researches (1).

Burton, Reed, and Flint (1) point out that there are considerable amounts of such mucoids present at the junction of the epidermis and the corium. They have also shown that removal of the mucoids by mucolytic enzymes causes unhairing. The mucolytic enzymes, such as pectinases, diastases, and elastase, are much more efficient in removing the interfibrillar substances than the ordinary lime-sulfide depilatories. These cementing substances contain hyaluronic acid and chondroitin sulfate as the principal nonproteinous constituents, which also may be responsible for the cohesion of the fibers, functioning as weak crosslinking agents. In the afore-mentioned experiments of Reed, the mucolytic enzymes unhaired fresh calfskins in 3 days. The hair was not damaged in this mild process, and the epidermis was detached in the form of continuous sheets.

The depilatory enzymes, which are the active agents in the sweating method of unhairing, an obsolete method still used on sheepskin, have had only limited use for certain types of light skins. The superiority of the liming method lies primarily in the conditioning effect of the calcium hydroxide on the collagen, in addition to its economy, safety, simplicity, and uniformity of action. In a clarifying investigation of the depilation of sheepskins with enzymes, Gillespie (4a) points out that there are apparently a number of distinct depilatory enzymes. First, there are those of *Aspergillus parasiticus* and some related molds which require a reducing agent and activation by zinc salts. A second group includes the enzymes of *A. oryzae*, which are familiar from the patent literature. They are highly effective without any activation but may be further activated by reducing agents. Finally, the enzymes of the pig pancreas are inactivated by reducing agents. Gillespie found that proteases and carbohydrases, including pectinases and diastases, are not mucolytic. They are devoid of depilatory power. He believes that contamination of the enzyme preparations mentioned with bacteria may have been responsible for the unhairing noted by Reed and his co-workers.

c. Keratolysis

In the regular keratolytic process employed in modern methods of unhairing skins and hides, the hide is treated in a saturated solution of calcium hydroxide, containing a large excess of lime and a small amount of a specific depilatory, generally sodium sulfide or hydrosulfide. Within a few hours or days, according to the degree to which the lime is sharpened with the depilatory, the hair roots are loosened or the hair is destroyed ("pulping"), and unhairing is thus accomplished.

Loosening of the hair is due to the chemical action of the OH and SH ions of the lime liquor on the hair root or the hair. The hair structure is weakened, and finally it disintegrates. The unhairing is due to the breakdown of the disulfide link of the amino acid cystine, which is characteristic of the keratins in wool and hair. This link is built into two polypeptide chains, forming a stabilizing crosslink between them:

$$\begin{array}{ccc} \diagup & & \diagdown \\ CO & & HN \\ \diagdown & & \diagup \\ \multicolumn{3}{c}{HC \cdot CH_2 \cdot S \cdot S \cdot CH_2 \cdot CH} \\ \diagup & & \diagdown \\ NH & & OC \\ \diagdown & & \diagup \end{array}$$

It was established by Stiasny (5), in the early part of this century, that both OH and SH ions are necessary for unhairing to occur. From the brilliant researches of Merrill (6) and the provocative ideas of Marriott (7), in his comprehensive investigations of the liming process, it was concluded that unhairing involves the reduction of the disulfide link. An important advance in our conception of keratolysis was thus recorded, which was in fact a remarkable concept at that time, when the role that cross-

linking plays in the stability of proteins was unknown. The idea of keratolysis as a reaction due to breaking of a covalent crosslink between protein
chains was hence a noteworthy event in protein chemistry. Merrill (6)
showed that a reducing agent such as stannous chloride used for pretreating
hide will catalyze the unhairing of hide subsequently treated in an alkaline
solution. The depilatory action of a great number of organic sulfur compounds has been extensively investigated by Turley and Windus (8) in a
series of important papers. In the original concept of unhairing, the first
reaction was thought to be a reduction of the —S—S— link to two SH—
groups. The freed keratin chains should then disintegrate by the action of
OH ions, resulting in the removal of the hair. However, further study of the
keratolytic reaction indicated that the first reaction involved in unhairing
is the breaking of the disulfide crosslink by the action of hydroxyl ions, and
that the action of the depilator depends on its ability to prevent the re-
formation of the —S—S— bridge or the formation of new crosslinks which
tend to stabilize the keratin molecule (9). The breaking of the disulfide
crosslink in alkaline solution is a straight hydrolysis, catalyzed by OH ions,
leading to the formation of a thiol and a sulfenic acid group (10):

$$\diagup\!\!\!\diagdown CH \cdot CH_2 \cdot S \cdot S \cdot CH_2 \cdot CH \diagup\!\!\!\diagdown \xrightarrow{\ H_2O\ } \diagup\!\!\!\diagdown CH \cdot CH_2 SOH + HS \cdot CH_2 \cdot CH \diagup\!\!\!\diagdown$$

Then the specific action of the unhairing agent enters. If only hydroxyl ions
are present, it is thought that the active groups formed by the splitting of
the —S—S— bond react further, with formation of new crosslinks between
adjacent protein chains. Among the many reaction mechanisms proposed,
experimental evidence has been given for the formation of the —$CH_2 \cdot S \cdot$
CH_2— link (in lanthionine). Cuthbertson and Phillips (11) have shown
that 0.38 N barium hydroxide solution will convert about half of the disulfide links into lanthionine in less than 1 hour's time at room temperature.
Potassium cyanide in neutral solution can convert all the cystine of wool
to lanthionine. It appears that the lanthionine formation is one of the
principal reactions leading to new crosslinks, although the mechanism of
its formation is still not settled. The formation of such crosslinks in alkali
treated hair would explain the immunization reaction, i.e., the fact that
skin soaked in alkaline solution will not readily unhair in the subsequent
unhairing solution (12). Lime solution is more effective than sodium hydroxide solution of corresponding pH in producing this effect. It has been
suggested by McKay (13) that the reactions occurring when hair is immersed in a solution of calcium hydroxide in the absence of sulfide are as
follows.

The first step of the hydrolysis of the disulfide link is given above. This is followed by the formation of metallic links through calcium: $CH \cdot CH_2 \cdot S \cdot O \cdot Ca \cdot S \cdot CH_2 \cdot CH$. The vital role played by the divalent metal was demonstrated by McKay. Hairs were immersed in a solution of 0.01 N sodium hydroxide and then in a solution of the same sodium hydroxide made 0.01 M in $CaCl_2$. The hair was not immunized in the solution of 0.02 M calcium hydroxide. On the other hand, hair treated in the sodium hydroxide solution containing calcium was immunized. It was shown that a certain minimum alkalinity is necessary for the immunization reaction (not reached by 0.02 M $Ca(OH)_2$). In the presence of the necessary degree of alkalinity, very small concentrations of divalent ions are able to immunize hair. In other words, provided that conditions are favorable for the formation of bridges, very few such crosslinks are required to effect immunization. This is somewhat similar to the effect of bridging collagen chains in tanning. The very stable state of the combination of calcium with keratin is shown by the fact that the thoroughly washed immunized hair, after boiling in several changes of decinormal hydrochloric acid, still contained calcium which probably is present in an un-ionized form. It has been found that the calcium and magnesium ions are able to function as crosslinks between protein molecules, thereby increasing their molecular weights (14).

As already mentioned, the role of the depilator is considered to prevent the secondary formation of crosslinks by its interaction with the sulfenic acid group formed in the initial hydroxyl-governed cleavage of the —S—S— link, which is a straight hydrolytic reaction. Many reducing agents possess this property, the most important technically being the alkali sulfides, primarily sodium sulfide (hydrosulfide). Other agents used or proposed are cyanides (7, 15), salts of thioglycolic acid (16) (the active constituent of some cold permanent wave preparations), sulfites, and aliphatic amines (17). The reaction mechanisms of many of these agents have been postulated, but they lack the necessary experimental foundation.

In summary, it can be said that keratolysis consists in two reactions: (1) hydrolysis of the disulfide link and (2) inactivation of the groups freed in the first reaction. This depends on the hydroxyl ion concentration, and the second step on the concentration of the unhairing agent (in the case of sodium sulfide, on the concentration of the SH ions).

In spite of the marked progress in our knowledge of the nature of depilation and keratolysis during the last two decades, many details of these difficult problems still await a satisfactory explanation.

d. Effects on collagen

The effect of lime, and of alkali generally, on collagen has been discussed in earlier chapters, and also the effect of such solutions on hide during the liming process. Therefore, a brief summary will suffice here. In addition to the purely chemical changes, such as deamidation and the minor destruction of the arginine residue, with possible cleavage of some peptide bonds, yielding polypeptides to the solution, one important function of the liming process should be mentioned. That is the "opening up" of the fiber structure, making it accessible and permeable to large molecules. This process may involve the breaking of crosslinks in the form of chondroitin sulfate (18). Another important reaction is the activation of ionic groups by the breaking up of the salt links through hydrolysis of the charged amino groups by the hydroxyl ions, which on prolonged liming (swelling) partly involves irreversible changes. Indirectly, interchain links of the hydrogen bond type are disrupted by the swelling. The increase in the number of carboxylic groups resulting from the deamidation process connotes greater ionic reactivity. This is proved by the fact that the binding capacity of collagen for electrolytes and tanning agents, both chromium salts and vegetable tannins, is increased. This was first demonstrated and conceived as ionic and coordinate reactions by Widen and the author in the early 1920's (19). The reactivity of collagen is further favored by the physical alterations in the hide caused by the liming, and also by chemical changes in the nonionic protein groups, since the swelling of hide leads to the rupture of some of the coordinate (hydrogen) bonds between adjacent protein chains (lowered cohesion of the hide) (19). These hydrogen bonds are not completely re-formed in the subsequent deliming process, which reduces the swelling by establishing neutral reaction of the hide. The peptide bond is therefore made more accessible to various agents.

2. The Conversion of Collagen into Gelatin, and Its Molecular Structure

a. Isoelectric points

Gelatin is prepared by hydrolytic degradation of collagen, mainly derived from bovine skin tissue. The stock is usually given a thorough soaking in alkali (lime). It is then neutralized and extracted with water at 60°C. A less common method consists in treatment with acid at pH 3 to 3.5, followed by extraction of the stock, mainly pigskin. The two types of gelatin obtained—ordinary alkali-treated gelatin, and acid-extracted gelatin, a specialty of limited use—possess different isoelectric points. The former is isoelectric at pH 4.7, the point of the classical gelatin; the latter at pH about 9. As is evident from the earlier discussion of the effect of alkali on the chemical constitution of collagen, with regard to deamidation and breakdown of the arginine residue, the location of the isoelectric point of limed gelatin at lower pH values is exactly what would be expected. The original isoelectric point of native collagen is not appreciably changed by the mild acid pretreatment. From the historical point of view it is of interest to point out that the first suggestion that native collagen and alkali-treated (limed) collagen have different isoelectric points was made by the investigators of gelatin. Kraemer should be given credit for stating the fact that, according to their previous history, gelatins are isoelectric at pH about 5 or 8; the former value is characteristic of regular calfskin gelatin (limed), and the higher value of acid-pretreated pigskin gelatin (20). Briefer and Cohen (21) carried the work further. They used the opalescence method for location of the isoelectric point; the technique already employed by Kraemer and by Kraemer and Dexter (22). These workers state that there are two types of gelatin, with isoelectric points at pH 4.7 and 8, the type produced depending on the method of preparation.

The final answer to this perplexing problem of gelatins with two distinct isoelectric points was given independently by Beek and Soakne (23) and by Highberger (24) in 1938 in their investigations of the effect of liming and alkali treatment of collagen on its isoelectric point. Their explanation is now generally accepted. This outstanding work has been discussed earlier. It should be mentioned that, as far back as 1930, Sheppard and Houck (25) confirmed the fact that alkali-treated and acid-treated pigskins give different types of gelatin. Other papers on this subject indicated that the importance of the method of preparation was gradually being realized. In fact, with reference to their isoelectric state the two types of gelatin are directly related to their collagen precursors, native collagen and limed collagen.

Probably the most convenient and reliable method of estimating the isoionic point of gelatin, due to Ward and his associates (26), consists in passing the gelatin solution through a mixed bed of cationic and anionic exchange resins (Amberlites IR 120 and 400) to remove the salts. The pH value of the filtered solution coincides with the isoionic point, which coincides with the isoelectric point. This method has been very helpful in the preparation of deionized gelatin. Ward found the alkali-processed type of gelatin to be isoelectric at pH 4.85 to 5.1, and the acid-processed pigskin gelatin at pH 9.3.

b. Conversion of collagen to gelatin

An important point in the manufacture of gelatin, particularly for its quality, e.g., gel strength and yield, is the extent and the condition of the lime soak which usually lasts for several weeks. It has been claimed by Küntzel and Koepff (27) that by application of heat before the lime treatment of the gelatin stock, the period of pretreatment can be shortened considerably without impairing the quality of the gelatin produced. The idea goes back to the well-known fact that shrunken (heat-denatured) collagen is more susceptible to alkali than is normal pelt. However, the results of investigations of Ames (28) were in complete disagreement with the claim of Küntzel and Koepff, a very poor grade of gelatin being obtained.

It should also be possible to make use of the lyotropic function of neutral salts, such as calcium chloride, to shorten the period of the lime soak in the degradation of collagen. Küntzel and Koepff (27) found that by the addition of calcium chloride to the liming bath the time of pretreatment could be shortened and the quality of the gelatin improved. After checking these experiments by a series of comprehensive investigations Ames (28) concluded that the claims of Küntzel and Koepff were incorrect. The gelatin obtained was poor in jelly strength and dull in color. What appears to happen to a batch of glue stock in a bath of lime containing large amounts of calcium chloride is that the calcium chloride causes the lime to attack the surface of the skin fibers vigorously, while the center remains unaltered and therefore difficult to extract. According to Ames, better results are obtained by the addition of sodium sulfate to solutions of sodium hydroxide instead of lime for the lengthy soaking of gelatin. It was found that the neutral sulfate depressed the swelling in the soak. The stock was then more accessible to lime, and its penetration facilitated. Washing of the alkali-treated stock caused it to swell greatly. This salt effect is just opposite to that produced by calcium chloride, as recommended by Küntzel and Koepff.

There are three methods of preparing gelatin, each of which is a definite type with a characteristic isoelectric point and nitrogen content. Extraction of stock treated for a long time in alkaline solution results in gelatin with an isoelectric point at pH 4.7. A second type is produced by extracting the precursor in the presence of acid, when the gelatin is isoelectric at pH 8 to 9. The third form is prepared by heating the precursor with water. It gives instable gelatin, which is isoelectric at pH 5 to 6 (28).

In the comprehensive researches of Ames (28) on the preparation of gelatin, the following main points are of interest in this connection. The collagen precursor is brought to swell in the alkaline soak, in which the accessory proteins are removed from collagen. The isoelectric point of collagen moves from the region of pH 8 to pH 5 during the alkali treatment, mainly owing to deamidation. Collagen gradually becomes more susceptible to hydrolysis with hot water. However, alkali brings about only one stage of the transformation, since *heat* is always required to effect the change from collagen into gelatin. The treated collagen shrinks in warm water (60°C.) and then dissolves as gelatin, the rate of dissolution depending on the length of the period of soak. The jelly strength of the gelatin is greatest for shortest time of extraction. For gelatin extracted in the presence of acids, the precursor does not require any soaking beyond what is required for complete penetration of the acid through the material. Provided that the collagen has not received an alkali pretreatment, a gelatin of definite composition and a constant isoelectric point will be obtained. When acid is used to extract partly limed collagen, the gelatin will show a variable nitrogen content and the location of the isoelectric point will be governed by the degree of liming. The readiness with which collagen is converted into gelatin appears to be determined by the rate of extraction and the ability of the gelatin to form firm gels. Optimal values are reached at the same time that the isoelectric point attains its minimum pH. This indicates a certain relationship between loss in ammonia (deamidation) and the rate of conversion.

It appears that salt linkages and hydrogen bonds are too easily broken to account for the transformation of collagen into gelatin (28). In addition to the rupture of the afore-mentioned types of crosslinks, the experimental findings favor the view that in the collagen–gelatin transformation some rather stable crosslinks are broken (28). The following types of bonds are indicated to be involved in the conversion: the hydroxy-keto-imide link; an ester bond, possibly the one formed between the hydroxy and carboxyl groups; and finally a crosslink to which the carboxyl group contributes, with the guanidyl group as a possible partner (28a). In view of the fact that acid-processed gelatin contains the same amount of amide groups as its precursor, native collagen, the amide group is probably not involved to any considerable extent in the conversion of collagen into gelatin.

c. Structure and molecular weight

When collagen is treated in alkaline solutions of pH > 11 salt links are broken quite rapidly. Crosslinks in which amide and guanidyl groups participate are apparently much more difficult to break. There is no indication that peptide bonds are hydrolyzed in a lime soak of reasonable length, since collagen, although swollen, is practically insoluble. Application of heat causes a spatial rearrangement and also cleavage of a few keto-imide links at certain points, resulting in the formation of gelatin. Thus, there are two main stages in the making of gelatin out of collagen: (*1*) the soaking period, with its principal function of breaking certain interchain crosslinks; (*2*) the extraction with heat applied, in which the protein chains are freed and split to some extent. Furthermore, shrinkage with internal re-arrangement of chains is also indicated. It appears safe to conclude that, if both processes are carried out carefully under strict control a substance of definite composition and properties will be the final outcome.

It is generally assumed that, by the hot extraction of presoaked collagen for the dissolution of gelatin the polypeptide chains are separated and broken into shorter chains along their length. Hence, the molecules of gelatin should take on a form similar to that present in heat-denatured collagen. In the investigations of Scatchard and Oncley and their co-workers (29) on gelatin from ossein, the average molecular weight of the degraded gelatin obtained from the parent gelatin by the action of hot water indicated that those bonds which were spaced about 1200 amino acid residues apart on the collagen chains were more easily broken than the others. In the preparation of gelatin, these labile bonds are probably hydrolyzed first, producing a parent molecule of gelatin whose molecular weight is of the order of 110,000. The other bonds are randomly ruptured, at a slower rate, yielding an assortment of gelatin molecules of widely differing lengths, ranging from the parent molecules to polypeptides and amino acids. By controlled degradation, fractions of molecular weight ranging from 15,000 to 45,000 were obtained.

From the ultracentrifugal measurements of Signer and Mosimann (30) on gelatin fractionated by alcohol precipitation in the presence of urea, two fractions were found to have molecular weights of 16,000 to 18,000, showing good homogeneity. For the fractions of lowest solubilities, the molecular weight was of the order of 90,000 and 150,000. Pouradier (31) showed a value of 64,000 for the gelatin in his investigations. Indications point to molecular weights as high as 100,000 to 150,000 for high-grade gelatins. The larger molecules are neither fully extended peptide chains, nor compact spherical molecules, nor randomly coiled chains.

If the parent molecule of gelatin is a compact ellipsoid of revolution, its axial ratio is about 47. For the parent molecule with a molecular weight of 110,000, the dimensions calculated for an elongated ellipsoid were 800 Å. in length and 17 Å. in width (29). On the other hand, if the molecule has the form of a coiled chain, the coiling will not be at random but will extend largely in one direction. Thus, gelatin molecules are probably highly elongated and of widely differing lengths. It seems possible that they associate by means of van der Waals forces or weaker types of hydrogen bonds to gels (32). Many of the properties of gels can be explained on the basis of a network structure formed by the junction of the elongated molecules at widely separated sites of attraction. The gel-forming bonds are probably broken by heat. The details of the association equilibrium and the chemical nature of the bonds are still uncertain. However, the fact that lyotropic agents, such as concentrated solutions of urea and alkali metal thiocyanates, inhibit the gel formation favors the view that hydrogen bonds, probably located at the peptide bonds mainly, are the main forces responsible for gel formation. This explanation was first advanced by Meyer (33). Robinson (34, 35) has found that lithium bromide and iodide prevent gel formation also, noting further that these salts of a strongly lyotropic nature prevent the change in specific optical rotation which occurs during gel formation (mutarotation).

The fractionation of gelatin into portions of reasonably uniform molecular weight is a necessary step in the estimation of the molecular weight and its fractional distribution. Two methods are mainly used. In the first, a coacervate of gelatin is obtained by adding ethanol to a gelatin solution. The coacervate contains the less soluble portions of the gelatin. This method has been developed by Pouradier and Venet (31) and used in their comprehensive studies of gelatin. It is noteworthy that gelatins with identical isoelectric point and similar molecular weight may differ considerably in the concentration of ethanol required for flocculation, which indicates that there is no direct connection between the molecular weight of gelatin and its tendency for flocculation. The second method, which was devised by Ward and his associates (35a), is based on the findings of Pankhurst (35b) that complexes of definite composition are formed between gelatin and sodium dodecyl sulfate, or similar detergents. Pankhurst suggested that the dodecyl anion is attached to the cationic protein group by means of the sulfate group (ionic valency) and further stabilized by van der Waals forces on the keto-imide group. This orientation of the detergent results in a gelatin molecule with a hydrophobic surface layer, which is of the hydrocarbon type. By addition of NaCl, in amounts yielding 0.4 to 1.0 M solution, successive fractionation of the solution is obtained. The gelatin in the coacervate formed is separated from the dodecyl sulfate by precipitation from 2:1 acetone–water, in which the sulfate is soluble. This method gives nearly the theoretical yield and has proved extremely useful for preparation of distinct fractions of gelatin. Pouradier and his coworkers have shown that the nitrogen content, the isoelectric point, and the acid-binding capacity do not vary appreciably from fraction to fraction for a single gelatin. The reason is probably that the chains of low molecular weight are merely shorter fragments of chains similar to those from which the large fragments are derived. These facts are in harmony with the view that, in forming gelatin, the collagen chains are cleaved at certain weak links, which are common in gelatin itself and break during further hydrolysis. Additional support of this view is supplied by the finding (35a) that the same N-terminal groups are found in the low- and the high-molecular fractions.

d. The sol and gel states

The viscosity of gelatin solutions and the rigidity of the gels are highly temperature-dependent. Above 35°C., the gelatin solutions show normal flow and the viscosity may be satisfactorily measured in the pH region in the vicinity of the isoelectric point. Below 20°C., gelatin exists in the gel form. Between these two temperatures, the gelatin solution may exist as a gel, as a visco-elastic liquid, or as a liquid showing anomalous viscosity, depending on the temperature and the thermal history.

Gelatin solutions of temperatures over 35°C. probably contain discrete molecules. In very concentrated solutions, the molecules may interfere with each other, but no permanent linking is set up. For the formation of the three-dimensional network of the gel, intermolecular forces are necessary, strong enough to maintain the rigidity, hydrogen bonds probably being the dominant type.

The viscosity of fractions of gelatin, in solution of 5 % strength and at 40°C., is a function of the dilute solution viscosity, irrespective of the isoelectric point of the gelatin. This proves the absence of aggregates in these conditions. No such relationship holds between the rigidities of the fractions and the dilute solution viscosity, even for gelatins with the same isoelectric point. Ward (35a) points out that some structural feature of the gelatin molecule—at present unknown—is involved in gel formation, and that for undegraded gelatin it is more important than the molecular weight.

By the researches on the fundamental properties of gelatin, carried out by Ward and his associates at the British Gelatine and Glue Research Association, our knowledge of the nature, behavior, and properties of gelatin has been greatly extended. It is evident from these researches that many of the fundamental properties of gelatin sols and gels are independent of the molecular weight of the gelatin. Thus, for instance, the rigidity of fractions of gelatin gels at 0 to 10°C. is independent of the reduced viscosity and hence of the molecular weight. At higher temperatures or at low concentration, the molecular weight enters as an additional factor.

It has been shown by the Ward group (35a) and the Pouradier team that the melting point of gels from fractions of different gelatins does not depend only on their molecular weight or reduced viscosity. Another property which is not controlled by the molecular weight and not directly related to differences in the isoelectric state of the gelatin is the threshold concentration of ethanol, at which turbidity of the gelatin solution appears. As to the stress relaxation of gelatin gels, measurements of the dynamic and static moduli demonstrate the absence of relaxation times from 10^{-3} to 10^2 seconds, since the two moduli are identical. The instantaneous rigidity is not changed by the relaxation process. Probably the gelatin molecules detach themselves from stressed positions and reattach themselves in an unstressed position. The new bonds formed should then be of the same type as those present in the original gelatin. These findings support the thesis that the gelatin gel does not form a static system but a dynamic one, even in the absence of stress, solution and redeposition occurring steadily. The increase of the rigidity on keeping (aging) probably involves such re-arrangements.

e. Configuration of the gelatin molecule in the sol and gel states

In the discussion of the configuration of collagen, it was shown that in ordinary collagen the hydrogen bonds are formed between the protein chains mainly, whereas in thermally contracted collagen the hydrogen bonds are visualized as intrachain links. It has also been shown that some degree of reversibility between the two forms is indicated on stretching of the denatured and shrunk collagen fiber. It is interesting to find that gelatin gels show thermal shrinkage also (36). In the last few years, the problem of the configuration of gelatin in the gel and the sol state has been investigated by Robinson (35, 37), from the point of view of the α-β transformation concept of Ambrose and Elliott, which already has been discussed.

Robinson and Bott (35) found that films of gelatin prepared by hot evaporation are in a different form from those prepared through the intermediate gel state. Since cold-evaporated gelatin is, according to X-ray evidence, in the collagen type of fold, it is evident that hot-evaporated gelatin is in a different fold, probably one in which the hydrogen bonds are *intra*molecular. Hot-evaporated gelatin would thus form a less rigid film than cold-evaporated gelatin which contains *inter*molecular hydrogen bonds and is thus able to form stable films.

Robinson (37) further showed that Smith's theory (38) of gelatin existing in two forms, the sol and the gel states, with a melting point at approximately 35°C., is principally valid. Smith's concept of the interconversion of the two forms was suggested as an explanation of the mutarotation of gelatin. It played a considerable role in Wilson's early discussion of the two isoelectric points of gelatin and collagen and also in the theorization on the mechanism of vegetable tannage. Smith found that at temperatures above 35°C. the specific rotation of gelatin remains constant (the sol form), but on cooling, the gel state with very large specific rotation is formed. Robinson's findings fully support the concept of Smith, since the mutarotation can be correlated with the data from the spectra and the dichroism of the polarized infrared light, which disclose the different configurations of the polypeptide chains of the sol and gel forms.

Solutions of gelatin of 5% strength were evaporated at 55°C. and at 18°C. Conditions of evaporation were chosen that would give films of suitable thickness for determination of their specific rotation and infrared dichroism. Cold-evaporated gelatin gives the collagen diagram, distinctly different from the α and β configurations, and, when suitably oriented, the infrared dichroism characteristic for collagen.

From data on the specific rotation and from the infrared absorption spectra, Robinson (37) concluded that gelatin in aqueous solution exists at temperatures $>35°C$. as single molecules in a configuration which cannot form interchain hydrogen bonds in solution. At lower temperatures the polypeptide chain acquires a configuration which can form interchain hydrogen bonds.

The hot-evaporated film showed no infrared dichroism at 3330 cm.$^{-1}$, which is observed with collagen and cold-evaporated gelatin film (for the NH-stretching frequency). The specific rotation was $-128°$. The corresponding cold-evaporated film showed the 3330-cm.$^{-1}$ NH-stretching frequency characteristic for the collagen fold, and a specific rotation of $-262°$. The two forms are interconvertible, differing in the nature of the polypeptide fold. The cold-formed gel is similar to the β form with interchain hydrogen bonds; the hot form corresponds in certain ways to the α form with intrachain hydrogen bonds. This difference in the type of stabilizing bond between gelatin films formed by cold and hot evaporation of gelatin solution also explains Bradbury and Martin's (36) finding that the film of the cold form has greater tensile strength than the film formed from hot solution. This concept of two interconvertible forms of gelatin should also explain the finding of Pinoir and Pouradier (39) that a film of gelatin which has been evaporated at 60°C., when placed in water at 10°C., did not dissolve, but commenced to swell. On the other hand, it dissolved completely at 25°C. By estimating the uniplanar diffusion, Robinson was able to prove that the conversion of the hot-evaporated form to the cold form took place. It should also be mentioned that another factor is involved which has been known from the time of Gerngross and Katz's pioneering work on stretched films of gelatin, i.e., the fact that the cold form is more crystalline than the hot form. However, as Robinson points out, the existence of two forms of gelatin with different chain configurations is the logical explanation of the changes in specific rotation, and particularly for the altered infrared absorption which is common for the crystalline and amorphous regions of the proteins.

By measuring the *intrinsic* viscosity of isoelectric gelatin (P_I 5.1) at 35°C. in gelatin solutions of sufficiently high concentration so that it may function as its own buffer, it is possible to ascertain the contribution of the individual gelatin molecule to the viscosity of the solution for certain ranges of pH and salt concentrations. Stainsby (40) employed this method, which is particularly suited for the study of molecules of aniso-dimensional shape, and obtained data which indicate the following main features. At the isoionic point, the gelatin chain configuration is contracted by the attractive forces between the balanced charges along each molecule (salt links), together with possible weaker internal hydrogen bonding. It is a coiled macromolecule. If the molecule is considered as a rigid ellipsoid, the ratio of length to diameter is about 25. The addition of neutral salts to the isoionic solution reduces the forces between the charged sites of the chain and results in molecular extension. Thus, by the addition of acid or alkali, a net positive or negative charge along the chain is produced. The excess charges repel and cause molecular extension. This explanation is similar to the ideas expressed by Kuhn and Katchalsky (41) concerning the form of simple polyelectrolytes as a function of their pH value. The form of the chains of gelatin, for instance at pH $\cong 4$ with extended chains and at pH 5 with contracted chains, also has a definite effect on the type of crosslink formed by fixation of chromium salts at these pH values, as Pouradier and his co-workers (42) have shown (inter- and intrachain crosslinking, respectively).

f. Photographic gelatin

Only a brief note on the use of gelatin in photographic emulsions will be given (43). Gelatin has several functions, acting (1) as a protective colloid to maintain the dispersion of the silver halides, probably due to surface reactions; (2) as a mechanical support for the silver halide; (3) as a factor affecting the sensitivity of the silver; and (4) as a remover of the halogen liberated by the action of light on the silver halide.

A very interesting and highly important problem is the effect of gelatin on the sensitivity of the silver halide grains (43). It has been known for a long time that only certain types of gelatin are suitable for photographic films. In the 1920's, considerable research was carried out to determine the secret of "good" photographic gelatin, the photographic chemist becoming more and more convinced that a sensitizing substance must be present. Sheppard and Hudson (44) made a thorough search for this substance, investigating the various stages in the process of gelatin manufacture from the raw hide to the final product. It was found that the acid liquors used for *deliming* the alkali-swollen hide showed an appreciable sensitizing power. The sludge obtained was examined by a complicated scheme of extraction and precipitation. It was indicated that the unknown substance, "gelatin X," was allyl mustard oil or some compound closely related to it. It became apparent that only the mere presence of sulfur, *per se*, was not sufficient and that the sensitizer was intensively active, one part in one million parts of gelatin exerting a measurable effect on speed of emulsion. The substance was finally isolated in pure form from the deliming of skins and shown to be allyl isothiocyanate or allyl thiocarbamide. The first stage in sensitizing is the conversions of the allyl mustard oil to a thiocarbamide by means of ammonia. The thiocarbamide forms an addition compound:

$$(\text{AgBr})_n \left[\begin{array}{c} \text{NHR} \\ / \\ \text{C}{=}\text{S} \\ \backslash \\ \text{NH}_2 \end{array} \right]$$

which is converted into silver sulfide during the making of the emulsion. The silver sulfide on the silver halide grains increases the sensitivity of the film. Sheppard (45) established definitely the importance of the *alien* sulfur compounds in gelatin. It became evident that the amount of the labile sulfur in gelatin is of the greatest importance for its photographic properties.

The discovery of the function of the sulfur compounds present as impurities in gelatin and the importance of the labile sulfur did not, however, completely solve the riddle of the different behavior of gelatins in making of emulsions. The labile sulfur of gelatin exists in various forms, some of which increase the sensitivity, whereas others produce fog, a dichroic effect. Furthermore, the presence of antifogging and desensitizing substances, probably imidazoles, is indicated. Thus, apart from the content of free sulfhydryl compounds and labile sulfur, the presence of the thio compounds mentioned and compounds of the type of imidazoles will govern the photographic properties of gelatin.

The nature of the reactions in the permanent hardening (tanning) of gelatin films for photographic purpose will be dealt with later in connection with the various tanning processes in the monograph on tanning.

In the researches of Elöd and his numerous pupils (46), Küntzel (47), Page (48), Pouradier and his associates (42), and the present author (49) regarding the nature of tanning processes, gelatin gels or solutions have been employed with great advantage, particularly in investigations for which the elimination of the topochemical and steric complication of two-phase systems is desirable or even necessary.

References

1. Reed, R., J. Soc. Leather Trades Chem. **37**, 75 (1953); Burton, D., Reed, R., and Flint, F. O., *ibid.* **37**, 82 (1953); Burton, D., and Reed, R., *ibid.* **37**, 13 (1953).
2. Rudall, K. M., *in* "Fibrous Proteins," p. 21. Society of Dyers and Colourists, Leeds, 1946.
3. Gustavson, K. H., J. Soc. Leather Trades Chem. **33**, 162 (1949).
4. Kritzinger, C. C., J. Am. Leather Chem. Assoc. **43**, 675 (1948).
4a. Gillespie, J. M., J. Soc. Leather Trades Chem. **37**, 344 (1953).
5. Stiasny, E., Gerber **1906**, 200, 214; J. Intern. Soc. Leather Trades Chem. **3**, 129 (1919).
6. Merrill, H. B., J. Am. Leather Chem. Assoc. **22**, 230 (1927); Ind. Eng. Chem. **17**, 36 (1925).

7. Marriott, R. H., *J. Intern. Soc. Leather Trades Chem.* **12**, 216, 281, 342 (1928).
8. Turley, H. G., and Windus, W., *J. Am. Leather Chem. Assoc.*, **33**, 246 (1938); **36**, 603 (1941); *in* "Stiasny Festschrift," p. 396. Roether, Darmstadt, 1937.
9. See Bowes, J. H., *in* "Progress in Leather Science," Vol. 1, pp. 158–192. BLMRA, London, 1946.
10. Speakman, J. B., *Nature* **122**, 930 (1933); *J. Soc. Dyers Colourists* **52**, 335 (1936); Speakman, J. B., and Whewell, C. S., *J. Soc. Dyers Colourists* **52**, 380 (1936).
11. Cuthbertson, W. R., and Phillips, H., *Biochem. J.* **39**, 7 (1945).
12. Marriott, R. H., *J. Intern. Soc. Leather Trades Chem.* **12**, 216, 281, 392 (1928); Speakman, J. B., and Whewell, C. S., *J. Soc. Dyers Colourists* **52**, 380 (1936).
13. McKay, R., *J. Soc. Leather Trades Chem.* **35**, 382 (1951).
14. See Brohult, S., Dissertation, Uppsala, pp. 37–38, 1940; *J. Phys. & Colloid Chem.* **51**, 206 (1947).
15. Windus, W., and Turley, H. G., *J. Am. Leather Chem. Assoc.* **36**, 603 (1941); Goeller, H. G., *J. Intern. Soc. Leather Trades Chem.* **18**, 388 (1934); Theis, E. R., and Blum, W. A., *J. Am. Leather Chem. Assoc.* **38**, 68 (1943).
16. Michaelis, L., *J. Am. Leather Chem. Assoc.* **30**, 557 (1935).
17. McLaughlin, G. D., Highberger, J. H., and Moore, E. K., *J. Am. Leather Chem. Assoc.* **22**, 345 (1927).
18. Bowes, J. H., and Kenten, R. H., *Biochem. J.* **46**, 1 (1950).
19. Gustavson, K. H., and Widen, P. J., *Collegium* **1926**, 562; Gustavson, K. H., *in* "Handbuch der Gerbereichemie" (W. Grassmann, ed.), Vol. II, Part 2, pp. 189–192. Springer, Vienna, 1939.
20. Kraemer, E. O., *Colloid Symposium Monograph* **4**, 102 (1926).
21. Briefer, M., and Cohen, J., *Ind. Eng. Chem.* **20**, 408 (1928); Briefer, M., *Ind. Eng. Chem.* **21**, 266 (1929).
22. Kraemer, E. O., and Dexter, S. T., *J. Phys. Chem.* **31**, 764 (1927); Kraemer, E. O., and Fanselow, J. R., *ibid.* **29**, 1169 (1925).
23. Beek, J., Jr., and Sookne, A. M., *J. Research Natl. Bur. Standards* **21**, 117 (1938); *J. Am. Leather Chem. Assoc.* **33**, 621 (1938).
24. Highberger, J. H., *J. Am. Chem. Soc.*, **61**, 2302 (1939).
25. Sheppard, S. E., and Houck, R. C., *J. Phys. Chem.* **34**, 2187 (1930).
26. Janus, J. W., Kenchington, A. N., and Ward, A. G., *Research* **4**, 247 (1951).
27. Küntzel, A., and Koepff, H., *Collegium* **1938**, 433.
28. Ames, W. M., *J. Soc. Chem. Ind.* **63**, 200, 234, 277 (1944).
28a. Gustavson, K. H., *Svensk Kem. Tidskr.* **67**, 115 (1955).
29. Scatchard, G., Oncley, J. L., Williams, J. W., and Brown, A., *J. Am. Chem. Soc.* **66**, 1980 (1944).
30. Signer, R., and Mosimann, H., *The Svedberg Mem. Vol.* 464 1944.
31. Pouradier, J., and Venet, A. M., *J. chim. phys.* **47**, 11 (1950).
32. Ferry, J. D., *Advances in Protein Chem.* **4**, 2 (1948).
33. Meyer, K. H., "Natural and Synthetic High Polymers," Interscience, New York, 1942.
34. *Cf.* Ambrose, E. J., Bamford, C. H., Elliott, A., and Hanby, W. E., *Nature* **167**, 264 (1951); and ref. 35.
35. Robinson, C., and Bott, M. J., *Nature* **168**, 325 (1951).
35a. Stainsby, G., Saunders, P. R., and Ward, A. G., *J. Polymer Sci.* **12**, 325 (1954); Ward, A. G., *Brit. J. Appl. Phys.* **5**, 85 (1954).
35b. Pankhurst, K. G. A., "Surface Chemistry," p. 109. Butterworths, London, 1949; Pankhurst, K. G. A., and Smith, R. C. M., *Trans. Faraday Soc.* **40**, 565 (1944); **41**, 630 (1945).

36. Bradbury, E., and Martin, G., *Proc. Roy. Soc.*, **A214**, 183 (1952).
37. Robinson, C., *in* "Nature and Structure of Collagen" (J. T. Randall ed.), pp. 96–105. Butterworths, London, 1953.
38. Smith, C. R., *J. Am. Chem. Soc.* **41**, 135 (1919); for an excellent review see ref. 32; Kraemer, E. O., and Fanselow, J. R., *J. Phys. Chem.* **29**, 1169 (1925); Ferry, J. D., and Eldridge, J. E., *ibid.* **53**, 184 (1949).
39. Pinoir, R., and Pouradier, J., *Compt. rend.* **227**, 190 (1948).
40. Stainsby, G., *Nature* **169**, 662 (1952).
41. Kuhn, W., *Experientia* **5**, 318 (1949); Kuhn W., Küntzle, O., and Katchalsky, A., *J. Polymer Sci.* **5**, 283 (1950); Katchalsky, A., *Experientia* **5**, 319 (1949); *J. Polymer Sci.* **7**, 393 (1951); *Trans. Faraday Soc.* **47**, 1360 (1951); *Endeavour* **12**, 90 (1953).
42. Pouradier, J., Roman, J., Venet, A., Chateu, H., and Accary, A., *Bull. Soc. Chim.* **19**, 928 (1952).
43. See Mees, C. E. K., "Theory of the Photographic Process," pp. 86–100. Macmillan, New York, 1942.
44. Sheppard, S. E., *Phot. J.* **65**, 380 (1925); Sheppard, S. E., and Hudson, J. H., *Ind. Eng. Chem. Anal. Ed.* **2**, 73 (1930).
45. Sheppard, S. E., *Science et inds. phot.* **7**, 361 (1936).
46. Elöd, E., and Schachowskoy, T., *Collegium* **1933**, 701; **1934**, 414; *Kolloid Z.* **72**, 67 (1935); and particularly *Kolloid-Beih.* **51**, 1, 122 (1939); Elöd, E., and Cantor, T., *Collegium* **1934**, 568.
47. Küntzel, A., and Boensel, H., *Collegium* **1936**, 576; Küntzel, A., *Kolloid-Z.* **97**, 99 (1941).
48. Page, R. O., *J. Intern. Soc. Leather Trades Chem.* **28**, 168 (1944).
49. Gustavson, K. H., *J. Am. Leather Chem. Assoc.* **48**, 559 (1953).

CHAPTER 13

Some Physicochemical Aspects of the Reactions of Collagen with Tanning Agents

An outline of some recent physicochemical developments for the characterization of the reactions of collagen with its most important and best-known moieties, the tanning agents, provides an appropriate termination to these discussions on the behavior of collagen. At the same time, it may serve as a bridge for approaching the problems encountered in the diversified processes of tanning. The actual issues concern: (1) the thermodynamic constants; (2) the important contributions of the monolayer technique to the general problem of tannage; (3) the long-period spacings of tanned collagen; and finally (4) the mechanism of the diffusion of tanning agents through the hide structure.

1. THERMODYNAMIC CHARACTERIZATION OF TANNING AGENTS

The changes in the three principal thermodynamic constants of collagen —the heat of activation, the entropy of activation, and the free energy of activation—after its interaction with various agents can be used to evaluate the degree of order or disorder produced in the collagen which forms the substrate of such systems. From measurements of the rate of shrinkage of kangaroo tail tendon at two or three temperatures, closely located in the range just below the temperature of instantaneous shrinkage, and by application of the theory of absolute reaction rates to the data, the half-shrinkage time being the primary figure, Weir (1) has determined the effect of a number of agents on the activation constants of tendon collagen. The values of ΔS, ΔH, and ΔF_{60} (the free energy of activation at 60°C.) for a number of systems are given in Table 35.

As noted in the discussion of thermal shrinkage, ΔF_{60} is a measure of the hydrothermal stability of the collagen, being directly related to the temperature of shrinkage. The following points are of particular interest. The tanning potency of the bifunctional disulfochloride and the lack of tanning faculty of the corresponding unifunctional cyclohexane derivative have been stressed in another connection. The data from these two compounds illustrate the absolute requirement that the tanning agent be bifunctional. Although most of the mineral tanning agents listed increase the $T_s(\Delta F_{60})$, aluminum and molybdenum salts being exceptional in that respect, all of them except chromium lower the ΔH and ΔS. If the size of the molecular

TABLE 35

THE EFFECT OF TANNAGE ON ACTIVATION CONSTANTS OF TENDON COLLAGEN (1)

Tannage	Heat of activation (ΔH), kcal./ mole	Entropy of activation (ΔS), cal./ mole/ degree	Free energy of activation at 60°C. (ΔF_{60}), kcal./mole
Untreated (blank)	141	349	24.7
Zirconium	137	307	35.1
Iron	119	282	25.2
Aluminum	82	172	24.8
Uranium	102	231	25.3
Vanadium	118	281	25.2
Tungsten	110	253	25.5
Polymetaphosphate	129	311	25.5
Molybdenum	119	284	24.7
Copper	141	340	28.0
Mercuri	120	276	28.7
Cyclohexane monosulfonyl chloride	145	361	24.9
Cyclohexane disulfonyl chloride	217	573	26.4
Chromium, 0.06% Cr_2O_3	160	404	26.5
0.13% Cr_2O_3	203	522	28.5
0.51% Cr_2O_3	323	962	36.1
1.02% Cr_2O_3	390	1041	44.1
1.98% Cr_2O_3	325	840	45.2
Glyoxal	288	760	34.6
Quinone	271	710	35.9

Note: Vegetable tannage could not be included because of lack of uniform penetration of the tendon by the tannins.

unit of the collagen chains involved in the shrinkage is assumed to be constant, it follows that the values of ΔH and ΔS measure the degree of crosslinking. Then, according to the figures of the table, most tanning agents do not function as crosslinking agents. Among the agents listed, only chromium salts and the bifunctional organic tanning agents should be able to crosslink the collagen chains. It seems to the author of this book questionable that changes in the heat of activation should be the sole criterion in the formation of crosslinks.

2. THE CONTRIBUTIONS OF THE MONOLAYER TECHNIQUE TO THE PROBLEM OF TANNAGE

The introduction of the monolayer technique in the investigation of tanning systems is due to Rideal and Schulman and their co-workers.

These researches have been continued and extended by Schulman, Gorter, and Pankhurst, and their co-workers. The surface layer reactions are actually models for the essential chemistry of the reactions of tanning agents with single protein chains, the various steric factors of macro, micro, and submicro elements being eliminated.

Schulman and Rideal (2), and Cockbain and Schulman (3) injected an aqueous solution of tannic acid under a preformed monolayer of gliadin. The tannic acid molecule did not penetrate the protein monolayer but anchored itself to the polar head groups of the long-chain amines and of the proteins, forming the undersurface of the monolayer. This fixation of the tannin to the protein monolayer is accompanied by a change in the phase boundary potential and in the rigidity or viscosity of the film. Rideal and his co-workers found on examination of various films that the changes of the properties of the films formed varied considerably for various polyphenols. Gallic acid reacted only slowly and weakly with the gliadin monolayer, but tannic acid reacted rapidly, even in very dilute solutions. The tanned monolayer was no longer elastic and behaved more like a pellicle or skin, which was stable to protein-dispersing agents. It may be concluded that the tannic acid is attached by more than one hydroxyl group to the amino groups of the protein, and thus links the system together by multipoint contact. Gallic acid was found not to be a tanning agent. It is interesting to note that the Rideal group found that 4,4'-dihydroxystilbenes behave in a similar manner, possessing tanning power. An important point in the work of Rideal and Schulman is the finding that long-chain amines are tanned by tannic acid, since the amino group is the sole reactive group in these compounds. Thus, this is evidence for the functioning of the amino group as a tannin-binding site, which fact, when extended to proteins, such as collagen, is of importance for our concept of the mechanism of vegetable tannage. Gorter and Blokker (4) investigated the same system by spreading a gliadin monolayer on the surface of a dilute solution of tannic acid. By the formation of a less compressible and more rigid film, and by a considerable reduction of the surface potential, about 100 millivolts, the occurrence of tanning reactions was indicated.

Ellis and Pankhurst (5), who were the first to prepare monolayers of collagen, have studied the effect of various tanning agents on the collagen film by measuring the changes in surface pressure, Π, surface viscosity, η, and surface potential, ΔV, of the film on tanning (6). The tanning agents studied included vegetable tannins, polyphenols, syntans of the sulfo-acid type, quinone, and chromium salts. The results of these investigations, as well as those of Schulman and Dogan (7), on the reaction of salts of heavy metals on fatty acids, amines, and globular proteins, are of utmost importance for understanding the tanning mechanism. The great sensitivity

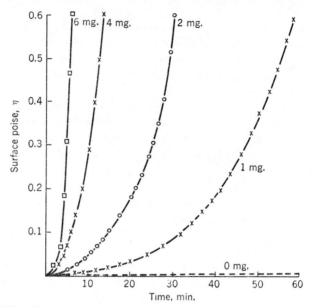

FIG. 40. The effect of mimosa tannin (in milligrams per liter) on the surface viscosity of the collagen monolayer, as a function of time.

of this technique is well illustrated by the curves in Fig. 40, which show the effect of mimosa tannins on the viscosity of the collagen monolayer at pH 4, at concentrations of this tannin from 1 to 6 mg. per liter. Even such a minute amount of tannin as that present in a solution containing 1 mg. per liter has a drastic effect on the surface viscosity-time curve. Synthetic tannins consisting of sulfonated polyphenols produced a similar but lower rise in the surface viscosity. The findings of Ellis and Pankhurst, which illustrate the factor of the molecular size of various agents, are particularly worthy of mention. Simple structures, such as phenol, resorcinol, catechol, pyrogallol, hydroquinone, gallic acid, benzoquinone, and cathechin, do not increase the viscosity of the collagen monolayer, which implies complete lack of tanning faculty. Benzoquinone and catechin, used in the form of pure, freshly prepared samples (monomers), have no tanning effect even in solutions of such high concentration as 60 mg. per liter.

The molecules of the compounds mentioned, all of which are polyfunctional with the exception of phenol, are not large enough to function as crosslinking agents by multipoint attachment to adjacent collagen chains. Evidently, they do not fulfill the spatial requirement. However, as is well known, ordinary laboratory samples of benzoquinone and cathechin show definite tanning potency. In order to explain this unexpected failure of the quinone monomer as a tanning agent, Ellis and Pankhurst investigated the time factor of the reaction, i.e., the effect of the aging of freshly sublimated benzoquinone. The results of their research are shown in Fig. 41. The curve for the quinone monomer shows that it has no effect on the surface viscosity; that is, it is devoid of tanning power. On aging of the product or of the solutions of the quinone, tanning properties are gradually developed, as shown by the curves. The polymerization of the quinone probably also involves oxidation for the formation of the network structure, schematically represented by Fig. 42. Similar experiments with freshly prepared catechin gave the same general results, indicating that the catechin monomer is not

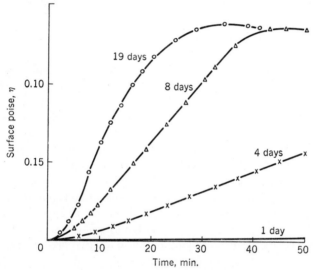

FIG. 41. The effect of benzoquinone, in solutions of different age (degree of polymerization), on the surface viscosity of the collagen monolayer, as a function of time.

sterically fit to bring about crosslinking of the collagen chains. After prolonged boiling of the catechin solution (20 to 40 hours), the curves of the surface viscosity indicate that considerable tanning action has developed. An interesting detail is that the oxidized form of quinone with —O— bridges, and with peripheral hydroxyl groups as the sole reactive groups (Fig. 42), will show variations in tanning power according to the size and the form of the molecule and the number of hydroxyl groups in the periphery. The larger and more symmetrical the polymer, the smaller will be the number of hydroxyl groups, and the further apart they will be. This implies an optimum size of the molecule beyond which the functional groups will be too far apart for crosslinking of adjacent protein chains. The limiting value of the surface viscosity found for polymerized quinone by Ellis and Pankhurst is in line with this view. Heated catechin solutions did not .

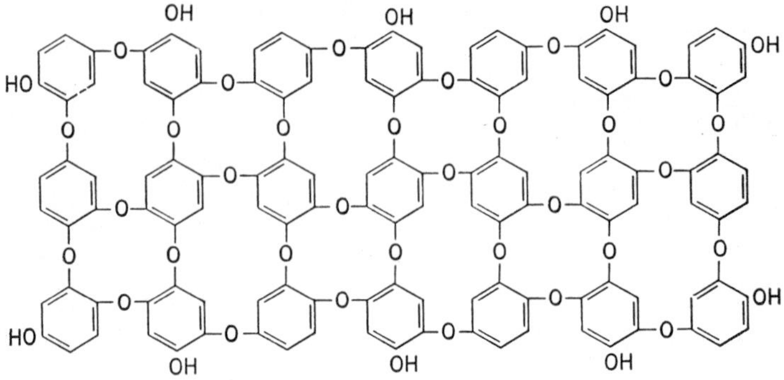

FIG. 42. Benzoquinone polymer.

show such a limiting value. This may be explained by the distribution of five hydroxyl groups on the three rings of the monomeric catechin, which on polymerization gives a molecule with functional hydroxyls distributed throughout the polymer and not confined to the periphery, as they are with polymerized benzoquinone.

These findings and those obtained in experiments with mimosa tannins are accounted for by the concept of multipoint attachments of the tanning agents to the collagen molecule. The fixation of vegetable tannins of the condensed type involves the keto-imide groups of collagen, the result being a closely packed continuum. Ellis and Pankhurst emphasize that as an absolute requirement a tanning agent should possess at least two reactive groups, spaced favorably for combination with two chains of the protein.

The behavior of basic chromium salts differs in many respects from that of the nonionic compounds discussed above. They do not condense the collagen monolayer, and neither does the sulfo-acid syntan. This difference is probably connected with the absence of closely packed aggregates. The results found with these ionic tanning agents suggest that the reaction occurs between the polyfunctional ions and oppositely charged groups of the collagen, in contrast to the behavior of the vegetable tannins (mimosa), which appear to be mainly associated with nonionic protein groups, primarily the keto-imide link. With all vegetable tanning agents, the surface viscosity of the collagen monolayer increases as the tanning proceeds.

Ellis and Pankhurst (6), in summarizing their important findings, stress the following points: It is indicated that the condensed type of vegetable tannins react with collagen predominantly by hydrogen bonding between the multifunctional tannin molecule and the —CO·NH— groups of the protein. At pH values exceeding 3, there is evidence of coulombic binding by means of the anionic groups of the tannin on the cationic groups of collagen. There is no evidence that this secondary type of reaction contributes to the tanning potency. However, there are experimental findings, which as far as this author can determine, prove tanning effects by this type of reaction in the pH range of natural mimosa tannins and sulfited quebracho extract, i.e., in the zone of pH 4.5 to 6.0. Ellis and Pankhurst further stress the fact that vegetable tannins increase the cohesion of the film considerably and convert the monolayer into a compact structure of high surface viscosity. On the other hand, tanning agents which mainly react by ionic valency forces, such as the cationic basic chromium salts and sulfo-acid anions, appear to act initially by coulombic forces with the oppositely charged side chains of collagen. This reaction results in a more open but also highly viscous network.

The investigations of Schulman and Dogan (7) on the interaction of ions of heavy metals (Cr, Fe, Al, Co, Cu, Zn, and Pb) with monolayers of fatty acids, long-chain hydrocarbon sulfo compounds, amino acids, polypeptides, and proteins are important contributions to our knowledge of the mechanism of mineral tannages. These researches demonstrate unequivocally that various steric factors and the hydrogen ion concentration of the systems play a governing role in controlling the interaction of the metal ions mentioned with ionic groups in oriented monolayers. The nature of the reaction is shown to be initially an attraction and association of the cationic basic chromium complexes to the carboxyl ions in the monolayers. Then, a link between the adlineated hydroxyl groups of the chromium complex is formed by hydrogen bonding, to build up a two-dimensional solid lattice. The work on the fatty acid monolayer–chromium salts is of special interest and highly informative with regard to the mechanism of chrome tanning, since the only ionic group present, and the only reactive group moveover, is the carboxyl. Schulman and Dogan found that fatty acid monolayers are made insoluble by chromium cations only at pH values at which the basic salts are formed. The reaction leads to solidification of the monolayers and is accompanied by a large increase in the area per molecule of fatty acid. The aggregates of these chrome soaps were analyzed. It was found that in straight fatty acids one ion of chromium is attached to one fatty acid molecule. However, if the area of fatty acid is increased by branch chain substitution, an additional chromium atom can be incorporated into the monolayer per fatty acid molecule. From these data, Schulman and Dogan conclude that the formation of these two-dimensional lattices is due to the interlinking of neighboring fatty acid chains by the chromium complex through hydrogen bonds attached to the hydroxyl groups of the chromium complex, on one end, and the ketonic groups in the carboxyl groups of the fatty acid, on the other end. The steric condition in the formation of these lattices of two-dimensional extension was found to vary considerably with each metal ion, chromium showing the greatest power, probably because of the ease with which it forms stable polymerization complexes.

Long-chain hydrocarbon amino acids behave similarly. It is important to note that the long-chain amine monolayers, which were shown to be reactive toward vegetable tannins in the early work of the Rideal school, are absolutely inert to the metal ions. This proves also that, by protolytic changes and removal of the proton by the basic groups of the amine, the basic complex formed exerts no tanning effect on the amine monolayer. The reason is that no charged carboxyl groups are present in the film for binding of the chromium complexes. The absolute requirement of the presence of carboxyl ions in the substrate (film) was beautifully proved by Schulman and Dogan. They studied proteins which, on the one hand, contain large amounts of carboxyl groups, such as serum albumin, and those which, on the other hand, are lacking in these groups, such as the prolamine gliadin, which carries numerous basic groups (amino). Serum albumin reacts with chromium ions in the same way as the fatty acid film, by means of the carboxyl groups, whereas the gliadin film is not affected at all by chromium salts. The cupric ion has little affinity for the carboxyl group of the globular protein, compared to its pronounced affinity for the imidazole group of the histidine residue. This specificity is shown by the failure of globular proteins which are rich in carboxyl ions but poor in histidine to bind copper. Indeed, the monolayer technique is superb for demonstrating the specificity of various protein groups for inorganic as well as for organic tanning agents.

The afore-mentioned nonreactivity of the gliadin devoid of carboxylic groups with cationic chromium complexes, and the great reactivity of the serum albumin, in which carboxyl groups are plentiful, are illustrated in Fig. 43. The curves show the effect of chrome alum on the surface pressure plotted against the spreading values of albumin films and of gliadin films, and also the time effect. Schulman and Dogan, in summarizing their findings on the reaction of ions of heavy metals with monolayers of proteins, point out that protein monolayers in which there is a carboxyl group in the protein molecule, such as serum albumin, but *not* gliadin, react in a manner directly analogous to that of the fatty acids, with the basic metal ions other than copper. These monolayers expand and solidify, with time effects as illustrated by Fig. 43, showing that the steric factor involved in the crosslinking between the hydroxyl group of the basic metal cation and the adjacent chain is important in the tanning of the protein chains. Copper, in direct contrast, does not crosslink proteins through their carboxyl groups but does through the imidazole group. It is possible that this failure of copper is in part connected with the inability of cupric ion to form compounds or polynuclear cations generally. It may be that basic copper ion can exist only in the monohydroxide form, whereas metal ions of tanning ability, such as the chromium cations, exist in the basic state in the di-

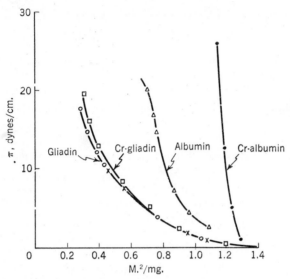

Fig. 43. The effect of chrome alum on the surface pressure of monolayers of gliadin and albumin.

TABLE 36

METAL ION-PROTEIN MONOLAYER INTERACTION

Substrate	Iron	Aluminum	Chromium	Copper
Long-chain tyrosine			+++	+++
Gliadin			0	++
Insulin			++	++
Methemoglobin			+	0
Serum albumin	+++	+++	+++	0
Gelatin (bulk)	+	++	+++	+
pH of optimum insolubility of gelatin films	2.3–3.2	4.0–6.0	3.5–5.0	4–5

hydroxide form as binuclear complexes, which makes them sterically fit to bridge the gap between the protein chains. In Table 36 the behavior of protein monolayers to salts of iron, aluminum, chromium, and copper are listed (7). The pH range of insolubility of the metal complexes with gelatin coincides rather closely with the pH range of interaction of the basic salt with the serum albumin monolayer. The researches of Schulman and Dogan add strength to the concept of crosslinking as the means of stabilizing proteins by tanning.

3. THE CONCEPT OF TANNING IN THE LIGHT OF ELECTRON-OPTICAL AND X-RAY METHODS

Electron micrographs as well as the small-angle X-ray diffraction pattern of intact collagen and tanned collagen indicate that the protofibrils which appear to be the individual polypeptide chains in most instances are arranged parallelly to the fibril axis in such a way as to align chemical features of the chains. The bands and interbands match transversally. It seems probable that the most prevalent side chains, those of the nonpolar groups, such as glycine, alanine, and the other simple monoamino acids, are evenly distributed over the whole segment of the chains. The interbands are generally considered to contain predominantly the bulky amino acids, such as the prolines; the bands are believed to accommodate the long, polar side chains, such as the residues of diamino and the dicarboxylic amino acids. It also appears likely that the interbands have a more compact fibrillar structure, providing the main stabilizing forces, the numerous hydrogen bonds, and that they are not easily penetrated, whereas the bands, with their long cationic and anionic side chains, present a more open structure and thus contain reactive groups more easily accessible to reacting substances, such as tanning agents.

Phosphotungstic acid, the commonly used stain for fibrils in electron microscopy, is in itself a tanning agent, a heteropolyacid. Hence, it is very interesting to find from the electron micrographs that phosphotungstic acid is confined to the band regions (Schmitt and Gross, 8). Small-angle diffraction diagrams obtained by Bear and his co-workers (9) have also been interpreted to indicate the entrance of phosphotungstic acid and also of the polymetaphosphate anion into the band level exclusively. These diagrams also furnish compelling arguments against the view that collagen fibrils consist of arrays of globular disks, or beadlike particles (10). Moreover, the largest spacing transverse to the fibril axis corresponds to 10 to 11 Å. in dry collagen, that is, the dimension of a single polypeptide chain.

Nutting and Borasky point out that the demonstration of an orderly arrangement of collagen fibrils at distances less than 100 Å. virtually precludes the existence of regions in the collagen fibril that are "amorphous" and "crystalline" (11) in the sense currently used in polymer physics. Hence, these investigators prefer to regard the collagen as an orderly structure, with the orientation less perfect in certain regions. Bear (10) has independently arrived at the same conclusion by a different technique. The main contribution of electronic methods to the general problem of tannage is therefore in ascertaining any disturbance in the cross-striation and changes in the distance of the mean length, the 640-Å. figure, due to penetration through, and incorporation of the tanning agent with, the collagen fibrils, provided that direct interaction with the protrofibril can take place (12).

It has long been a puzzle as to why the diagram of collagen obtained by the classical wide-angle X-ray method is not appreciably altered by incorporation of tanning agents with the collagen lattice (13–15). This was noticed in the early 1920's by Herzog (13), a pioneer investigator of proteins by X-ray diffraction, who suggested that failure to detect changes in the diagram of tanned collagen was due to the inability of the tanning agent to penetrate the intramicellar regions, the large molecules of these agents being able only to react intermicellarly. In the modern terminology of Schmitt and Bear, the intermicellar spaces would correspond to the bands, and the micelles to the interbands. As wide-angle X-ray diagram is produced by the highly ordered regions of the collagen chains, the interbands, which are not readily accessible to the tanning agents fixed by collagen, the negative findings of the classical X-ray studies as to the effect of tanning on the collagen structure is no longer a problem.

With the small-angle X-ray diagrams of collagen and leather, an all-over survey of the collagen fibril and the protofibrils became possible. Thus, changes in the repeating regions of imperfect order, the bands, are registered on the diagram. Bear's application of this new method to studies of the effect of tanning agents on the ultrafine structure of collagen has been outstanding. Significant differences have been found for collagen in the native and in the tanned state, although the interpretation of the altered diagrams presents the greatest hurdle. It is usually necessary to combine information derived from other sources, such as electron micrographs, with diffraction theory to reconstruct the diffraction system of the tanned collagen. As early as 1948, it was indicated from the electron-microscopic findings of Schmitt and Gross (8) that basic chromium salts are taken up at the band level chiefly, although some light penetration through the interband regions also takes place. The resolving of bands of chrome-tanned calfskin into six intraperiod bands, as shown in Fig. 13, was an important advance, discovered independently on chromed cowhide by Nutting and Borasky (11) in the same year. The intraperiod bands represent discontinuities of the electron density along the fibril. The presence of the doublets in the b region of the diagram (Fig. 13) is of particular interest. It is noteworthy that the same type of diagram was obtained by Bear by small-angle diffraction of chrome-tanned kangaroo tail tendon. This diagram shows the third, sixth, and ninth lines as extraordinarily prominent. The correlation of the results from the two methods may imply that the changes shown in

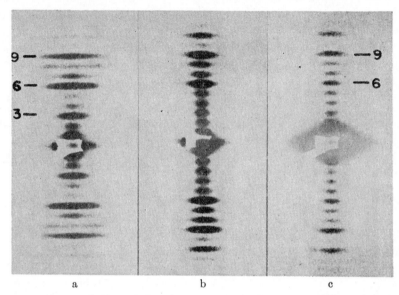

FIG. 44. Low-angle X-ray diffraction pattern of tendon, tanned with (a) chromium, (b) polymetaphosphate, and (c) quebracho extract. From R. S. Bear et al., J. Am. Leather Chem. Assoc. **46**, 129 (1951), Fig. 2.

these lines are located at the interband level. Bear found similar diffraction effects in collagen tanned with formaldehyde, polymetaphosphate, and vegetable tannins, although to a smaller extent. Figure 44 shows the diagrams from tendon tanned with (a) chrome, (b) polymetaphosphate, and (c) quebracho tannins. The heavy intensification of the third, sixth, and ninth layer lines of the chrome-tanned tendon, whose indices are multiples of three, is clearly shown. Bear et al. (9) suggest that some of the chromium may be introduced throughout the collagen fibril, as was already indicated by the electron micrographs of Schmitt and Gross (8), penetrating into the bands as well as the interbands. This view would account for the fact that tanned collagen can still absorb water normally at low humidity and also for the finding that wide-angle diffraction evidence of interband swelling is shown in the tanned collagen, a fact stressed by Bear (9, 10). A similar tendency seems to be characteristic for chrome-tanned collagen. Such behavior had been noticed in the early work of Bear on formaldehyde-treated rat-tail tendon and to a lesser degree in tendon heavily stained with phosphotungstic acid. The intraperiodicity of the collagen fibril is not appreciably changed by most tanning agents, provided that excessive amounts of the agents are not introduced, in which case the wide-angle diagrams are also changed. Excessive tanning may wedge apart the fibrillar structure, starting at bands. Formaldehyde tanning generally results in lowered periodicity (570 to 585 Å.), and Nutting and Borasky (11) report the main spacing of canaigre-tanned cowhide to be 575 to 600 Å., indicating that both tannages shrink the fibrils. The main contribution of electron optics to our knowledge of the nature of the changes involved in tanning is that tanning agents made up from small molecules, such as formaldehyde, and chromium salts, and even larger molecules, such as polymetaphosphate and heteropolyacids (phosphotungstic acid) react in the intrafibrillar regions with the protofibril, being attached mainly to the amino acid residues in the band regions. The chief difficulty lies in the translation of the changes in the layer lines into the specific amino acid residues involved in the tannage. So far, only in one case does such an interpretation appear to be justified. Bear et al. (9) observed that, by reacting collagen and deaminated collagen with polymetaphosphate, the deaminated collagen shows lower intensities of the sixth and ninth lines. The location of the lysine residues at one or more of these bands was suggested. Bear cautions against premature attempts to describe alterations in the small-angle diffraction in terms of chemical constitution, as envisaged by Kratky (16), who suggested that the distribution of lysine should profoundly alter the intensity of the eighth and ninth lines and, moreover, that the sixth line should be closely related to the distribution of the aspartic acid residue. Bear's findings are not in harmony with such a view. As Bear points out, however, it is not improbable that the bands of the collagen fibrils may contain ionic groups of high hydratability which would be readily accessible because of the open fibrillar structure at the bands. On the other hand, Bear (9) points to the possibility that the inaccessibility of the residues of hydroxyamino acids to chemical reagents without fibrillar disintegration is related to their presence at the orderly arranged, closely aligned interband regions. The fundamental discovery of the Zahn school (17) that the dinitrodibenzenesulfone forms *interchain* crosslinks with the ε-amino groups of collagen adds strength to Bear's concept of the accumulation of certain types of residues in the band and interband regions. A valuable contribution to the changes of collagen during its processing before and in the tanning, as revealed by the electron microscope, has been made by Borasky and Rogers (12).

4. DIFFUSION OF TANNING AGENTS THROUGH THE SKIN

The rate of diffusion of the tanning agents through the hide substrate is a problem belonging to the general features of tanning processes and will therefore be briefly discussed here. It involves an exceedingly complicated set of problems, pertaining to the physical state of the substrate, whether swollen or flaccid, and its compactness, the availability and accessibility of reactive protein groups of different types, the size of the molecule of the tanning agent, and its degree of affinity for the various protein groups involved in the particular tannage.

On visual examination, a piece of pelt may appear to be completely penetrated by the tanning agent, and sectional analysis may show the tanning agent to be evenly distributed throughout the various strata of the leather. However, this finding does not allow the conclusion to be drawn that the tanning agent has penetrated the fibrils and interacted with the protofibrils. Thus, the micro- and submicropenetration may be grossly incomplete. By means of electron-optical methods, the occurrence of this fibrillar case-hardening can be ascertained.

For the investigation of the rate of diffusion of tanning agents through the hide substrate, and the study of the laws governing the diffusion process, purified vegetable tannins are eminently suitable, since they consist of relatively large particles (molecular weights of 1000 to 2000, generally), and their method of combination with collagen is rather simple. The rate of diffusion and the progress of tanning is usually estimated by following the movement of the sharp boundary generally formed between the tanned and untanned part by taking sections at intervals, staining the slide with bichromate, and measuring the distance covered under the microscope. With this technique, Stather and Laufmann (18) found that the rate of diffusion of a number of vegetable tanning materials is proportional to the square root of time, $D = k \cdot \sqrt{t}$, and also that the diffusion coefficient is directly proportional to the square root of the concentration of the vegetable tannins.

Armstrong (19) has applied a pycnometric method in his investigations. It is thus possible to estimate the amount of tannins in one phase of a two-phase system, such as hide–tannin solution, and to follow the changes in tannin concentration from one phase to the other from the apparent mass of one phase immersed in the other. If ordinary pelt with its internal space filled with water is introduced into a solution of tannins, its initial apparent mass in that solution depends on the density of the tan solution. The tannins diffuse into the pelt, displacing the water, which results in an increase of the apparent mass. Thus, the amount of tannin taken up by the pelt should be a function of the apparent mass of the pelt and the density of the solution. This method makes continuous observation possible.

The diffusion of the tannins through the pelt gradually slows down, because part of the diffusing tannins combine with collagen. This type of a retarded diffusion process, a diffusion with attrition of the diffusate, has been theoretically treated by Hill and by Hermans (20). According to their formula, the speed of diffusion should be proportional to the square root of time and of concentration, as was first suggested by Bergmann, published by his co-worker Stather (18), and confirmed by Armstrong's comprehensive and informative investigation.

If a fully soaked piece of skin, consisting essentially of collagen fibers with water filling the interfibrillary space, is immersed in tan solution, its apparent mass will vary with the density of the solution. Also, as the tannin diffuses into the skin, it displaces water and the apparent mass increases.

It can be shown that the increase in apparent mass, Δm^* (corrected for changes in the density of the solution), is related to the amount m_{FT} of tan fixed by the collagen and the amount m_{ST} of tan in solution between the fibers:

$$\Delta m^* = k_{FT} \times m_{FT} + k_{ST} \times m_{ST}$$

where k_{FT} and k_{ST} are constants, depending on the type of tannin used, which can be experimentally determined. They represent the apparent mass in water of unit mass of tan.

As tannin diffuses into the skin (Fig. 45), it becomes fixed, and this slows

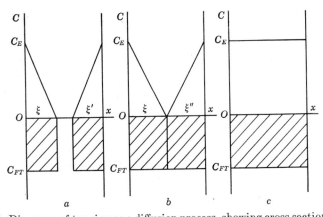

FIG. 45. Diagrams of tanning as a diffusion process, showing cross sections through the skin normal to its surface at different times. The axis OX represents distances measured normally from the surface; OC represents the concentration axis, for C_{ST} above OX and for C_{FT} below OX. ξ is the distance of the tanned/untanned boundary from the grain layer, and ξ' is that from the flesh layer (in practice, ξ is generally greater than ξ'). The end of stage I is shown in b; the end of stage II in c. With skin, the phase is separated by two parallel planes, at the flesh and grain sides, respectively. Thus there will be two boundaries moving toward each other until they meet. The period up to that time, which is the period when most of the tan is fixed, may be called the first stage of tanning. At the end of this stage, the concentration of tan in solution in the piece falls linearly from C_E on the outside to zero at the meeting plane of the boundaries. Thereafter there is a diffusion of tan until the concentration inside is uniform and equal to C_E; this period may be called the second stage of tanning. Subsequently, and perhaps concurrently, there may be a further deposit of tan, which represents the third stage of tanning.

down the diffusion. The theory of this type of diffusion process has been developed by Hill and by Hermans and predicts the formation of sharp boundaries, which, if the external tan concentration is constant, move over a distance ξ proportional to the square root of time and to the external concentration. Furthermore, m_{FT} is proportional to ξ, and, also, the concentration of tan in solution in the piece falls in a linear way from the external value at the surface of the skin to zero at the moving boundary, so that m_{ST} is also proportional to ξ and hence to m_{FT}. Thus, Δm^* is proportional to the total amount of tan in the piece and should also be proportional to the square root of time.

Figure 45 depicts the process. It is seen that tanning occurs in two stages. During the first stage two boundaries move until they meet each other. During the second there is a simple diffusion of tan until the internal concentration is uniform throughout the skin and equal to the external, the amount of tan in solution in the piece being then twice that at the end of the first stage.

By plotting Δm^* against the square root of time for skin in a mimosa solution (0.12 g. per milliliter) of pH 3.8 (Fig. 46), a graph is obtained which is in good agreement with the theory. Three inflexion points are shown—one during the first day (probably due to diffusion through the smaller side of the piece used), after which a straight line relationship holds; another after ten days, A, marking the end of the first stage; and a final one at 25 days,

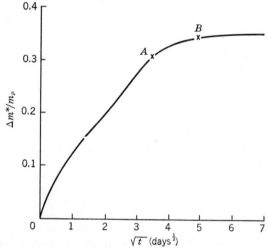

FIG. 46. Graph of $\Delta m_1^*/m_p$ against the square root of time for the same pieces as in Fig. 45. Point A marks the estimated end of the first stage of tanning; point B marks the end of the second stage.

B, marking the end of the second stage, the value of m^* remaining constant thereafter.

If tannic acid is used instead of mimosa tannins, Δm^* does not reach equilibrium until after 40 days, and calculations indicate that there is a continuous deposition of tan occurring even during the second stage.

As the external concentration of the tan solution is increased, it would be expected that the final internal concentration and hence the final amount of tannin in solution in the piece, m_{FT} , would increase and that m_{ST} would remain constant or possibly increase. With tannic acid, however, as the concentration is increased the final values of Δm^* for pieces of skin of the same protein content reach a limit which implies that either $m_{ST} + m_{FT}$ has limiting values, or that, if m_{ST} increases continuously with the external concentration, then when the external concentration is increased beyond a certain value (about 0.26 g. per milliliter) the amount of tanic acid fixed decreases with increasing concentration.

Among the many interesting results in Armstrong's paper, it was found that tanning with tannic acid is a more complicated process than with mimosa tannins, from the point of view of the diffusion process. This is probably due to the fact that mimosa tannins are preponderantly hydrogen-bonded on the keto-imide groups of collagen, whereas the reaction of tannic acid with the hide protein involves also the ionic (basic) groups of the protein. The most important aspect of Armstrong's contribution is its verification of the square root interrelationship of the rate of diffusion with time and concentration by a novel and convenient method not requiring an extensive set of measurements.

It is obvious from our scanty and superficial knowledge of the diffusion of agents through fibrous proteins and protein gels that a real insight into the mechanism of the diffusion and penetration of tanning agents in the fibrillar and lower structural levels is lacking. The issue is complicated by effects due to different degrees of stability of the compounds formed, and hence, in addition to the molecular size, the general state of valency participation enters heavily in the final equation. An example is provided by a comparison of the slow penetration of a vegetable tannin, such as quebracho (probable molecular weight of 1000 to 2000), through compact heavy hide, which for complete penetration will take weeks, with the rapid penetration of polymetaphosphoric acid (mean molecular weight of 3000 to 4000) and a high-molecular fraction of lignosulfonic acid (mean molecular weight of 4000 to 6000), which will be a matter of a few days. The quebracho molecule is uncharged, whereas the other two agents are strong polyelectrolytes. Similar differences are known in the diffusion of dyestuffs through leather, the molecular weight being a secondary factor compared to the chemical spec-

ificity (Otto, 21). The excellent discussions of Vickerstaff (22) and of
Speakman (23) regarding the influence of the affinity of the dyestuff for
the substrate and of its chemical nature (wool) on the rate of penetration of
dyestuffs should be consulted.

It appears that a study of the diffusion of dyestuffs through hide and
leather would be more promising than the use of vegetable tannins and
would give results easier to interpret, particularly if one type is used. This
may be done by varying the number and position of the sulfonic acid groups
or other substituents and by applying the modern methods of measuring
diffusion in gels, for instance the technique devised by Sylvén and his group
(24), to measure the diffusion rates of various substances in bovine *nucleus
pulposus*, or the method of Jelley and Pontius (25). They have studied the
diffusion of dyes through gelatin gels. The diffusion is arrested by plunging
the specimen into a solid carbon dioxide–alcohol bath at $-80°C.$ to freeze
the water. After freeze-drying, the cross-sectioned sample is examined in a
microdensitometer for estimation of the profile of diffused dye. Investigations of the diffusion of four magenta 3-azobenzanthrone dyes of closely
related structure demonstrated the governing importance of the structure
of the dye molecule. Even minor changes in the molecular structure greatly
alter the rate of diffusion and the diffusion profile. Otto's investigations
showed similar results. The most important finding of Jelley and Pontius is
their demonstration that the equilibrium concentration of the dye in the
gel is much greater than that of the dye in the bath, in some instances about
two hundred times as great. The presence of intermicellar solutions with
greatly enriched contents of tanning agents, compared to that of the external solution, throws some doubt on the attempts to explain the micellar
tanning systems on the basis of the concentrations of the tanning bath.

An excellent example of the importance of the number of electric charges
on the molecule for the rate of diffusion of a dyestuff through neutral skin
(pelt) is given in Otto's investigation of the monoazo dyestuff, Fast Red
AV, with one sulfo group in the molecule, and the corresponding dyestuff
molecules with two, three, and four sulfo groups per molecule. The general
type of the naphthalenediazonaphthol of this class of dyestuff is shown by
the following model:

According to Otto (21), the degrees of penetration of the mono-, bi-, tri-,
and tetrasulfonic acids of these dyestuffs, used in solutions of 0.05 M

TABLE 37

THE REACTION OF FAST RED DYES WITH HIDE POWDER AND POLYAMIDE

Type of Dye	Number of Sulfo Groups	pH	T_s of Treated Hide	Degree of Penetration Through Substrate, % of Its Thickness	
				Hide	Polyamide
Fast Red AV	1	2.7	69	7	15
Fast Red E	2	2.5	66	20	25
Naphthol Red SE	3	2.2	62	50	55
Ponceau	4	2.1	60	60	70

strength, through pelt and through a modified polyamide, are as given in Table 37. The penetration of the naphthaleneazonaphthol compounds increases with the number of sulfo acid groups in the molecule for both the collagen and the polyamide, which proves that the size of the molecule is of secondary importance. In the case of collagen, a substrate with numerous ionic groups, the attraction of the freed cationic groups of the protein for the polyacid anion would be expected to be favored by increasing numbers of sulfo acid groups introduced in the molecule. It might be some type of a "zipper" effect which would accelerate the penetration considerably. Only a part of the sulfo acid groups is probably involved in direct valency interaction with the cationic protein groups; the rest of the anionic groups, with their protons attracted by the carboxyl ions of collagen, may be compensated by the freed cationic groups of collagen electrostatically ("long-range effect"). This explanation cannot be applied to the polyamide data, which run parallel to those from the hide, since the ionic groups of the polyamide amount only to 5 to 10% of those of collagen. Hence, with the nonpolar polyamide other forces are probably involved. Otto (26) suggests that the weak valency forces associated with the keto-imide group of the back

bone of the polyamide are directed toward certain groups such as the CH

of the resonating structure. This effect of the π electron is considered to be responsible for the ireversibility of the dyestuff fixation. If the ionic forces are increased, i.e., the number of sulfo groups per molecule, the activity of the π electron is lowered and the dyestuff will tend to reversible interaction with the substrate. Nevertheless in both systems, the diffusion is governed primarily by the affinity of the diffusing molecule for the substrate. Otto emphasizes that an accumulation of ionic groups in the dyestuff molecule tends to shield the weakly polar valency forces (π electrons), making them less active. The future development of the theoretical fundamentals of diffusion of tanning agents through hide will probably be in line with the approach introduced by Otto in his studies on the interaction of aromatic compounds with skin and leather. His researches have revolutionized our ideas of the mechanism of the dyeing of leather and the nature of the compounds formed in the irreversible fixation of dyestuffs by collagen.

REFERENCES

1. Weir, C. E., *J. Soc. Leather Trades Chem.* **36**, 155 (1952).
2. Schulman, J. H., and Rideal, E., *Proc. Roy. Soc.* **B122**, 29, 46 (1937).
3. Cockbain, E. G., and Schulman, J. H., *Trans. Faraday Soc.* **35**, 1266 (1939).
4. Gorter, E., and Blokker, A., *Proc. Koninkl. Ned. Akad. Wetenschap.* **45**, 228, 335 (1942).
5. Ellis, S. C., and Pankhurst, K. G. A., *Nature* **163**, 600 (1949); *Trans. Faraday Soc.* **50**, 82 (1954).
6. Ellis, S. C., and Pankhurst, K. G. A., *Discussions Faraday Soc.* **No. 16**, 170 (1954).
7. Schulman, J. H., and Dogan, M. Z., *Discussions Faraday Soc.* **No. 16**, 158 (1954).
8. Schmitt, F. O., and Gross, J., *J. Am. Leather Chem. Assoc.* **43**, 658 (1948).
9. Bear, R. S., Bolduan, O. E. A., and Salo, T. P., *J. Am. Leather Chem. Assoc.* **46**, 124 (1951); see also *ibid.* **46**, 107 (1951).
10. Bear, R. S., *Advances in Protein Chem.* **7**, 69 (1952).
11. Nutting, G. C., and Borasky, R., *J. Am. Leather Chem. Assoc.* **43**, 96 (1948).
12. Borasky, R., and Rogers, J. S., *J. Am. Leather Chem. Assoc.* **47**, 312 (1952).
13. Herzog, R. O., *Kolloid-Z.* **41**, 277 (1927).
14. Highberger, J. H., and Kersten, H. J., *J. Am. Leather Chem. Assoc.* **33**, 16 (1938).
15. Astbury, W. T., *J. Intern. Soc. Leather Trades Chem.* **24**, 69 (1940).
16. Kratky, O., *J. Polymer Sci.* **3**, 195 (1948).
17. Zahn, H., and Wegerle, D., *Das Leder* **5**, 121 (1954).
18. Stather, F., and Laufmann, K., *Collegium* **1935**, 420.
19. Armstrong, D. M. G., *Discussions Faraday Soc.* **No. 16**, 45 (1954).
20. Hill, A. V., *Proc. Roy. Soc.* **B104**, 39 (1929); Hermans, J. J., *J. Colloid Sci.* **2**, 387 (1947).
21. Otto, G., *Das Leder* **4**, 1 (1953).
22. Vickerstaff, T., "Physical Chemistry of Dyeing," pp. 396–398, and particularly pp. 345–346. Oliver and Boyd, London, 1950.
23. Speakman, J. B., and Smith, A., *J. Soc. Dyers Colourists* **52**, 121 (1936).
24. Paulson, S., Sylvén, B., Hirsch, G., and Snellman, O., *Biochim. et Biophys. Acta* **7**, 207 (1951).
25. Jelley, E. E., and Pontius, R. B., *J. Phot. Sci.* **2**, 16 (1954).
26. Otto, G., *Das Leder* **4**, 193 (1953).

Author Index

Numbers in italics indicate the page on which the reference is listed in the bibliography at the end of each chapter.

A

Abderhalden, E., 3, 5, *26*, *27*, 176, 200
Abramson, H. A., 89, *101*
Accary, A., 13, *28*, 233, *244*, 291, 292, *294*
Adam, N. K., 24, *29*
Adams, R. S., 108, 109, *131*
Adler, J., 192, *201*,
Aggeew, N., 227, *244*
Alexander, P., 19, *28*, 47, *52*, 136, 137, 238, 239, *245*
Alge, A., 143, 145, *154*
Ambrose, E. J., 13, 18, *28*, 35, *51*, 58, 60, *84*, 93, *101*, 287, 289, *293*
Ames, W. M., 103, *131*, 137, *153*, 284, 285, *293*
Anders, G., 48, *52*
Anderson, H., 263, *275*
Ang, K. P., 251, 252, 253, 258, *258*
Anson, M. L., 18, *28*, 221, *243*
Armstrong, D. M. G., 111, 115, *132*, 308, 309, 311, *314*
Armstrong, S. H., 125, *132*
Astbury, W. T., 1, *26*, 35, 45, 48, 49, *51*, *52*, 55, 56, 57, 58, 59, 60, 69, 80, 83, *84*, *86*, 133, *153*, 176, *201*, 211, *243*, 305, *314*
Atkin, W. R., 24, *29*, 93, *101*, 106, 110, *131*, *132*, 172, 190, *200*, *243*, 248, *258*
Ayers, J., 41, *51*, 135, *153*

B

Baddiley, J., 251, *258*
Baehr, G., 78, 86
Bailey, K., 35, *51*, 58, 59, *84*, 100, *101*
Balfe, M. P., 159, *170*, 172, *200*, 206, 228, *243*, *244*
Baló, J., 80, *86*, 266, *275*
Bamford, C. H., 14, *28*, 287, *293*
Bancroft, W. D., 207, *243*, 247, *258*
Banga, I., 80, *86*, 266, *275*
Batzer, H., 184, *201*
Baudouy, C., 73, *85*
Bear, R. S., 33, 34, 35, 45, 47, *51*, 54, 55, 56, 57, 59, 60, 61, 62, 63, 64, 65, 66, 67,
68, 69, 70, 71, *84*, *85*, 199, 200, *201*, 212, 236, *243*, 304, 305, 306, 307, *314*
Becker, E., 48, *52*
Beek, J. Jr., 77, *86*, 94, 97, *101*, 283, *293*
Belden, B. C., 247, *258*
Bergmann, M., 6, *27*, 37, 48, 49, *52*, 74, *85*, 176, *200*, *201*, 256, *259*, 261, 262, 263, 264, 265, 267, 268, 270, 272, *275*, *276*, 308
Bergström, S., 97, *101*
Beveridge, J. M. R., 38, 44, *51*
Biscoe, J., 56, *84*
Bjorksten, J., 79, *86*
Blanc-Jean, G., 136, *153*
Blackburn, S., 254, *258*
Block, R. J., 7, *27*
Blokker, A., 24, 25, *29*, 297, *314*
Blum, W. A., 109, *132*, 281, *293*
Boedtker, H., 75, *85*
Boensel, H., 292, *294*
Bolam, T. R., *170*
Bolduan, O. E. A., 62, *84*, 304, 306, *314*
Borasky, R., 68, 69, *85*, 136, *153*, 198, 199, *201*, 212, 214, 215, 218, *243*, 304, 305, 307, *314*
Bott, M. J., 287, 289, *293*
Bowes, J. H., 9, 25, *28*, *29*, 38, 39, 42, 43, 48, *51*, *52*, 76, 77, *86*, 95, 96, 98, 99, 100, *101*, 111, 113, 131, 132, 155, *170*, 206, 234, *244*, 247, 250, 254, 256, *258*, 280, 282, *293*
Bradbury, E., 289, 290, *294*
Bragg, W. L., 35, *51*, 60, *84*
Brand, E., 48, 49, *52*
Bradfield, J., 78, *86*
Branson, H. R., 17, *28*
Braybooks, W. E., 24, *29*, 172, 190, *200*
Briefer, M., 94, *101*, 283, *293*
Brill, R., 53, 84
Brockway, L. O., 185, *201*
Brohult, S., 281, 293
Brown, A., 286, *293*
Brown, G. L., 8, *27*, *28*, 76, *86*
Brown, L., 14, 28
Browne, A. R., 203, 236, *242*

315

318   AUTHOR INDEX

Subject Index

A

Absorption spectra, 35–36
Acetates, effect on collagen, 188
Acetic acid,
  anomalous behavior on ionization, 186
  dimerization constant of, 186
  dimerization of, 185–186
  effect of concentrated solutions on collagen, 121–124, 187–189
  lyotropic effect on the reactivity of collagen treated by, 189
  -pretreated collagen, reactivity to tanning agents, 188–190
  resonance in the molecule of, 186
  solubilization of collagen by solutions of, 187
Acetone, for dehydration of collagen, 164, 248, 251
Acetylation of proteins, 251–254
Acid amide groups, 95
Acid and base binding,
  by collagen, 104–121
  by gelatin, 104–105
  by keratin, 36, 58
Activation energy, 215–216, 265
Adipose layer and tissue, 31–32
Adsorption methods for protein analysis, 7
Affinity
  of acids for collagen, 106–120
  of acids for keratin, 115, 127–129
  of anions for collagen, 127–130
  of anions for keratin, 128
Albumins, crosslinking by formaldehyde, 232–233
Alcohol-heated, shrunk collagen, 206
Alcohols, action on collagen, 205–206
Alkali,
  action on collagen, 96–100, 282
  combination, with collagen, 112–113
    with proteins generally, 21–22
Alkylation of keratin, 238–240
Amide groups, types of, 95
Amino acids, 4–5
Amino acids,
  aliphatic, 4–5, 39
  aromatic, 4–5, 39

basic, 5, 39
C-terminal groups, methods of estimation, 9
composition of, 4–5
chromatography of, 7–8
common types of, 4–5, 39
  alanine, 4
  arginine, 5
  aspartic acid, 4
  cysteine, 5
  cystine, 5
  glutamic acid, 4
  glycine, 4
  histidine, 4
  hydroxylysine, 42
  hydroxyproline, 5
  isoleucine, 4
  leucine, 4
  lysine, 5
  methionine, 5
  phenylalanine, 4
  proline, 5
  serine, 4
  threonine, 4
  tryptophan, 4
  tyrosine, 4
  valine, 4
dicarboxylic, 4, 99
  estimation by chromatographic method by Moore and Stein, 7
  decarboxylase technique of Gale, 8
  electrodialysis, 8
  isotopic dilution method, 8
  microbiological assay, 8
  paper chromatography, 7–8
  paper electrophoresis, 8
fractionation of, 7–8
hydroxyl containing, 42–44
interatomic distances in, 15–16
ionization, 20–21
ionization constants of ionic groups of, see Proteins,
isolation of, 7–8
isoelectric point of, 92
N-terminal groups, estimation by Sanger reagent, 9, 250
nonpolar, 2

trated solutions of acetic acid, 189

by collagen pretreated in solution of lyotropic agents, 178–190

by collagen pretreated in solutions of sodium perchlorate, 183

by collagen pretreated in solutions of swelling agents, 189

by gelatin at different pH values, 234

by heat-denatured collagen, 221–222

by neutral salt pretreated collagen, 180, 183

function of the hydroxy group of collagen in the fixation of,

non-ionic chromium complexes, 47, 181

sulfito-chromium complexes, 46, 180–181

hydrothermal stabilization of collagen, 227–228

independence of fixation of cationic complexes by non-ionic groups of collagen, 181

interaction with albumin monolayers, 303

with fatty acid monolayers, 301–302

with gelatin monolayers, 303

with gliadin monolayers, 303

with protein monolayers, 301–304

minimum amount required for tanning, 235

reaction of anionic chromium salts, 180, 183, 189, 222

of cationic chromium salts, 180, 183, 189, 222

of non-ionic chromium salts, 178, 180, 183, 189, 222

secondary changes in combination with collagen, 231–232

stability of chromium salts fixed by collagen, 231

stabilization of collagen by, 242

steric factors in fixation, 234–235

use for indicating type of reactions of collagen, 178–181

Chymotrypsin, 261–263

Citrulline, formation from arginine residues, 96

Clapeyron-Clasius equation, 151

Classification,

of proteins, 1, 35, 58

of collagens, 82–84

Clostridium histolyticum, collagenase from, 266

Clostridium welchii, collagenase from, 266

Coacervates, in fractionation of gelatin, 287

Collagen,

acetylation, 251–254

acid binding capacity, 105, 107, 112

acid extracted skin, 73–76

action of collagenase on, 266

of proteinases on, 165, 267–270

alkali binding capacity, 105, 112

amide groups in, 95

hydrolysis by alkali, 94–97

amino acid content, 39

architecture of, 53

ascorbic acid and formation of, 77–78

axial repeating period, 60

backbone spacing in X-ray diagram, 59

band regions, 61–62

biochemical aspects of, 77–79

birefringence of fibers, 71, 72

of fibers of tanned, 72

proof of inter- and intramicellar reaction by, 72

reversal of, 72

bovine skin, 31–32

break-down products on alkali treatment of, 98–100

calf-skin, 45

carbohydrate content of, 77, 81

characterization of, 82–83

chemical composition, 39–41

chondroitin sulfate, 42–43, 81–82

citrate-extracted, 73–77

classification of, 35, 82–83

cod fish skin, 43–47

cohesion of, 71, 141–142

coiling of molecular chains, 67

configuration of, 53–60

contraction, 202–227

conversion to gelatin, 283–285

coordinative reactions of, 123, 178, 181, 184

crosslinking of peptide chains in, 133–138

evidence for, 236–237

steric factors in, 234–235